T0175366

Cardiac Imaging

A CORE REVIEW

Second Edition

Cardiac Imaging

A CORE REVIEW

Second Edition

Editors

Jean Jeudy, MD

Staff Radiologist, Cardiothoracic Imaging
Department of Diagnostic Radiology and Nuclear
  Medicine
University of Maryland School of Medicine
Baltimore, Maryland

Sachin Malik, MD

Section Chief, Thoracic and Cardiovascular Imaging
VA Palo Alto Healthcare System
Palo Alto, California
Clinical Assistant Professor (Affiliated)
Cardiovascular Imaging
Stanford University Medical Center

Stanford, California

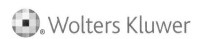. Wolters Kluwer

Philadelphia • Baltimore • New York • London
Buenos Aires • Hong Kong • Sydney • Tokyo

Acquisitions Editor: Nicole Dernoski
Development Editor: Eric McDermott
Editorial Coordinator: Vinoth Ezhumalai
Marketing Manager: Kirsten Watrud
Production Project Manager: Catherine Ott
Design Coordinator: Stephen Druding
Manufacturing Coordinator: Beth Welsh
Prepress Vendor: Straive

Second Edition

Copyright © 2022 Wolters Kluwer

1st edition Copyright © 2016 by Wolters Kluwer. All rights reserved. This book is protected by copyright. No part of this book may be reproduced or transmitted in any form or by any means, including as photocopies or scanned-in or other electronic copies, or utilized by any information storage and retrieval system without written permission from the copyright owner, except for brief quotations embodied in critical articles and reviews. Materials appearing in this book prepared by individuals as part of their official duties as U.S. government employees are not covered by the above-mentioned copyright. To request permission, please contact Wolters Kluwer at Two Commerce Square, 2001 Market Street, Philadelphia, PA 19103, via email at permissions@lww.com, or via our website at shop.lww.com (products and services).

9 8 7 6 5 4 3 2 1

Printed in China

Cataloging-in-Publication Data available on request from the Publisher

ISBN: 978-1-9751-4799-0

This work is provided "as is," and the publisher disclaims any and all warranties, express or implied, including any warranties as to accuracy, comprehensiveness, or currency of the content of this work.

This work is no substitute for individual patient assessment based upon healthcare professionals' examination of each patient and consideration of, among other things, age, weight, gender, current or prior medical conditions, medication history, laboratory data and other factors unique to the patient. The publisher does not provide medical advice or guidance and this work is merely a reference tool. Healthcare professionals, and not the publisher, are solely responsible for the use of this work including all medical judgments and for any resulting diagnosis and treatments.

Given continuous, rapid advances in medical science and health information, independent professional verification of medical diagnoses, indications, appropriate pharmaceutical selections and dosages, and treatment options should be made and healthcare professionals should consult a variety of sources. When prescribing medication, healthcare professionals are advised to consult the product information sheet (the manufacturer's package insert) accompanying each drug to verify, among other things, conditions of use, warnings and side effects and identify any changes in dosage schedule or contraindications, particularly if the medication to be administered is new, infrequently used or has a narrow therapeutic range. To the maximum extent permitted under applicable law, no responsibility is assumed by the publisher for any injury and/or damage to persons or property, as a matter of products liability, negligence law or otherwise, or from any reference to or use by any person of this work.

shop.lww.com

CCS0921

CONTRIBUTORS

Joe Y. Hsu, MD

Cardiac Radiologist
Diagnostic Imaging
Kaiser Permanente Los Angeles Medical Center
Los Angeles, California

Nancy Pham, MD

Assistant Professor
Department of Radiology
University of California, Los Angeles
Los Angeles, California

Brian Pogatchnik, MD

Clinical Instructor
Cardiovascular and Thoracic Imaging
Stanford University Medical Center
Stanford, California

Alan Ropp, MD, MS

Diagnostic Radiologist—Thoracic Imager
Diagnostic Radiology and Medical Imaging
University of Virginia
Charlottesville, Virginia

Amar B. Shah, MD, MPA

Associate Professor of Radiology
Department of Radiology
Zucker School of Medicine at Hofstra/Northwell Health
Manhasset, New York

Jody Shen, MD

Clinical Instructor
Cardiovascular and Thoracic Imaging
Stanford University Medical Center
Stanford, California

The second edition of the *Cardiac Imaging: A Core Review* builds on the success of the first edition by covering the essential aspects of cardiac imaging in a manner that serves as a guide for residents to assess their knowledge and review the material in a format that is like the ABR core examination. Similar to the first edition, the print copy of the *Cardiac Imaging: A Core Review, 2nd edition* still contains 300 questions with approximately one-third of the questions being new. Some questions from the print copy of the first edition are still available but have been moved to the eBook of *Cardiac Imaging: A Core Review, 2nd edition*.

The co-editors, Dr. Jean Jeudy and Dr. Sachin Malik have done an excellent job in producing a book that exemplifies the philosophy and goals of the *Core Review Series*. They meticulously worked on covering key topics on cardiac imaging along with quality images. The questions have been divided logically into chapters to make it easy for learners to work on particular topics as needed. The questions are multiple-choice with each question having a single best answer. There is a brief post-question rationale as to why the correct answer is correct and why the other plausible answer choices are incorrect. There are also references provided for each question to allow one to delve more deeply into a specific subject matter.

The intent of the *Core Review Series* is to provide the resident, fellow, or practicing physician a review of the important conceptual, factual, and practical aspects of a subject with multiple choice questions written in a format similar to the ABR core examination. The *Core Review Series* is not intended to be exhaustive but to provide material likely to be tested on the ABR core exam and that would be required in clinical practice.

As the series editor and founder of the *Core Review Series*, it has been rewarding to not only be a co-editor of one of the books in this series but to bring together and work with so many talented individuals in the profession of radiology across the country. This series represents countless hours of work by so many individuals that it would not have come together without their participation. It has been very gratifying to receive so many positive comments from residents of the impact they feel the series has made in their board preparation. The *Core Review Series* has become a trusted board exam resource for radiology residents.

I would like to thank Dr. Jeudy and Dr. Malik for their dedication to the series and for doing an exceptional job on the second edition. I believe *Cardiac Imaging: A Core Review, 2nd edition* will serve as a valuable resource for residents during their board preparation and a useful reference for fellows and practicing radiologists.

Biren A. Shah, MD, FACR
Professor of Radiology
Wayne State University School of Medicine
Associate Residency Program Director
Section Chief, Breast Imaging
Detroit Medical Center

In 2011, the American Board of Radiology (ABR) introduced a new phase in board certification for diagnostic radiology residents. A new all-encompassing core examination was implemented, which was image rich, computer-based, and aimed to challenge residents to prove their comprehensive knowledge across the entire field of diagnostic radiology.

The goal of the format was to emphasize higher-level comprehension of subject matter including synthesis of information, differential diagnosis, and management decisions. The examination continues to evolve with 2021 being the first time administering a completely remote computer-based examination allowing for secure delivery of the examination from home.

Since the early transition to the new format, the number of available resources has changed, while the quality of review material still varies. With the benefit of our clinical and educational experience, our goal with this book has been to maintain a refined source of material reflecting the level of comprehensive information that residents will encounter on the core examination. The questions provided in this book are grouped into key subtopics in cardiac imaging. Many cases are image based, and a subset offer higher-order questions where the user must commit to an answer before advancing to the following associated question.

The curation of examination questions remains an arduous process. Study material must be reviewed for clarity, accuracy, and relevance. References must be relevant and reflect current clinical understanding and practices. In organizing our content, we have strived to provide you with the most comprehensive and complete knowledge base. The psychometric integrity of the questions in this book reflect the same standards of the ABR, ensuring residents will have quality questions to study from.

We hope that this book serves not only as a key resource for the initial qualifying examination but also as a practical guide preparing for the ABR's Certifying examination and Maintenance of Certification (MOC) examination. We hope you pass with flying colors!

Thank you to the many individuals who without their contributions and support, this book would not have been written. Additionally, we extend tremendous thanks to the staff at Lippincott Williams & Wilkins for providing this opportunity and beneficial help along the way. Finally, we are deeply grateful to our families and loved ones, who have encouraged us through long hours of work and supported us each step along the way.

Best regards for a productive career in this dynamic specialty.

Jean Jeudy, MD
Sachin Malik, MD

CONTENTS

Contributors   v
Series Foreword   vii
Preface   ix

1 Basics of Imaging: Radiography, CT, and MR 1
Nancy Pham, MD, Joe Y. Hsu, MD, Amar B. Shah, MD, MPA, Jean Jeudy, MD, and Sachin Malik, MD

2 Normal Anatomy, Including Variants, Encountered on Radiography, CT, and MR 15
Joe Y. Hsu, MD, Amar B. Shah, MD, MPA, and Sachin Malik, MD

3 Physiologic Aspects of Cardiac Imaging 35
Amar B. Shah, MD, MPA and Jean Jeudy, MD

4 Ischemic Heart Disease 57
Brian Pogatchnik, MD, Amar B. Shah, MD, MPA, and Sachin Malik, MD

5 Cardiomyopathy 82
Jean Jeudy, MD and Sachin Malik, MD

6 Cardiac Masses 116
Joe Y. Hsu, MD and Jean Jeudy, MD

7 Valvular Disease 145
Jean Jeudy, MD and Sachin Malik, MD

8 Pericardial Disease 168
Alan Ropp, MD, MS, Amar B. Shah, MD, MPA, and Jean Jeudy, MD

9 Congenital Heart Disease 188

Joe Y. Hsu, MD and Jean Jeudy, MD

10 Acquired Disease of the Thoracic
Aorta and Great Vessels 220

Joe Y. Hsu, MD, Amar B. Shah, MD, MPA,
and Jean Jeudy, MD

11 Devices and Postoperative
Appearance 242

Jody Shen, MD, Joe Y. Hsu, MD, Amar B. Shah, MD, MPA,
Jean Jeudy, MD, and Sachin Malik, MD

Index   265

1 Basics of Imaging: Radiography, CT, and MR

Nancy Pham, MD • Joe Y. Hsu, MD • Amar B. Shah, MD, MPA • Jean Jeudy, MD • Sachin Malik, MD

QUESTIONS

1 What is the purpose of double-inversion recovery in black blood imaging?

A. To improve blood pool signal
B. To suppress fat
C. To suppress blood flow
D. To improve temporal resolution

2 With conventional filtered back projection (FBP), what is the relationship of tube current to noise?

A. Directly proportional
B. Inversely proportional
C. No direct relationship
D. Exponentially proportional

3 A patient is coming back for a follow-up CT. You looked at a prior CT, and it was very noisy. What parameter can you change on the follow-up CT to reduce the noise by a factor of 2 (assuming filtered back projection was used)?

A. Increase the effective mAs by a factor of 2.
B. Increase the effective mAs by a factor of 4.
C. Decrease the kVp by 40%.
D. Decrease the kVp by 20%.

4 In filtered back projection, changing the type of reconstruction algorithm/ kernel can affect the spatial resolution and what else?

A. Radiation dose
B. Image noise
C. Temporal resolution

5 How is dose length product (DLP) related to scan length?

A. It is not related.
B. It is directly proportional.
C. It is inversely proportional.

6 A 32-year-old male with chest pain, diffuse ST elevations on electrocardiogram, and elevated troponin is referred for cardiac MRI after a left heart catheterization revealed normal coronary arteries. What accounts for the finding highlighted by the arrows in the images below?

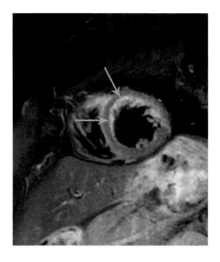
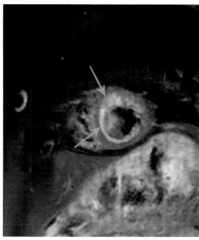
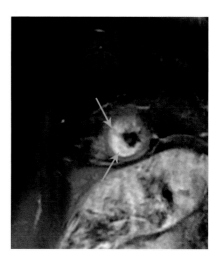

A. Myocardial edema
B. Myocardial fibrosis
C. Incomplete blood suppression
D. Incomplete myocardial nulling

7 The image below is from a phase-contrast image in a patient with suspected aortic stenosis. Which of the following statements is most accurate about the image?

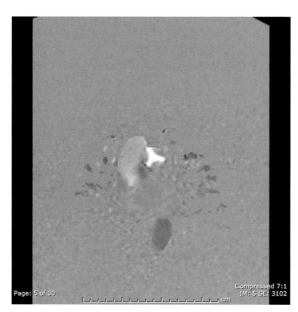

A. The velocity-encoding gradient was set too low.
B. The image shows no net phase shift of the blood.
C. Bipolar gradients were applied to obtain the image.
D. There is stenosis of flow across the valve.

8 How does one calculate an estimated effective dose in millisieverts?

   A. Multiply the dose length product by a conversion factor.

   B. Divide the dose length product by a conversion factor.

   C. Multiply the CT volume dose index by a conversion factor.

   D. Divide the CT volume dose index by a conversion factor.

9 In a patient with contraindication to beta-blockers, which medication can be given to slow the heart rate?

   A. Atenolol

   B. Nitroglycerin

   C. Verapamil

   D. Sildenafil

10 A patient arrives for a coronary CT angiography examination. Prior to giving sublingual nitroglycerine, you explain to the patient that a possible side effect is headache. Which of the following is a relative contraindication?

   A. Hypotension

   B. Obesity

   C. Diabetes

   D. Dyslipidemia

11 Increasing which of the following parameters would fix the artifact seen in the MR image below?

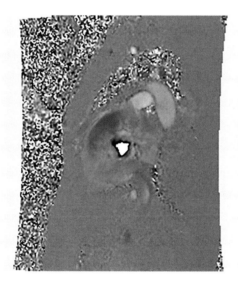

   A. Field of view

   B. Slice thickness

   C. Velocity-encoding gradient

   D. Bandwidth

12 Nephrogenic systemic fibrosis (NSF) is a systemic disease that has been associated with gadolinium deposition. What is a clinical feature of the disease?

   A. Facial scarring

   B. Pulmonary fibrosis

   C. Retroperitoneal fibrosis

   D. Skin thickening of the extremities

13 A change in contrast flow rate from 6 to 4 mL/sec would result in which of the following?

A. Initial increase and then decrease in arterial enhancement
B. Increase in iodine molecules given per time
C. No change in arterial enhancement
D. Reduced iodine flux

14 Which of the following images is a curved multiplanar reformation?

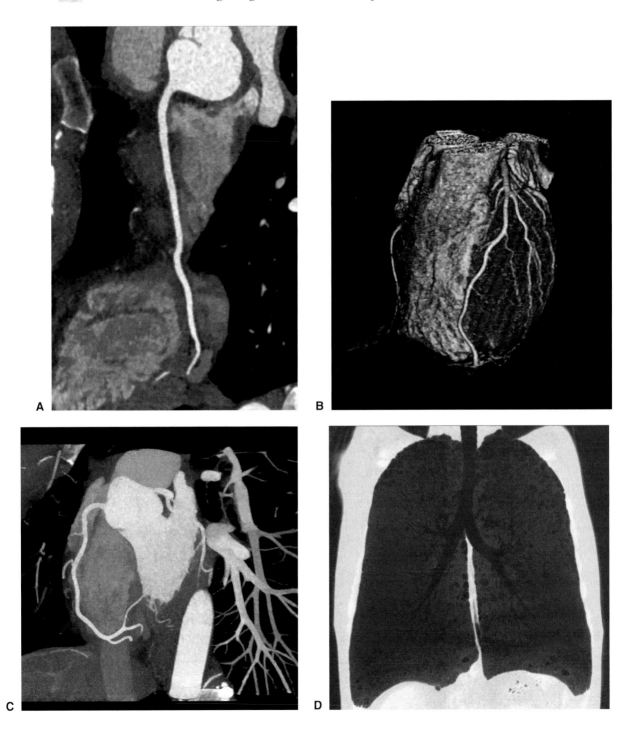

15 A new MRI technologist is being trained in cardiac MRI. Ten minutes after giving intravenous gadolinium contrast, the new technologist runs a time to inversion scout (TI scout) sequence to determine the best TI for the late gadolinium enhancement images. Based on the TI scout images below, which of the following TI values should the technologist choose to best null the myocardium?

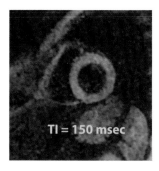 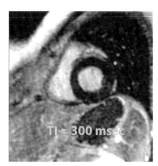 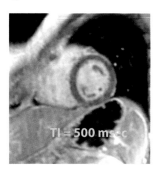 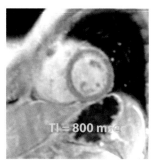

A. TI = 150 msec
B. TI = 300 msec
C. TI = 500 msec
D. TI = 800 msec

16 Your technologist completes a short-axis balanced steady-state free precession cardiac MRI (cMRI) sequence to calculate cardiac function. While scanning the apex of the heart, the technologist notices a mass in the liver with bright signal and asks you if this sequence can confidently characterize the lesion. Your response is which of the following?

A. Yes, since the sequence is only T2 weighted, the mass is a cyst.
B. Yes, it is a cyst since the sequence is not susceptible to calcification or metallic artifact.
C. No, the mass contains calcification, which accounts for its bright signal.
D. No, although the sequence has relative T2 weighting, it has both T2 and T1 properties.

17 Short-axis bright blood cine images through the base of the heart during diastole and systole are shown. Based on the artifact denoted by the arrows, what is the frequency encoding direction?

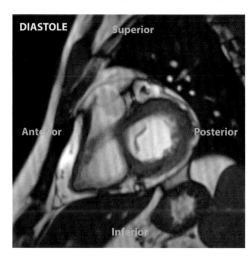 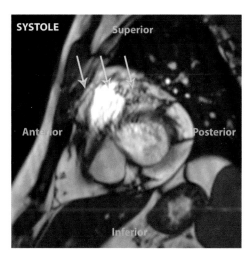

A. Anterior–posterior
B. Superior–inferior
C. Through plane
D. In plane

18 A patient with a cardiac pacemaker device arrives for a cardiac MRI. The technologist reviews the information card for the pacemaker device that the patient brought with him. The information card has the following logo seen below. What is the most appropriate action for the technologist to take in regard to scanning the patient?

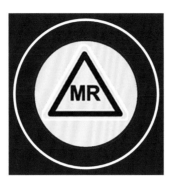

A. Do not scan the patient since the device is MR unsafe.

B. Scan the patient under very specific conditions since the device is MR conditional.

C. Scan the patient without any specific conditions since the device is MR safe.

19 Which of the below shows the ideal contrast bolus geometry?

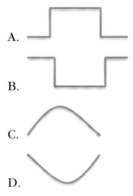

20 What is the most likely cause of transient interruption of the contrast bolus from an injection in the right antecubital fossa?

A. Increased flow from the IVC

B. Increased flow from the SVC

C. Increased flow from the brachiocephalic vein

D. Increased flow from the coronary sinus

21 What is the impact on the specific absorption rate (SAR) by a patient undergoing a scan on a 3T scanner compared to a 1.5T scanner assuming flip angle and TR are held constant?

A. Higher SAR

B. Lower SAR

C. No impact on SAR

D. Mixed impact on SAR

22 Which of the following patterns of pharmacokinetics is characteristic of gadolinium when administered to a patient with normal myocardium?

A. Intravascular injection—extracellular space

B. Intravascular injection—extracellular space–intracellular space

C. Intravascular injection—intracellular space–extracellular space

D. Intravascular injection—intracellular space

23   Why does gadolinium have paramagnetic properties when placed in a magnetic field?

A. Excess protons in the nucleus
B. Unpaired electrons in the outer shell
C. Uneven number of neutrons
D. Emission of positrons

24   A patient is undergoing screening by an MRI technologist for cardiac MRI. In which zone does this take place?

A. Zone 1
B. Zone 2
C. Zone 3
D. Zone 4

25   With balanced steady-state free precession sequences, what is the relationship of longitudinal magnetization (LM) to the transverse magnetization (TM)?

A. LM = TM
B. LM > TM
C. LM < TM

26   Which of the following images from a cardiac MRI is from a balanced steady-state free precession cine sequence?

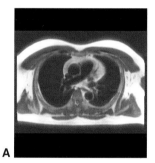 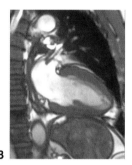 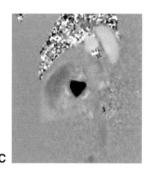 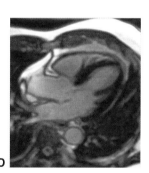

A   B   C   D

27   A 45-year-old male with a BMI of 27 undergoes a cardiac CTA (CCTA) in the emergency department. What instructions do you give your technologist to reduce radiation exposure?

A. Scan from the thoracic inlet to diaphragm.
B. Use a kVp of 100 rather than 120.
C. Use retrospective gating.
D. Do calcium scoring.

28   You perform a cardiac CTA (CCTA) using retrospective gating to evaluate cardiac function. In order to minimize dose, you use tube modulation. What best describes the effect of tube modulation?

A. Changes mAs based on BMI
B. Changes mAs depending on cardiac cycle
C. Maintains uniform mAs
D. Decreases mAs with arrhythmia

29   While at the MR scanner, the technologist increases the spatial resolution in the phase-encoding direction. Assuming no other parameter changes, this will result in which of the following?

A. Increase the acquisition time.
B. Decrease the field of view.
C. Increase the echo train length.
D. Decrease the number of excitations.

30 Which of the following images from a cardiac MR examination is obtained using a single inversion recovery pulse?

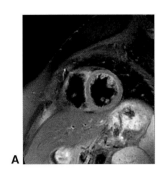 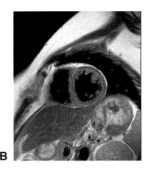 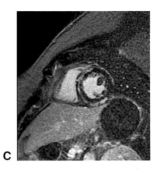 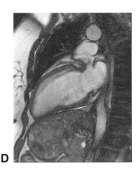

A   B   C   D

31 Increasing which of the following parameters during a coronary CTA will reduce the radiation dose (assuming no other changes)?

A. Pitch
B. kV
C. mA
D. Field of view

ANSWERS AND EXPLANATIONS

1 **Answer C.** Double-inversion recovery sequence in black blood cardiac imaging is designed to suppress the signal from blood flow.

Reference: Ginat DT, Fong MW, Tuttle DJ, et al. Cardiac imaging: part 1, MR pulse sequences, imaging planes, and basic anatomy. *AJR Am J Roentgenol* 2011;197(4):808–815. doi:10.2214/AJR.10.7231.

2 **Answer B.** With filtered back projection, tube current is inversely proportional to noise. That is, increasing the mA by factor of 4 will yield half the noise (1/square root of 4). Tube current determines the number of photons generated and noise.

Reference: Litmanovich DE, Tack DM, Shahrzad M, et al. Dose reduction in cardiothoracic CT: review of currently available methods. *Radiographics* 2014;34(6):1469–1489. doi:10.1148/rg.346140084.

3 **Answer B.** With filtered back projection, tube current is inversely proportional to noise. That is, increasing the mA by factor of 4 will yield half the noise (1/square root of 4). Relationship of kVp to noise is complex, but in general, decreasing the kVp will increase the noise if other factors are held constant.

Reference: Litmanovich DE, Tack DM, Shahrzad M, et al. Dose reduction in cardiothoracic CT: review of currently available methods. *Radiographics* 2014;34(6):1469–1489. doi:10.1148/rg.346140084.

4 **Answer B.** Reconstruction algorithm/kernel does not affect radiation dose since it is applied after the study is already obtained. It can affect spatial resolution and noise depending on which algorithm/kernel is used.

Reference: Litmanovich DE, Tack DM, Shahrzad M, et al. Dose reduction in cardiothoracic CT: review of currently available methods. *Radiographics* 2014;34(6):1469–1489. doi:10.1148/rg.346140084.

5 **Answer B.** DLP is obtained by multiplying the CTDIvol by the scan length; therefore, it is directly proportional.

Reference: Litmanovich DE, Tack DM, Shahrzad M, et al. Dose reduction in cardiothoracic CT: review of currently available methods. *Radiographics* 2014;34(6):1469–1489. doi:10.1148/rg.346140084.

6 **Answer C.** The images shown are short-axis double-inversion recovery black blood sequences. The "double" refers to the fact that there are two radiofrequency inversion pulses used to suppress the signal from blood. The first inversion pulse is nonselective meaning that it affects all hydrogen protons exposed to the transmit coil. The second inversion pulse is selective meaning that it only affects the hydrogen protons in the slice that is being imaged. Following the two inversion pulses, a preset amount of time passes (inversion time) and the image is then acquired. The image is acquired at the time that blood from outside the slice of interest has moved into the slice of interest and its magnetization has crossed zero (no signal at zero magnetization = dark blood). In the images shown, the arrows point to areas of increased signal intensity in the subendocardial portions of the left ventricular cavity, which get larger closer to the left ventricular apex (key point: not in the myocardium). This is because there is more stagnant blood flow in these areas so the blood is not completely replaced by the dark blood from outside the slice. Myocardial edema would show increased T2 signal intensity in the myocardium. Myocardial fibrosis would be best seen on late gadolinium enhancement images as areas of increased signal intensity. Myocardial nulling refers to setting an inversion time on late gadolinium enhancement images so that the myocardium is black.

Reference: Biglands JD. Cardiovascular magnetic resonance physics for clinicians: part I. *J Cardiovasc Magn Reson* 2010;12:71. doi:10.1186/1532-429X-12-71.

7 **Answer C.** Phase-contrast images are used to measure blood flow and velocity. In cardiac imaging, they are most commonly used to evaluate the peak velocity in cases of valve stenosis and the regurgitant fraction in cases of valve insufficiency. A bipolar gradient is applied, and results in stationary objects experiencing no net phase shift while moving objects will experience a phase shift proportional to their velocity, which yields signal. If the velocity-encoding gradient is set too high or low, aliasing will occur (which is not on the image below).

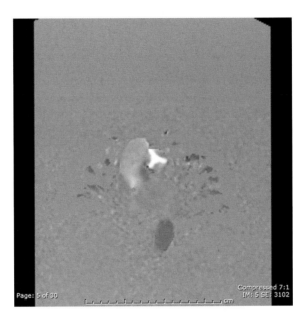

Reference: Lotz J, et al. Cardiovascular flow measurement with phase-contrast MR imaging: basic facts and implementation. *Radiographics* 2002;22(3):651–671.

8 **Answer A.** Effective dose gives a general population risk rather than patient-specific risk. It is obtained by multiplying the DLP by a conversion factor (f). The conversion factor is obtained by Monte Carlo simulation, and the best estimates (f) factor should be size specific.

Reference: Litmanovich DE, Tack DM, Shahrzad M, et al. Dose reduction in cardiothoracic CT: review of currently available methods. *Radiographics* 2014;34(6):1469–1489. doi:10.1148/rg.346140084.

9 **Answer C.** In patients with contraindication to beta-blocker (such as second-degree heart block, severe asthma, decompensated heart failure), a calcium channel blocker can be used. Verapamil is a calcium blocker agent. Atenolol is a beta-blocker so it should not be used if there is contraindication to beta-blocker. Nitroglycerin is used for vasodilatation of the coronaries and will not slow the heart rate. Sildenafil (Viagra) should not be used concurrently with nitroglycerin as it could cause severe hypotension.

Reference: Taylor CM, Blum A, Abbara S. Patient preparation and scanning techniques. *Radiol Clin North Am* 2010;48(4):675–686. doi:10.1016/j.rcl.2010.04.011.

10 **Answer A.** Hypotension is a contraindication to sublingual nitroglycerin (usually a systolic blood pressure of <90) because the medication can further lower blood pressure. Another important contraindication is if the patient has taken erectile dysfunction medication (i.e., sildenafil) in the past 24 to 48 hours. Obesity, diabetes, and dyslipidemia are not contraindications.

Reference: Taylor CM, Blum A, Abbara S. Patient preparation and scanning techniques. *Radiol Clin North Am* 2010;48(4):675–686. doi:10.1016/j.rcl.2010.04.011.

11 **Answer C.** The artifact shown is aliasing in the aortic valve. This artifact is seen with phase-contrast imaging, which in this example is being used to quantify flow through the aortic valve. Phase-contrast imaging uses bipolar gradients to measure the phase shift of stationary protons (staying in the slice) and moving protons (moving through the slice). The bipolar gradients are typically of equal but opposite polarity so stationary protons see no net phase shift, but moving protons demonstrates a net phase shift proportional to their velocity. The velocity-encoding gradient (VENC) is set prior to acquiring a phase-contrast image. The VENC determines the strength of the bipolar gradients, which essentially means the maximum velocity that can be detected. If the VENC is set below the true velocity of the moving blood, then aliasing occurs. Increasing the field of view, slice thickness, or bandwidth would not resolve the aliasing.

Reference: Lotz J, Meier C, Leppert A, et al. Cardiovascular flow measurement with phase-contrast MR imaging: basic facts and implementation. *Radiographics* 2002;22:651–671.

12 **Answer D.** NSF is characterized by thickening and hardening of the skin, which is symmetric and involves the upper and lower extremities. The skin can be nodular, and the disease process can involve the trunk; however, the face is usually spared.

Reference: Nainani N, Panesar M. Nephrogenic systemic fibrosis. *Am J Nephrol* 2009;29:1–9. doi:10.1159/000149628.

13 **Answer D.** The iodine flux is the number of iodine molecules administered per unit time and is related to the flow rate and the iodine concentration of the contrast agent. A higher flow rate will result in more molecules of iodine given per unit time and a greater amount of enhancement. Conversely, a decrease in flow rate will result in fewer molecules of iodine given per unit time and a reduced amount of enhancement.

Reference: Roberto P. *Multidetector-row CT angiography*. Springer Science & Business Media, 2006:44.

14 **Answer A.** Image A is a curved multiplanar reformation of the right coronary artery. This is a type of reconstruction created by centering the long axis of the imaging plane with a specific anatomic structure (in this case, the right coronary artery) in order to visualize the entire structure in one image. Image B is a 3-dimensional volume-rendered image. Image C is a maximum intensity projection image of the right coronary artery. This is a technique that projects the highest density voxel in a given slab onto a single image. Image D is a minimum intensity projection image of the lungs, which highlights the airways and emphysema. This is a technique that projects the lowest density voxel in a given slab onto a single image.

Reference: Cody DD. AAPM/RSNA physics tutorial for residents: topics in CT. Image processing in CT. *Radiographics* 2002;22(5):1255–1268.

15 **Answer B.** The myocardium is best nulled with a TI of 300 msec. The purpose of late gadolinium enhancement imaging is to visualize areas of myocardial

enhancement. This is best done by nulling the signal from normal myocardium so that areas of enhancement are relatively bright and easily visualized. At 150 msec, the blood is dark but not the myocardium. At both 500 and 800 msec, both the blood and myocardium are bright.

Reference: Biglands JD, Radjenovic A, Ridgway JP. Cardiovascular magnetic resonance physics for clinicians: part II. *J Cardiovasc Magn Reson* 2012;14:66. doi:10.1186/1532-429X-14-66.

16 **Answer D.** The balanced steady-state free precession sequence is a gradient echo sequence that is susceptible to metallic artifact and has weighted T2/T1 signal. While the sequence is relatively T2 weighted, it will also have T1 properties.

References: Bieri O, Scheffler K. Fundamentals of balanced steady state free precession MRI. *J Magn Reson Imaging* 2013;38:2–11. doi:10.1002/jmri.24163.

Chavan GB, Babyn PS, Jankharia BG, et al. Steady-state MR imaging sequences: physics, classification, and clinical applications. *Radiographics* 2008;28(4):1147–1160.

17 **Answer B.** The frequency encoding direction is superior–inferior. The artifact shown is a flow-related artifact caused by spins flowing out of the imaging plane, which is why it is most prominent during systole when there is the highest velocity forward flow through the main pulmonary artery. This artifact is seen in the anterior–posterior plane and occurs in the phase-encoding direction. Therefore, since the frequency encoding direction is opposite the phase-encoding direction, the answer is superior–inferior. In cardiac MRI, through plane and in plane generally refer to the direction of flow being assessed with phase-contrast imaging.

Reference: Saremi F, Grizzard JD, Kim RJ. Optimizing cardiac MR imaging: practical remedies for artifacts. *Radiographics* 2008;28(4):1161–1187.

18 **Answer B.** The yellow logo shown above is the logo for an MR conditional device. These devices may be scanned under very specific conditions. Examples include magnetic field strength, maximum spatial field gradient, dB/dt limitations, and SAR limits. The red logo shown below is for an MR unsafe device. These devices should not enter the MR scanner room. The green logo shown below is for an MR safe device. These devices may be scanned without any restrictions.

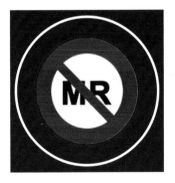 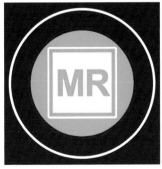

Reference: United States Food and Drug Administration. Understanding MRI Safety Labeling. fda.gov. April 23, 2020. https://www.fda.gov/media/101221/download

19 **Answer A.** Contrast bolus geometry is defined as the pattern of enhancement measured in a region of interest when looking at Hounsfield units versus time. In CT angiography, the ideal geometry is immediate and maximal enhancement that persists over time (steady state) of the study and does not change. However, this does not occur in the real world, typically one will get a rise in enhancement, short peak, and subsequent downslope.

Reference: Cademartiri F, van der Lugt A, Luccichenti G, et al. Parameters affecting bolus geometry in CTA: a review. *J Comp Assist Tomogr* 2002;26(4):598–607.

20 **Answer A.** Transient interruption of the contrast bolus occurs when deep inspiration increases central venous return from the IVC. This results in disruption of bolus and is most commonly witnessed during examinations for pulmonary embolism. As a result, the right ventricle and pulmonary artery will experience a decrease in attenuation compared to the SVC and can render the study nondiagnostic.

Reference: Wittram C, Yoo AJ. Transient interruption of contrast on CT pulmonary angiography: proof of mechanism. *J Thoracic Imaging* 2007;22(2):125–129.

21 **Answer A.** The higher field strength will contribute to a higher overall SAR. SAR is a function of field strength, flip angle, and TR. A doubling of the field strength or flip angle will lead to a 4× increase in the SAR.

Reference: Bitar R, Leung G, Perng R, et al. MR pulse sequences: what every radiologist wants to know but is afraid to ask. *Radiographics* 2006;26(2):513–537.

22 **Answer A.** When gadolinium is injected, it will be transported via systemic circulation to the myocardium. Upon reaching the myocardium, gadolinium will permeate the extracellular space; however, in healthy myocardium, there is no intracellular uptake. Infarcted myocardium has increased cell permeability, enlargement of the extravascular space, and, as a result, greater distribution and slower washout of gadolinium.

Reference: Edelman RR. Contrast-enhanced MR Imaging of the heart: overview of the literature. *Radiology* 2004;232(3):653–668.

23 **Answer B.** Gadolinium has paramagnetic properties due to unpaired outer shell electrons. When in a magnetic field, gadolinium becomes temporarily magnetized. The interaction between the outer shell of electrons and adjacent hydrogen nuclei leads to the T1-shortening properties of gadolinium.

Reference: Biglands JD, Radjenovic A, Ridgway JP. Cardiovascular magnetic resonance physics for clinicians: part II. *J Cardiovasc Magn Reson* 2012;14:66. doi:10.1186/1532-429X-14-66.

24 **Answer B.** The patient is screened in zone 2. In zone 1, there is no risk and the general public can enter the space. In zone 2, screening takes place. In zone 3, the magnetic field is sufficiently strong and can be hazardous to unscreened patients and personnel (console area). In zone 4, the magnetic field is strongest and all ferromagnetic objects must be excluded.

Reference: Kanal E, Barkovich AJ, Bell C, et al. ACR guidance document on MR safe practices: 2013. *Magn Reson Imaging* 2013;37:501–530.

25 **Answer A.** On balanced steady-state free precession sequence, a steady state is achieved by having the TR lower than the tissue T2 relaxation time. Since the TR is less than T2, there is not enough time for TM to decay before the next RF excitation pulse, resulting in the TM going back into the LM with the next excitation. At the same time, a portion of LM is flipped into the transverse plain.

Reference: Chavan GB, Babyn PS, Jankharia BG, et al. Steady-state MR imaging sequences: physics, classification, and clinical applications. *Radiographics* 2008;28(4):1147–1160.

26 **Answer B.** The image in B is a balanced steady-state free precession image of the heart in a two-chamber plane. In these images, the blood will appear bright and the tissue contrast will be a ratio of T2/T1. The image in A is a dark blood axial image through the chest. The image in C is the phase reconstruction from a phase-contrast image of the aortic valve. The image in D is a late gadolinium enhancement image of the heart in a three-chamber plane. Note how well the myocardium is nulled indicating optimal selection of the inversion time.

Reference: Biglands JD. Cardiovascular magnetic resonance physics for clinicians: part I. *J Cardiovasc Magn Reson* 2010;12:71. doi:10.1186/1532-429X-12-71.

27 **Answer B.** The patient can be scanned with a lower kVp based on the patient's body mass index. The scan length should be decreased (carina to diaphragm) and a lower mAs or auto mAs tool should be used to reduce dose. Retrospective gating will give more radiation than prospective ECG triggering. Doing a calcium score will add radiation from a noncontrast study.

Reference: Budoff M. Maximizing dose reductions with cardiac CT. *Int J Cardiovasc Imaging* 2009;25(Suppl 2):279–287.

28 **Answer B.** Patients who undergo retrospective gating will be imaged through systole and diastole. At low heart rates, tube modulation minimizes dose during systole but provides enough dose to calculate function and maximizes dose during diastole to evaluate the coronary arteries.

Reference: Mayo JR, Leipsic JA. Radiation does in cardiac CT. *AJR Am J Roentgenol* 2009;192:646–653.

29 **Answer A.** This change will increase the acquisition time because an increase in spatial resolution in the phase-encoding direction requires an increase in the number of phase-encoding steps. Image acquisition time = (repetition time × number of phase-encoding steps × number of excitations)/echo train length. Changing the spatial resolution alone does not change the field of view, echo train length, or number of excitations.

Reference: Biglands JD. Cardiovascular magnetic resonance physics for clinicians: part I. *J Cardiovasc Magn Reson* 2010;12:71. doi:10.1186/1532-429X-12-71.

30 **Answer C.** The image in C is a late gadolinium enhancement image. This image is obtained using a single radiofrequency inversion pulse used to null the myocardium. In this example, the image shows mesocardial/epicardial enhancement in the septal and inferior walls and epicardial enhancement in the lateral wall in a patient with myocarditis. The image in A is a T2-weighted dark blood image with spectral fat saturation. This image is obtained using two radiofrequency inversion pulses used to null the blood. It would have been reasonable to think this image was a dark blood image with inversion recovery fat saturation (also referred to as a "triple-IR" sequence), which uses three radiofrequency inversion pulses—one to null the fat and two to null the blood. However, while difficult, the incomplete fat saturation in the upper abdomen could clue you to the fact that this image used spectral fat saturation. Regardless, both sequences have more than one radiofrequency inversion pulse. The image in D is a balanced stead-state free precession image of the heart in a two-chamber plane, which does not use a typical 180-degree radiofrequency inversion pulse.

Reference: Biglands JD. Cardiovascular magnetic resonance physics for clinicians: part I. *J Cardiovasc Magn Reson* 2010;12:71. doi:10.1186/1532-429X-12-71.

31 **Answer A.** Increasing the pitch will reduce the radiation dose. Pitch is defined as the ratio of the table distance traveled in one full gantry rotation divided by the thickness of all the acquired slices. Conceptually, this means with a pitch of <1, the same area is irradiated more than once. As you increase the pitch, the same area is irradiated less, and hence, the radiation dose goes down. Increasing either the kV or mA will increase the radiation dose. Increasing the field of view does not affect the radiation dose.

Reference: Mayo JR, Leipsic JA. Radiation does in cardiac CT. *AJR Am J Roentgenol* 2009;192:646–653.

Normal Anatomy, Including Variants, Encountered on Radiography, CT, and MR

Joe Y. Hsu, MD • Amar B. Shah, MD, MPA • Sachin Malik, MD

QUESTIONS

1a What is the coronary artery dominance of this patient?

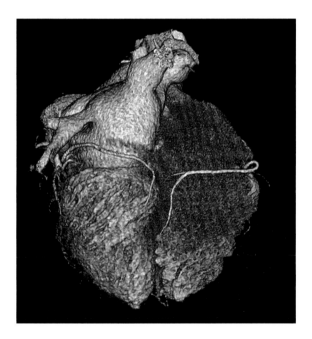

A. Left
B. Right
C. Codominant
D. Nondominant

1b How often is this type of anatomy present?
A. 10% to 20%
B. 40% to 50%
C. 80% to 90%

2   What is the normal relationship of the tricuspid and mitral valves?

A. They are located at the same level.
B. The tricuspid valve is more apically located than the mitral valve.
C. The mitral valve is more apically located than the tricuspid valve.

3   What is the normal relationship of the left pulmonary artery to the left mainstem bronchi?

A. Hyparterial
B. Eparterial
C. Isoarterial

4a   Which cardiac valve has not been surgically repaired in the images shown?

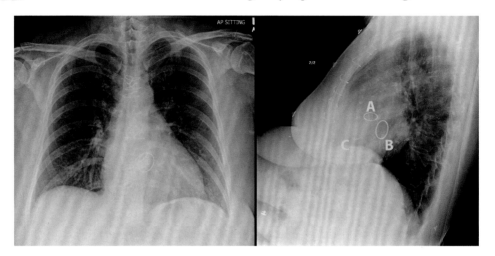

A. Pulmonic
B. Tricuspid
C. Mitral
D. Aortic

4b   Which letter on the lateral chest radiograph corresponds to the aortic valve?

A. A
B. B
C. C

5   Which of the following characteristics can help to identify the morphologic right ventricle in cases of congenital heart disease?

A. Moderator band
B. Papillary muscles only attached to the free wall
C. Bicuspid atrioventricular valve
D. Location of superior vena cava

6   What is the name of the valve at the ostium of the coronary sinus?

A. Eustachian
B. Thebesian
C. Vieussens
D. Marshall

7   This structure located in the right atrium is most likely which of the following?

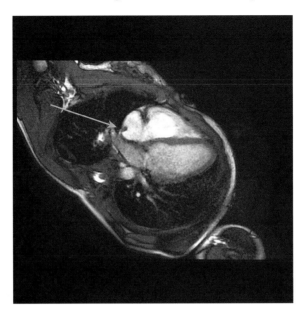

A. Crista terminalis
B. Thrombus
C. Myxoma
D. Central line

8   Which pulmonary vein is seen draining into the left atrium?

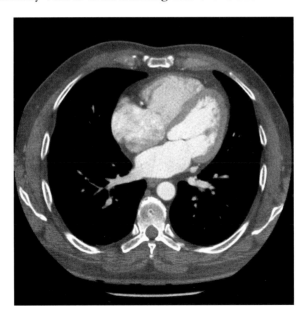

A. Right superior pulmonary vein
B. Right inferior pulmonary vein
C. Scimitar vein

9 Which of the following images shows a normal aortic valve during systole?

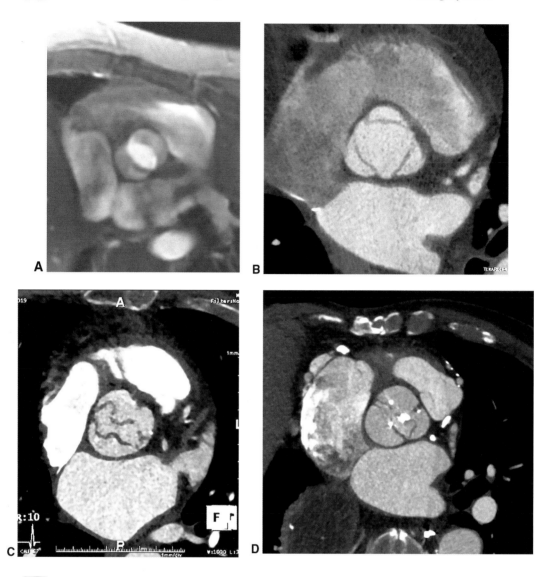

10 In what anatomic structure is the abnormality identified by the arrow located?

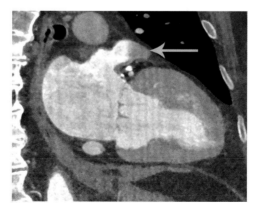

A. Aorta
B. Left atrial appendage
C. Pulmonary vein
D. Right atrium

11 The arrow points to what structure?

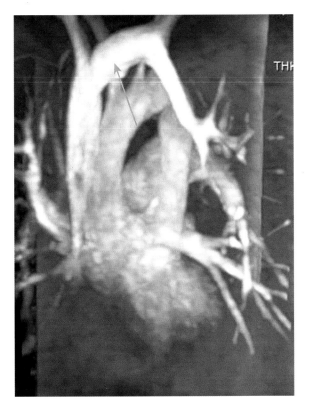

A. Aorta
B. Brachiocephalic vein
C. Left upper lobe pulmonary vein
D. Superior vena cava

12 The aortic root is defined as the space between which two letters in the image?

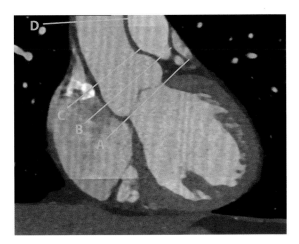

A. A and B
B. A and C
C. A and D
D. B and C

13 The vessel arising from the right coronary artery supplies which structure?

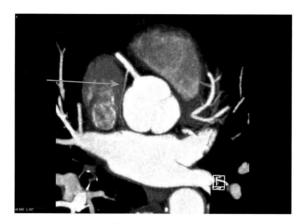

    A. Anterior wall of the right ventricle
    B. Infundibulum
    C. Left atrium
    D. Sinoatrial node

14 Which coronary artery typically supplies the structure identified by the arrow?

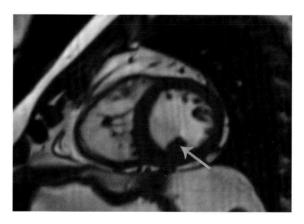

    A. Left anterior descending artery
    B. Left circumflex artery
    C. Obtuse marginal artery
    D. Right coronary artery

15 What structure is identified by the arrows?

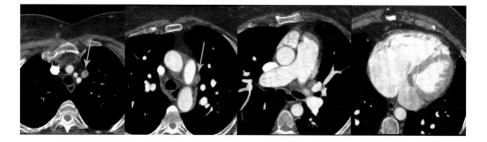

    A. Left superior vena cava
    B. Left superior anomalous pulmonary vein
    C. Left superior intercostal vein
    D. Aberrant left subclavian artery

16 What is the best description for this cardiac plane?

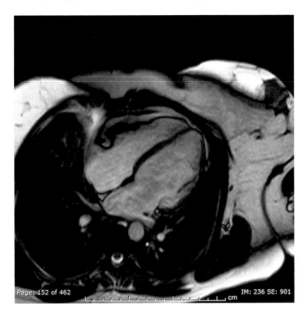

    A. Four-chamber plane
    B. Three-chamber plane
    C. Two-chamber plane
    D. Short-axis plane

17 The arrow points to which anatomic structure?

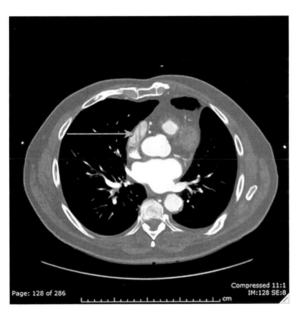

    A. Chiari network
    B. Eustachian valve
    C. Right atrial appendage
    D. Superior vena cava

18 The left ventricular wall identified by the arrow is supplied by which coronary artery?

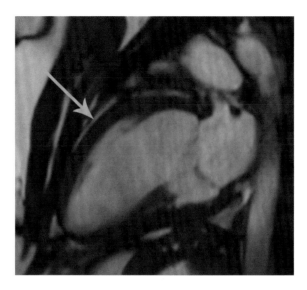

    A. Right coronary artery
    B. Posterior descending artery
    C. Left anterior descending artery
    D. Left circumflex artery

19 This image from a balanced steady-state free precession sequence shows a bicuspid aortic valve. What structure is indicated by the arrow?

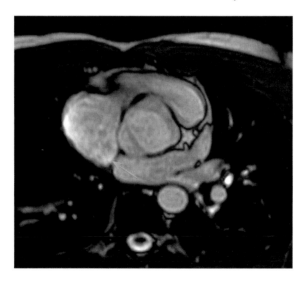

    A. Interatrial septum
    B. Noncoronary cusp
    C. Mitral attachment
    D. Crista terminalis

20 What structure is identified by the arrows?

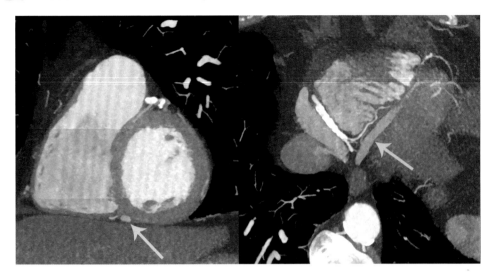

A. Coronary sinus
B. Middle cardiac vein
C. Great cardiac vein
D. Small cardiac vein

21 The arrow points to what structure?

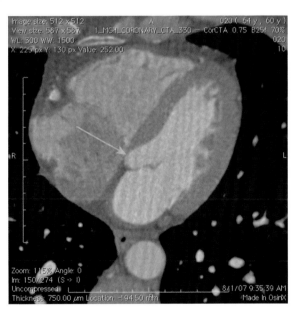

A. Fossa ovalis
B. Membranous septum
C. Mitral valve
D. Chordae tendineae

22 The arrow shows which coronary artery?

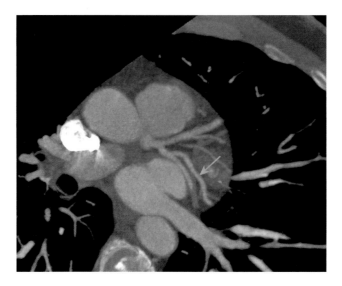

A. Circumflex
B. Diagonal
C. Left anterior descending
D. Obtuse marginal

23 The angiographic image below shows which coronary artery?

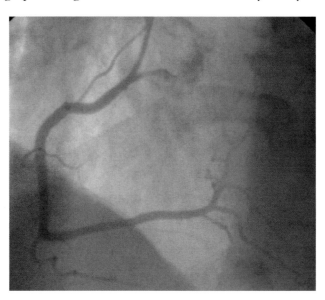

A. Right coronary artery
B. Left anterior descending
C. Left circumflex
D. Ramus intermedius

24 What structure is shown in the image?

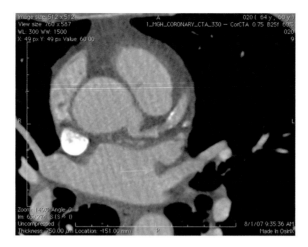

A. Inferior pulmonary vein
B. Left atrial appendage
C. Ligament of Marshall
D. Fossa ovalis

25 The angiogram from an RAO caudal position shows an arrow on which coronary artery?

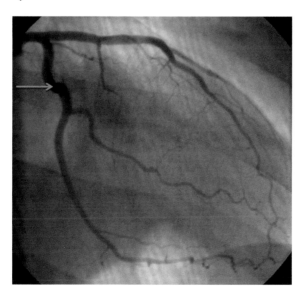

A. Right coronary artery
B. Left anterior descending
C. Left circumflex
D. Ramus intermedius

26 The arrow points to what anatomic structure?

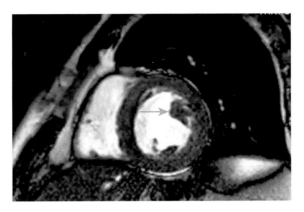

A. Anterolateral papillary muscle
B. Chordae tendineae
C. Lateral wall
D. Moderator band

27 An MR technologist-in-training is learning how to acquire the different cardiac planes. Prescribing the next scan across which of the following lines would get a three-chamber view of the heart?

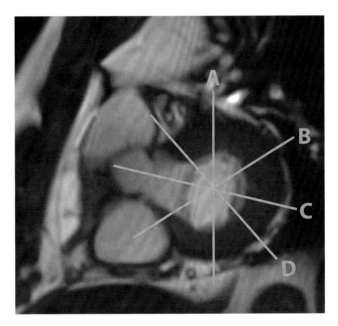

A. A
B. B
C. C
D. D

ANSWERS AND EXPLANATIONS

1a **Answer C.** Volume-rendered image shows a duplicated posterior descending artery supplied by both the right coronary and left circumflex arteries (arrows). This is consistent with codominant anatomy.

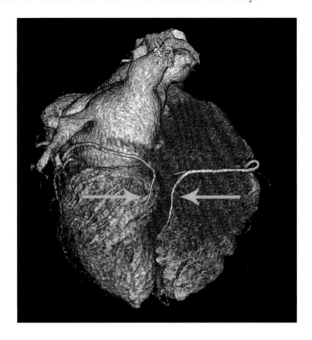

1b **Answer A.** Codominant anatomy occurs in roughly 10% to 20% of patients.

References: O'Brien JP, Srichai MB, Hecht EM, et al. Anatomy of the heart at multidetector CT: what the radiologist needs to know. *Radiographics* 2007;27(6):1569–1582. Review.

Pannu HK, Flohr TG, Corl FM, et al. Current concepts in multi-detector row CT evaluation of the coronary arteries: principles, techniques, and anatomy. *Radiographics* 2003;23: S111–S125. Review.

2 **Answer B.** The tricuspid valve is more apically located than the mitral valve. This can be helpful in identifying the valves/ventricles in patients with ventricular inversion. The AV valves (tricuspid and mitral) will go with their respective morphologic ventricles (tricuspid with morphologic RV, mitral with morphologic LV).

References: O'Brien JP, Srichai MB, Hecht EM, et al. Anatomy of the heart at multidetector CT: what the radiologist needs to know. *Radiographics* 2007;27(6):1569–1582. Review.

Schallert EK, Danton GH, Kardon R, et al. Describing congenital heart disease by using three-part segmental notation. *Radiographics* 2013;33(2):E33–E46. doi:10.1148/rg.332125086.

3 **Answer A.** Normal relationship of the left pulmonary artery to the left mainstem and left lobar bronchi is hyparterial (the bronchi is inferior to the artery). The normal relationship of the right pulmonary artery to the right superior lobar bronchus is eparterial (artery is inferior to the bronchus). This can be used when evaluating patients with situs anomalies to determine the right and left side.

References: Lapierre C, Déry J, et al. Segmental approach to imaging of congenital heart disease. *Radiographics* 2010;30(2):397–411. doi: 10.1148/rg.302095112. Review.

Schallert EK, Danton GH, Kardon R, et al. Describing congenital heart disease by using three-part segmental notation. *Radiographics* 2013;33(2):E33–E46. doi: 10.1148/rg.332125086.

4a **Answer A.** The pulmonic valve is the only valve that has not been surgically repaired. The patient has had a mechanical aortic valve repair, bioprosthetic mitral valve repair, and tricuspid valve annuloplasty.

References: Lapierre C, Déry J, Guérin R, et al. Segmental approach to imaging of congenital heart disease. *Radiographics* 2010;30(2):397–411. doi: 10.1148/rg.302095112. Review.

Schallert EK, Danton GH, Kardon R, et al. Describing congenital heart disease by using three-part segmental notation. *Radiographics* 2013;33(2):E33–E46. doi: 10.1148/rg.332125086.

4b **Answer A.** Letter A corresponds to the aortic valve. The most posteriorly located valve is the mitral valve (letter B). The pulmonic valve is the most superiorly located valve and is located anterior and superior to the aortic valve (letter P in the image denotes where a prosthetic pulmonic valve would be seen). The tricuspid valve is the most lateral right-sided valve (typically right of the spine on CXR; letter C).

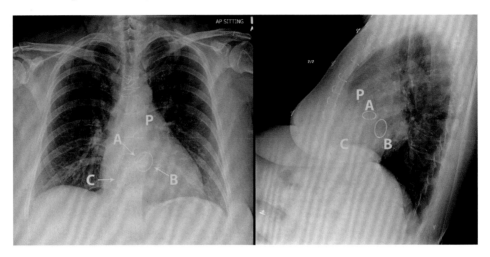

References: Lapierre C, Déry J, Guérin R, et al. Segmental approach to imaging of congenital heart disease. *Radiographics* 2010;30(2):397–411. doi: 10.1148/rg.302095112. Review.

Schallert EK, Danton GH, Kardon R, et al. Describing congenital heart disease by using three-part segmental notation. *Radiographics* 2013;33(2):E33–E46. doi: 10.1148/rg.332125086.

5 **Answer A.** The presence of a moderator band is one of several characteristics that help to identify the morphologic right ventricle in cases of congenital heart disease. Other characteristics include coarsened trabeculae, a tricuspid atrioventricular valve, papillary muscles attached to both the free and interventricular septal walls, and an outflow tract. One tip to help remember is by knowing that the valves follow the ventricles. The tricuspid valve follows the right ventricle and has three leaflets (hence tricuspid atrioventricular valve) and papillary muscles, which arise from the free and interventricular septal walls. The characteristics described in options B and C are to help identify the morphologic left ventricle. The location of the superior vena cava does not reliably help to identify the morphologic right ventricle.

Reference: Schallert EK, Danton GH, Kardon R, et al. Describing congenital heart disease by using three-part segmental notation. *Radiographics* 2013;33(2):E33–E46. doi: 10.1148/rg.332125086.

6 **Answer B.** The valve at the ostium of the coronary sinus is the thebesian valve. The eustachian valve is at the inferior vena cava. The Vieussens valve is at the junction of the coronary sinus and the great cardiac vein. The ligament of Marshall is the developmental remnant of the left superior vena cava.

Reference: Shah SS, Teague SD, Lu JC, et al. Imaging of the coronary sinus: normal anatomy and congenital abnormalities. *Radiographics* 2012;32(4):991–1008. doi:10.1148/rg. 324105220.

7 **Answer A.** This posterior right atrial structure is the crista terminalis, which is a muscular ridge separating the muscular and smooth portion of the right atrium. It can often be mistaken for a right atrial mass/thrombus but is a normal structure. While thrombus can be associated with the crista terminalis, it would typically be larger and associated with history of central line placement. Right atrial myxoma can occur in the posterior right atrial wall but are typically larger and along the interatrial septum.

Reference: Malik SB, Kwan D, Shah AB, et al. The right atrium: gateway to the heart—anatomic and pathologic imaging findings. *Radiographics* 2015;35(1):14–31. doi:10.1148/rg. 351130010.

8 **Answer B.** The vein seen draining into the left atrium is the right inferior pulmonary vein. This can be determined due to the fact that inferior pulmonary veins drain the lower lobe, which is posteriorly located. Therefore, any vein that is approaching from the posterior lung will be draining the lower lobe and thus inferiorly located. Any vein draining anteriorly would be the superior pulmonary veins. The scimitar vein typically will drain into the right atrium/IVC.

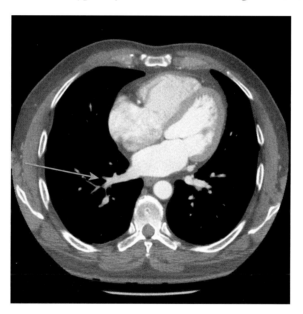

Reference: Porres DV, Morenza OP, Pallisa E, et al. Learning from the pulmonary veins. *Radiographics* 2013;33(4):999–1022. doi: 10.1148/rg.334125043. Review.

9 **Answer B.** The valve shown in image B is a normal trileaflet aortic valve. The three leaflets are named the left, right, and noncoronary leaflets. The right leaflet is the most anterior, and the noncoronary leaflet abuts the interatrial septum. The image in A is the magnitude reconstruction from a phase contrast image through the aortic valve, which shows a bicuspid aortic valve. The image in C shows incomplete opening of a thickened bicuspid aortic valve. The image in D shows a mildly thickened and calcified bicuspid aortic valve with a fused raphe between the left and right cusps.

Reference: Sievers HH, Schmidtke C. A classification system for the bicuspid aortic valve from 304 surgical specimens. *J Thorac Cardiovasc Surg* 2007;133(5):1226–1233.

10 **Answer B.** A two-chamber view of the heart from a CT angiography is shown. The arrow points to a filling defect in the left atrial appendage. On this arterial phase image, the differential for the filling defect is a thrombus or slow flow. Delayed images can be very useful in distinguishing between the two since slow flow would be expected to fill in on delayed images. However, particularly in patients with severe left atrial enlargement and atrial fibrillation, even delayed images may not be able to definitively distinguish between the two. Transesophageal echocardiography remains the gold standard for the assessment of left atrial appendage thrombus.

Reference: Garcia MJ. Detection of left atrial appendage thrombus by cardiac computed tomography. A word of caution. *J Am Coll Cardiol* 2009;2(1):77–79. doi:10.1016/j.jcmg. 2008.10.003.

11 **Answer B.** Patient has left upper lobe anomalous pulmonary venous return (arrow on the right). The anomalous vein drains into the left brachiocephalic vein and subsequently to the SVC and right atrium. The pattern of drainage creates a left-to-right shunt.

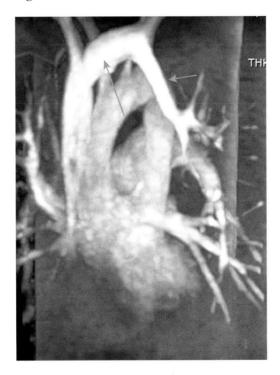

Reference: Dillman JR, Yarram SG, Hernandez RJ. Imaging of pulmonary venous developmental anomalies. *AJR Am J Roentgenol* 2009;192(5):1272–1285.

12 **Answer B.** The aortic root is defined as the space between A and C in the image. A corresponds to the aortic annulus. B corresponds to the sinuses of Valsalva. C corresponds to the sinotubular junction. D corresponds to the ascending thoracic aorta.

Reference: Charitos EI, Seivers HH. Anatomy of the aortic root: implications for valve-sparing surgery. *Ann Cardiothorac Surg* 2012;2(1):53–56.

13 **Answer D.** The sinoatrial nodal artery most commonly arises from the RCA and courses toward the interatrial septum. The artery can also arise from the left circumflex coronary artery.

Reference: Kini S, Bis, KG, Weaver L. Normal and variant coronary arterial and venous anatomy on high resolution CT angiography. *AJR Am J Roentgenol* 2007;188(6):1665–1674.

14 **Answer D.** A short-axis bright blood image through the mid left ventricle is shown. The arrow identifies the posteromedial papillary muscle. There are two papillary muscles in the left ventricle, the anterolateral and posteromedial papillary muscles. The anterolateral papillary muscle (seen in the image as the thick muscle bundle along the lateral wall of the left ventricle) has a shared blood supply from the left anterior descending and left circumflex coronary artery. The posteromedial papillary muscle is supplied by the right coronary artery (in right dominant patients) and is more prone to rupture following myocardial infarction given its single vascular supply.

References: Czarnecki A, Thakrar A, Fang T, et al. Acute severe mitral regurgitation: consideration of papillary muscle architecture. *Cardiovasc Ultrasound* 2008;6:5.

Fradley MG, Picard MH. Rupture of the posteromedial papillary muscle leading to partial flail of the anterior mitral leaflet. *Circulation* 2011;123(9):1044–1045.

15 **Answer A.** The arrows in the sequential superior to inferior axial images from a CT angiogram of the chest show a left superior vena cava (SVC). The inferior most image shows the typical finding of an enlarged coronary sinus, which is where the left SVC drains. A persistent left SVC is the most common congenital thoracic venous anomaly. The right SVC may be absent, small, or normal with or without a bridging vein. In this case, the right SVC is normal. This is not a left superior anomalous pulmonary vein, which would commonly drain into the left brachiocephalic vein and not the coronary sinus. The left superior intercostal vein, also referred to as an "aortic nipple" on chest radiograph, courses over the aortic arch. An aberrant left subclavian artery would arise from a right-sided arch and take a retroesophageal course. In addition, unless occluded, it would be expected to have the same level of contrast enhancement as the aorta in the images shown.

Reference: Sonavane SK, Milner DM, Singh SP, et al. Comprehensive imaging review of the superior vena cava. *Radiographics* 2015;35:1873–1892.

16 **Answer A.** This is a four-chamber plane, which shows the right atrium, right ventricle, left atrium, and left ventricle. The plane allows for evaluation of the mitral and tricuspid valves and to evaluate the right ventricular free wall, interventricular septum, and lateral wall of the left ventricle.

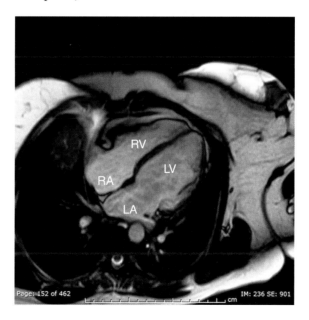

Reference: Nasif MS, Oliveira AC Jr, Carvalho AC, et al. Cardiac magnetic resonance and its anatomical planes: How do I do it? *Arq Bras Cardiol* 2010;95(6):756–763.

17 **Answer C.** The structure represents the right atrial appendage. The right atrial appendage extends anteriorly from the right atrium and contains multiple pectinate muscles. It is adjacent to the ascending aorta to the right of the midline and will maintain a broad conical shape. The right atrial appendage can be associated as a nidus of arrhythmia and can serve as a target for pacing.

Reference: Manolis AS, Varriale P, Baptist SJ. Necropsy study of right atrial appendage: morphology and measurements. *Clin Cardiol* 1988;11:788–792.

18 **Answer C.** This is a bright blood two-chamber view of the heart. The arrows points at the anterior wall. The anterior wall is supplied by the left anterior descending artery. The left anterior descending artery typically supplies the basal to mid anterior and anteroseptal walls, apical septal wall, apical anterior wall, and apex. The right coronary artery typically supplies the basal to mid inferior and inferoseptal walls. The apical inferior wall can be supplied by either the left anterior descending artery or posterior descending artery. The left circumflex artery typically supplies the basal to mid inferolateral and anterolateral walls and apical lateral walls.

Reference: Cerquiera MD, et al. Standardized myocardial segmentation and nomenclature for tomographic imaging of the heart: a statement for healthcare professionals from the Cardiac Imaging Committee of the Council on Clinical Cardiology of the American Heart Association. *Circulation* 2002;105:539–542.

19 **Answer A.** The arrow is pointing to the interatrial septum. The interatrial septum is directed toward the noncoronary cusp. In the below image, the left coronary cusp and right coronary cusp are fused.

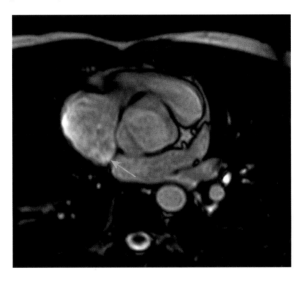

Reference: Ziad FI, John MM, Douglas PZ. *Clinical arrhythmology and electrophysiology: A companion to Braunwald's heart disease series.* Saunders W.B., 2018:582.

20 **Answer B.** The arrows in the image identify the middle cardiac vein. This vein is also referred to as the inferior interventricular or posterior interventricular vein. This vein courses through the posterior interventricular groove and eventually drains into the coronary sinus. The coronary sinus drains directly into the right atrium. The distal end is demarcated by the thebesian valve. The great cardiac vein courses in the left atrioventricular groove and almost always drains into the coronary sinus. The small cardiac vein is present in 30% to 50% of patients, receives blood from portions of the right ventricle, and most often drains into the coronary sinus.

Reference: Saremi F, et al. Coronary veins: comprehensive CT-anatomic classification and review of variants and clinical implications. *Radiographics* 2012;32:E1–E32.

21 Answer B. The interventricular septum contains two components, a membranous segment and a muscular segment. The majority of the septum is the muscular segment, which separates the right and left ventricle from each other. The most superior and posterior segment of the septum is the membranous portion, which is at the base of the heart between the inlet and outlet components of the muscular septum and inferior to the right and noncoronary cusps of the aortic valve.

Reference: Minette MS, Sahn DJ. Ventricular septal defects. *Circulation* 2006;114(20): 2190–2197.

22 Answer D. The image shows the left main coronary artery with a normal bifurcation into the left anterior descending (LAD) and left circumflex coronary artery (LCx). The first obtuse margin division is shown to arise from the LCx. The obtuse marginal divisions typically supply the inferolateral wall.

Reference: Kini SKG, Bis KG, Weaver L. Normal and variant coronary arterial and venous anatomy on high-resolution CT angiography. *Am J Roentgenol* 2007;188(6):1665–1674.

23 Answer A. The coronary artery is the right coronary artery and gives rise to the PDA and PLV divisions (blue and red arrows) and the conus branch (yellow arrow). The view above is a "c" view of the right coronary artery, which can be obtained from CTA datasets through using multiplanar reformatting to mimic the angiographic left anterior oblique (LAO) view.

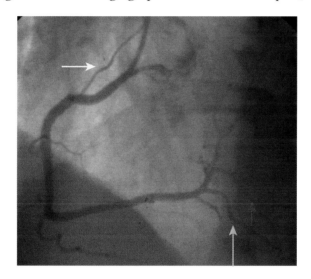

Reference: Kern M. Angiographic projections made simple: an easy guide to understanding oblique views. *Cath Lab Digest* 2011;19(8).

24 Answer C. This structure represents the ligament of Marshall. The ligament of Marshall is a normal structure which is positioned between the left atrial appendage ostium and the left superior pulmonary vein. It is the embryonic residua of the left-sided SVC and if enlarged can mimic a mass or thrombus.

Reference: Ho SY, Cabrera JA, Sanchez-Quintana D. Advances in arrhythmia and electrophysiology: left atrial anatomy revisited. *Circ Arrhythm Electrophysiol* 2012;5:220–228. doi:10.1161/CIRCEP.111.962720

25 Answer C. This RAO caudal position shows the left main bifurcating into the left circumflex and left anterior descending coronary artery. The blue arrow shows the left circumflex coronary artery, while the green arrow shows the LAD. The obtuse marginal and diagonal divisions are highlighted in yellow and red, respectively.

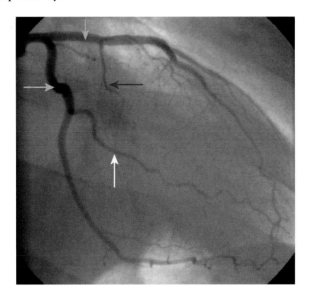

26 **Answer A.** The left ventricle has two papillary muscles, the anterolateral and posteromedial papillary muscles. The arrow points to the anterolateral papillary muscle. The mitral valve attaches to the papillary muscle via the thin fibrous chordae tendineae.

Reference: Moore KL, Dalley AF, Agur AM. *Clinically oriented anatomy*, 3rd ed. Baltimore, MD: Lippincott Williams & Wilkins, 2007.

27 **Answer C.** The image shown is a left ventricular short axis bright blood image at the level of the mitral valve. Scanning across line C would acquire a three-chamber view of the heart. This line transects the center of the mitral valve and the center of the aortic valve, which is partially seen on this slice. Line A would acquire a two-chamber view of the heart. Line B would acquire a four-chamber view of the heart. Line D is not a standard cardiac plane.

Reference: Nasif MS, Oliveira AC Jr, Carvalho AC, et al. Cardiac magnetic resonance and its anatomical planes: how do I do it? *Arq Bras Cardiol* 2010;95(6):756–763.

3 Physiologic Aspects of Cardiac Imaging

Amar B. Shah, MD, MPA • Jean Jeudy, MD

QUESTIONS

1. Decreased cardiac preload will occur with which of the following physiologic changes?

    A. Increased ventricular compliance
    B. Increased venous return
    C. Decreased atrial contractility
    D. Decreased heart rate

2. Which of the following diastolic parameters is being evaluated in the image?

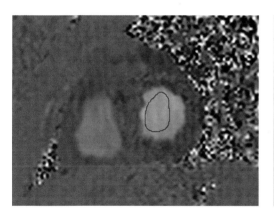 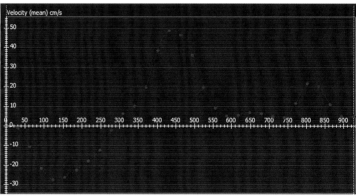

    A. E/A wave
    B. Tissue velocity
    C. Longitudinal ventricular strain
    D. Mitral insufficiency

3. At which point of the cardiac phase is the mitral valve open?

    A. Isovolumic relaxation
    B. Ventricular filling
    C. Isovolumic contraction
    D. Ventricular ejection

4   When measuring LV wall thickness, which of the following would be most consistent with intensive athletic conditioning?

A. 7 mm end systole
B. 10 mm end diastole
C. 14 mm end systole
D. 19 mm end diastole

5   A patient presents for evaluation of aortic stenosis by MR. Previous echo reports severe aortic stenosis with the gradient across the valve measured to be 36 mm Hg. What would be the most appropriate VENC to evaluate the valve?

A. 9 cm/sec
B. 30 cm/sec
C. 90 cm/sec
D. 300 cm/sec

6   A patient is being evaluated for heart failure. Cardiac MR is performed at 1.5T with inclusion of T1 parametric mapping. The global native T1 value = 1300 msec. After administration of contrast, the myocardium demonstrates a T1 mapping value of 200 msec.
What physiologic change in ECV has occurred between time points?

A. Increased ECV from baseline with underlying myocardial fibrosis
B. No change in ECV with underlying myocardial fibrosis
C. Increased ECV from baseline with no underlying myocardial fibrosis
D. No change in ECV with no underlying fibrosis

7   The below image is from a patient's previous retrospective ECG-gated coronary CTA. The technician asks your opinion of the study and what improvements would you recommend for this study.

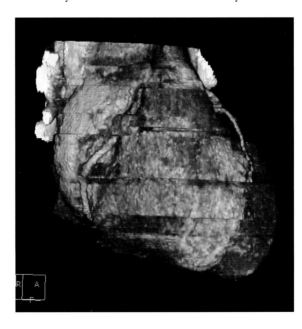

A. Consider evaluating ECG for editing.
B. Coach patient breathing before study.
C. Prospective triggering would have resulted in less motion.
D. Check nitroglycerin has dissolved before scanning.

8 A patient presents with a familial history of hypertension and coronary artery disease. The referring clinician is requesting a quantitative measure of left ventricular mass as well as evaluation of the coronaries. Which phase of the R–R interval would be most appropriate?

A. 0%

B. 20%

C. 60%

D. 80%

9 A patient had a cardiac MR from an outside facility. The study is good quality and reveals normal cardiac function. Unfortunately, phase-contrast imaging was not performed. The referring clinician is asking if there is evidence for an intracardiac shunt. How well can we make an estimate?

A. No way to determine shunt

B. Compare SVC and IVC diameters.

C. Evaluate for insufficiency jets from mitral and tricuspid valve.

D. Compare stroke volumes of both ventricles.

10 A patient presents with a history of aortic coarctation and 20 mm Hg gradient across the region of narrowing. Phase contrast was performed in the region of coarctation. Which estimated velocity most closely matches the true severity?

A. 240 cm/sec

B. 220 cm/sec

C. 160 cm/sec

D. 80 cm/sec

11a A 50-year-old male underwent a gated cardiac CTA (CCTA) acquisition using a 64-slice CT scanner. The gray box shows the only phase of the cardiac cycle during which images were obtained. What characterizes this phase of the cardiac cycle?

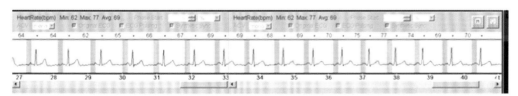

A. Atrial relaxation

B. Open mitral valve

C. Closed tricuspid valve

D. Ventricular contraction

11b A 50-year-old male underwent a gated cardiac CTA (CCTA) acquisition using a 64-slice CT scanner. The gray box shows the only phase of the cardiac cycle during which images were obtained. Why would the images be obtained using such an approach?

A. Allows ejection fraction to be calculated

B. Improves temporal resolution

C. Lower impact of elevated heart rate

D. Reduces radiation dose

11c Patients undergoing a cardiac CTA (CCTA) can receive a lower radiation dose through which of the following strategies?

A. Decreasing the pitch
B. Employing retrospective gating
C. Increasing mAs
D. Reducing kVp

12a The abnormality in the image is associated with which of the following?

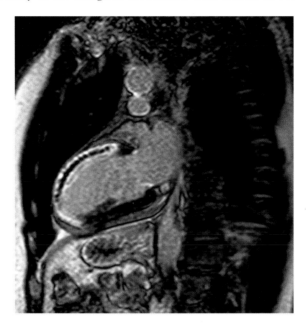

A. An ejection fraction >55%
B. Elongated mitral valve leaflet
C. Left ventricular wall thickening
D. Wall motion abnormalities

12b A severely decreased left ventricular systolic ejection fraction measures less than which value?

A. 55%
B. 50%
C. 45%
D. 40%
E. 35%

13 Which of the following describes isovolumetric contraction of the ventricles?

A. Corresponds to the trough of the QRS complex
B. The mitral and tricuspid valves are open.
C. Ventricular pressure increases.
D. Ventricular volume decreases.

14a Given the image below, which of the following findings would be expected?

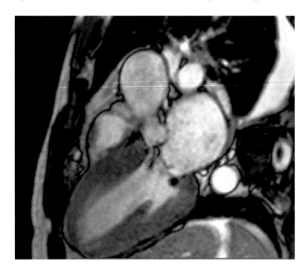

    A. Decreased left ventricular filling pressure
    B. Dilated ascending aorta
    C. Narrowing of the left ventricular outflow tract
    D. Thickening of the aortic valve leaflets

14b Which of the following physiologic changes occurs in the left heart in hypertrophic obstructive cardiomyopathy (HOCM)?
    A. Decreased myocardial mass
    B. Elevated left atrial pressure
    C. Increased left ventricular compliance
    D. Decreased atrial kick

15 Which of the following conditions increases the ventricular preload?
    A. Decreased atrial contraction
    B. Decreased ventricular compliance
    C. Deep inspiration
    D. Elevated heart rate
    E. Ligating an arterial–venous fistula
    F. Reduced atrial pressure

16 Aliasing on phase-contrast cardiac MRI occurs if the angular phase shift is
    A. >120 degrees and the velocity within that pixel is then misregistered
    B. >150 degrees and the velocity within that pixel is then misregistered
    C. >180 degrees and the velocity within that pixel is then misregistered
    D. >210 degrees and the velocity within that pixel is then misregistered

17 In preparation for a cardiac CTA, a patient was administered 100 mg of metoprolol via an oral tablet. Which of the following describes the mechanism of metoprolol?
    A. Increases the heart rate
    B. Stimulates the beta-1 receptors
    C. Exerts positive inotropic effects
    D. It is a cardioselective beta-blocker.

18a Which of the following criteria would indicate treatment for the condition shown in the image?

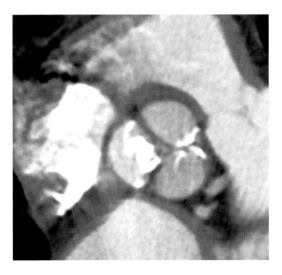

    A. A valve area of 1.3 cm²

    B. A valve calcium score of 2,000

    C. A velocity gradient of 45 mm Hg

    D. A velocity jet of 3 m/sec

    E. A bicuspid valve

18b The above patient has aortic stenosis and underwent a cardiac MRI. The velocity across the valve was calculated to measure 150 cm/sec. Given the velocity, what is the estimated pressure gradient?

    A. 5.5 mm Hg

    B. 6 mm Hg

    C. 8 mm Hg

    D. 9 mm Hg

19a The below image was obtained in diastole. Which of the following describes the underlying process?

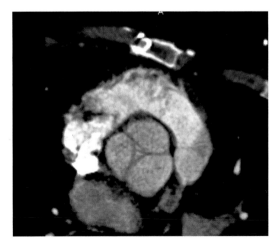

    A. Aortic stenosis

    B. Bicuspid aortic valve

    C. Increased end-diastolic volume

    D. Pulmonic insufficiency

    E. Pulmonic stenosis

19b Aortic insufficiency can be quantified using phase-contrast MRI. Which of the below indicates severe aortic insufficiency?

A. A bicuspid aortic valve

B. A dilated left ventricle measuring 6.5 cm

C. A regurgitant volume of 65 mL

D. An aortic valve area of 0.9 cm²

20a The following artifact is caused by

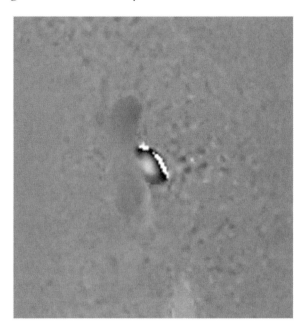

A. Incorrect inversion time

B. Incorrect encoding velocity

C. Incomplete fat saturation

D. Too high temporal resolution

E. Too low spatial resolution

20b A phase-contrast cardiac MRI (CMRI) sequence produces two sets of images. What set of images are produced by the phase-contrast acquisition?

A. Magnitude image and phase velocity map

B. Magnitude image and volume map

C. Magnitude image and velocity gradient map

D. Magnitude image and pressure gradient map

21 A patient is given intravenous beta-blockers in preparation for a cardiac CTA. What is the impact of this agent on the Frank-Starling curve?

A. Shifts the Frank-Starling curve upward and to the right

B. Shifts the Frank-Starling curve downward and to the right

C. Shifts the Frank-Starling curve upward and to the left

D. Shifts the Frank-Starling curve downward and to the left

22a A patient underwent a coronary venogram, and it showed abnormal connection between the coronary sinus and which structure?

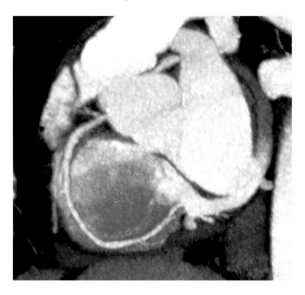

    A. Left atrium
    B. Left circumflex coronary artery
    C. Right atrium
    D. Inferior vena cava

22b The patient underwent a cardiac MRI to determine the left to right shunt. The calculated Qp/Qs was 1.2. What is the next step?

    A. No further treatment
    B. Percutaneous cardiac intervention
    C. Surgical treatment
    D. Stress echocardiogram

23 A patient underwent a cardiac CCTA secondary to an abnormal nuclear medicine stress test. The stress test showed a perfusion defect involving which vascular territory (territories)?

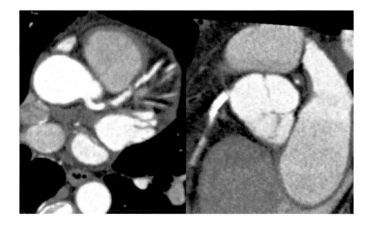

    A. Left anterior descending coronary artery
    B. Left circumflex coronary artery
    C. Left anterior descending coronary artery and left circumflex coronary artery
    D. Left circumflex and right coronary arteries
    E. Left circumflex coronary artery, left anterior descending coronary artery, and right coronary artery

24a A patient presents to the emergency room with atypical chest pain and persistent hiccups. Which anatomic territory is potentially affected?

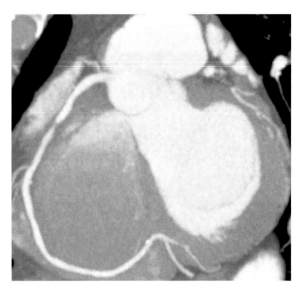

    A. Left anterior descending coronary artery
    B. Left circumflex coronary artery
    C. Right coronary artery
    D. No culprit lesion identified

24b What amount of narrowing in cardiac CTA indicates flow-limiting stenosis in a nonostial segment of the coronary artery?

    A. 40%
    B. 50%
    C. 60%
    D. 70%

25 Sublingual nitroglycerin (SL NTG) is administered during a cardiac CTA (CCTA). The patient experiences headaches after it is administered and asks to speak to a physician to explain why they were given the medication. What explanation do you give to the patient regarding the benefits of SL NTG use?

    A. Decreases motion of the coronary arteries
    B. Improves visualization of the coronary arteries
    C. Improves ventricular function
    D. Reduces radiation exposure

26 A patient with a history of atypical chest pain, severe asthma, and type 2 diabetes arrives for a cardiac CTA with a resting heart rate of 50 beats/min. The patient took sildenafil within the last 24 hours. A fellow asks if sublingual nitroglycerin (SL NTG) can be administered to the patient. Your response is

    A. No, due to hypotension
    B. No, it can induce arrhythmia.
    C. No, it increases the preload.
    D. No, due to respiratory arrest

27 You complete a cardiac MRI (CMRI) and need to report the ejection fraction. The end-systolic volume is 40 mL. The end-diastolic volume is 100 mL. The stroke volume is 60 mL. The myocardial mass is 65 g. The automated computer system reports an error and you must manually calculate the ejection fraction. What is the ejection fraction?

A. 40%
B. 55%
C. 60%
D. 65%
E. 70%

28 Atrial fibrillation is the most common cardiac arrhythmia. Patients with atrial fibrillation have ectopic electrical-stimulating foci that overwhelm the function of what normal cardiac structure?

A. Atrioventricular node
B. Bundle of His
C. Purkinje fibers
D. Sinoatrial node

29 A patient is referred for a cardiac MRI (CMRI) to determine the left ventricular myocardial mass. How is myocardial mass calculated?

A. (Epicardial myocardial volume − endocardial myocardial volume) × specific density of myocardium
B. (Endomyocardial volume − epicardial myocardial volume) × specific density of myocardium
C. (Epicardial myocardial volume) × specific density of myocardium
D. (Endocardial myocardial volume) × specific density of myocardium

30 Which of the following best describes diastolic dysfunction?

A. Cardiac MRI is advantageous compared to echocardiography in establishing the diagnosis.
B. Left ventricular filling rate decreases early in the disease process.
C. Left atrial size is normal.
D. Systolic ejection fraction is reduced.

31 A 55-year-old male undergoes a cardiac MRI (CMRI) and the left ventricular size is measured. What is the minimum value at which the cavity is considered to be dilated?

A. 4.8 cm
B. 5.3 cm
C. 5.8 cm
D. 6.3 cm

32 A 55-year-old male undergoes a cardiac MRI (CMRI) to quantify his aortic insufficiency. Which of the following will be expected?

A. Preserved stroke volume
B. Increased preload
C. Decreased cavity size
D. Preserved afterload
E. No change in isovolumetric relaxation

33a A patient underwent a gated cardiac CTA (CCTA) that showed a mass. Based on the image, what is the effect of the mass?

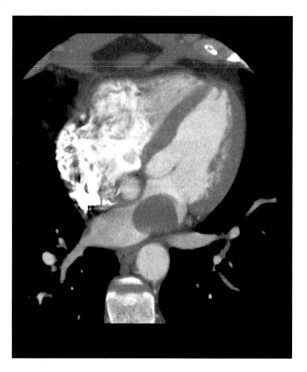

A. Obstructed left ventricular outflow tract
B. Obstructed pulmonary vein
C. Obstructed SVC
D. Obstructed tricuspid valve

33b The mass obstructed the pulmonary vein inflow and lead to pulmonary edema. Which of the following values indicates a normal pulmonary venous wedge pressure?

A. 10 mm Hg
B. 20 mm Hg
C. 30 mm Hg
D. 40 mm Hg

34 A 28-year-old competitive cyclist arrives for a cardiac MRI (CMRI). Which morphologic changes in the heart are expected?

A. Decrease in cavity size and wall thickness
B. Increase in cavity size and wall thickness
C. Increase in cavity size and decrease in wall thickness
D. No change in cavity size and wall thickness

ANSWERS AND EXPLANATIONS

1 **Answer C.** Preload reflects the resting length of cardiac myocytes just prior to left ventricular contraction (end diastole) and is also termed left ventricular end-diastolic pressure (LVEDP).

When venous return to the heart is increased, LVEDP and ventricular volumes are increased, which stretches the sarcomeres, thereby increasing their preload. Increased preload increases stroke volume, whereas decreased preload decreases stroke volume by altering the force of contraction of the cardiac muscle.

Increased venous return and increased ventricular compliance leads to increased ventricular filling and LV stroke volume, enhancing preload. Decreased atrial contractility leads to decreased ventricular filling and subsequently decreased preload. Hypovolemia would also decrease ventricular filling and subsequently decrease preload.

A decrease in heart rate allows for increased left ventricular filling time that subsequently leads to an increase in preload conditions.

Reference: Bonow RO, Mann DL, Zipes DP, et al., (eds). *Braunwald's heart disease: a textbook of cardiovascular medicine*, 9th ed. Philadelphia, PA: Elsevier Saunders, 2012:2048.

2 **Answer A.** Primary measurements of transmitral inflow include rapid early filling phase, designated the E wave, and late diastolic filling associated with atrial contraction, designated the A wave.

The E wave reflects the LA pressure in early diastole and occurs immediately following mitral valve opening. The A-wave velocity is affected by LA pressure and LV compliance at the end of diastole. In stiff ventricles, the A wave is smaller and also of shorter duration.

General classification of diastolic function is based predominantly on the pattern of mitral inflow as determined by the relative heights of the E and A waves (E:A ratio), their peak velocities, and the rate of deceleration of the E wave.

References: Caudron J, Fares J, Bauer F, et al. Evaluation of left ventricular diastolic function with cardiac MR imaging. *Radiographics.* 2011;31(1):239–259.

Solomon SD, Bulwer B, (eds). *Essential echocardiography: a practical handbook with DVD.* Totowa, NJ: Humana Press, 2007.

3 **Answer B.** The cardiac cycle is defined as one complete sequence of cardiac filling, cardiac muscle excitation and contraction with ejection of blood and muscle relaxation (diastole and systole). The events of the cycle can be divided into a recurring series of intervals and valve movements:

1. SYSTOLE
    a. Atrial contraction
    b. Mitral valve closes
    c. Ventricular isovolumetric contraction—both valves are closed
    d. Aortic valve opens
    e. Rapid ventricular ejection
    f. Slow ventricular ejection
    g. Aortic valve closes

2. DIASTOLE
   a. Ventricular isovolumetric relaxation occurs—both valves are closed
   b. Mitral valve opens
   c. Ventricular filling
   d. Diastasis—initial passive filling of the heart's ventricles has slowed, but before the atria contraction starting the cycle again

Reference: Mohrman DE, Heller LJ. *Cardiovascular physiology*, 9th ed. New York, NY: McGraw-Hill Education, 2018:304.

4 **Answer D.** Normal left ventricular wall thickness is typically <10 mm in thickness. Participation in intense, repetitive physical activities is known to alter the structural characteristics of the heart with varying degrees of concentric or eccentric hypertrophy depending on the form of training. These changes have been coined the "athlete's heart."

There is an overlap between this type of physiologic cardiac hypertrophy and mild forms of hypertrophic cardiomyopathy (HCM). The athlete's heart shows an eccentric biventricular hypertrophy with wall thicknesses between 12 and 15 mm and a moderately dilated left ventricle. HCM is commonly characterized by asymmetric left ventricular hypertrophy with a reduced LV diameter. LV wall thickness greater than 17 mm is highly suggestive of HCM.

Physiologic hypertrophy is consistent with a normal diastolic function with even increased early diastolic filling. In the setting of HCM, diastolic dysfunction occurs in the majority of patients and is therefore inconsistent with an athlete's heart.

References: Lauschke J, Maisch B. Athlete's heart or hypertrophic cardiomyopathy? *Clin Res Cardiol* 2009;98(2):80–88.

Pluim BM, Zwinderman AH, van der Laarse A, et al. The athlete's heart. A meta-analysis of cardiac structure and function. *Circulation* 2000;101:336–344.

5 **Answer D.** The Bernoulli principle allows us to determine the pressure gradient across valvular stenosis based on the sum of kinetic and pressure energy of blood flowing in a system.

The simplified Bernoulli equation ($P = 4v^2$) allows us to determine the instantaneous pressure gradient across a valve, using the maximum velocity of flow in meters/sec.

For the given scenario:
- $4v^2 = 36$ mm Hg
- $v^2 = 36/4 = 9$
- $v = 3$ m/sec
- $= 300$ cm/sec (remember to convert!)

Reference: Saikrishnan N, Kumar G, Sawaya FJ, et al. Accurate assessment of aortic stenosis: a review of diagnostic modalities and hemodynamics. *Circulation* 2014;129(2):244–253.

6 **Answer B.** T1 mapping is an **MRI technique** that allows quantification of the longitudinal magnetic relaxation of tissues such as the myocardium. Measurement of native and postcontrast myocardial and blood T1 values allows estimation of the extent of the interstitial myocardial space via the calculation of the fraction of the myocardial extracellular volume fraction (ECV)

$$ECV = (1 - \text{hematocrit}) \times (\Delta R1 \text{myocardium} / \Delta R1 \text{blood})$$

The ECV fraction is a direct measurement of the myocardial interstitium and thus a surrogate marker of processes such as myocardial fibrosis and abnormal infiltrative processes. An increase in ECV fraction correlates with expansion of the extracellular matrix within the myocardium.

Although we use pre- and postcontrast information to derive the ECV, there is no physiologic change in the ECV during the evaluation.

Meta-analysis of the studies report mean native T1 values of 1,150 msec and mean of ECV < 30% at field strength of 1.5 T. The native T1 value in this instance (1,300 msec) would indicate significant expansion of ECV suggesting significant interstitial fibrosis or myocardial infiltration.

References: Gottbrecht M, Kramer CM, Salerno M. Native T1 and extracellular volume measurements by cardiac MRI in healthy adults: a meta-analysis. *Radiology* 2019;290(2): 317–326.

Reiter G, Reiter C, Kräuter C, et al. Cardiac magnetic resonance T1 mapping. Part 1: aspects of acquisition and evaluation. *Eur J Radiol* 2018;109:223–234.

7 **Answer A.** The provided image demonstrates extensive stair-step artifact of the volume-rendered reconstruction due to ectopic rhythm during the study acquisition. ECG-gated cardiac CT examinations can be compromised by rhythm irregularities such as atrial fibrillation and premature beats.

Retrospective ECG-gated image reconstruction allows for reconstruction of images at any point in the cardiac cycle, providing the opportunity to seek out and use the phase with the least motion. The scanner syncs the cardiac cycle based on the R wave of the ECG. Occasionally, noise or abnormal beats on the ECG signal can be mistakenly considered by the scanner to be an R wave. Although these "extra syncs" do not represent actual R waves, images will be reconstructed into arbitrary reconstruction phases, resulting in cardiac displacement artifacts.

Through ECG editing, the temporal windows within the cardiac cycle can be manual modified, enabling correction and compensation for the artifacts produced by the consequence of heart rhythm irregularities. Extraneous "syncs" can be either deleted or disabled, instructing the reconstruction algorithm to ignore that extraneous signal and choose a more appropriate reconstruction. Additionally, the need to either add new syncs or move existing syncs may also be necessary to improve the diagnostic quality of studies.

Abnormalities with breath holds cause more global displacement artifacts and cannot be corrected with similar techniques. Prospective triggering captures only as small portion of the ECG cycle and does not allow for ECG editing.

References: Leschka S, Scheffel H, Desbiolles L, et al. Image quality and reconstruction intervals of dual-source CT coronary angiography: recommendations for ECG-pulsing windowing. *Invest Radiol* 2007;42(8):543–549.

Matsutani H, Sano T, Kondo T, et al. ECG-edit function in multidetector-row computed tomography coronary arteriography for patients with arrhythmias. *Circ J.* 2008;72(7): 1071–1078.

8 **Answer D.** Left ventricular (LV) mass is a well-established measure that independently predicts adverse cardiovascular events and premature death. Regression of left ventricular hypertrophy in patients with hypertension treated with antihypertensive medication, or after aortic valve replacement in patients with severe aortic valve stenosis, has been associated with improved cardiovascular outcomes.

LV mass is quantified on cardiac MRI from end-diastolic phase images of short-axis cine SSFP stack by drawing endocardial and epicardial contours. Using the modified Simpson rule, myocardial volume is obtained and multiplying this by myocardial density (1.05 g/mL) provides the myocardial mass. Systolic phase correlates to 30% to 40% of the cardiac cycle, whereas diastole correlates to the 70% to 80% phases of the cardiac cycle, which makes answer D the most appropriate.

References: Budoff MJ, Shinbane JS, (eds). *Cardiac CT imaging: diagnosis of cardiovascular disease*. London: Springer, 2010.

Levy D, Garrison RJ, Savage DD, et al. Left ventricular mass and incidence of coronary heart disease in an elderly cohort. The Framingham Heart Study. *Ann Intern Med* 1989;110:101–107.

Verdecchia P, Schillaci G, Borgioni C, et al. Prognostic significance of serial changes in left ventricular mass in essential hypertension. *Circulation* 1998;97:48–54.

9   Answer D. Cardiovascular shunts may be assessed in imaging by ventricular volume and aortic and pulmonary flow measurements.

In the absence of a shunt, right ventricular stroke volume (RVSV) should be equal to left ventricular stroke volume (LVSV). Similarly, aortic and pulmonary flow velocity measurements should also be equal. So, in total, both ventricular stroke volumes should equal the net forward flow per beat in the ascending aorta or the main pulmonary artery in a normal heart, without shunting or regurgitation

In the scenario above, assessment of RVSV and LVSV should provide a reasonable estimate of whether a significant shunt is present. Evaluation of cardiac morphology, abnormal intracardiac jets, and extracardiac anatomy would also be integral in the evaluation. The presence of valvular insufficiency would make determination difficult but consideration of supporting findings would be helpful.

Reference: Devos D, Kilner P. Calculations of cardiovascular shunts and regurgitation using magnetic resonance ventricular volume and aortic and pulmonary flow measurements. *Eur Radiol* 2010;20(2):410–421.

10   Answer B. Using the simplified Bernoulli equation: $\Delta P = 4v^2$

- $4v^2 = 20$ mm Hg
- $v^2 = 5$ mm Hg
- $v = 2.24$ m/sec
- $v = 224$ cm/sec

Reference: Varaprasathan GA, Araoz PA, Higgins CB, et al. Quantification of flow dynamics in congenital heart disease: applications of velocity-encoded cine MR imaging. *Radiographics* 2002;22(4):895–905; discussion 905–906.

11a   Answer B. The image shows the EKG tracing from a cardiac CTA acquisition. The gray box corresponds to late ventricular diastole, just prior to ventricular contraction. During late diastole, the mitral and tricuspid valves are open. During the late phase of diastole, the atrial has a minimal contraction allowing to fill the ventricles. The ventricles contract during systole, which corresponds to the QRS complex.

Reference: Klabunde R. *Cardiovascular physiology concepts*. Philadelphia, PA: Lippincott Williams & Wilkins, 2011:62–63. ISBN-10: 1451113846.

11b   Answer D. The patient was imaged using prospective triggering in order to reduce the radiation dose. During prospective triggering, only a short segment of the cardiac cycle, usually diastole, is imaged resulting in no imaging in the remainder of the cardiac cycle and as a result no radiation being given. This method contrasts to retrospective gating during which the entire cardiac cycle is imaged resulting in a higher radiation dose since both systole and diastole are imaged.

References: Hirai N, et al. Prospective versus retrospective ECG-gated 64-detector coronary CT angiography: assessment of image quality, stenosis, and radiation dose. *Radiology* 2008;248(2):424–430. doi:10.1148/radiol.2482071804.

Menke J, et al. Head-to-head comparison of prospectively triggered vs retrospectively gated coronary computed tomography angiography: meta-analysis of diagnostic accuracy, image quality, and radiation dose. *Am Heart J* 2013;165(2):154–163. doi:10.1016/j.ahj.2012.10.026.

11c   **Answer D.** Radiation dose can be reduced by decreasing the mAs, decreasing the kVp, using prospective triggering, and reducing the scan length. Reducing the pitch will increase the amount of radiation to the imaged area.

References: Labounty TM, et al. Coronary CT angiography of patients with a normal body mass index using 80 kVp versus 100 kVp: a prospective, multicenter, multivendor randomized trial. *AJR Am J Roentgenol* 2011;197(5):W860–W867. doi:10.2214/AJR.11.6787.

Leipsic J, et al. A prospective randomized controlled trial to assess the diagnostic performance of reduced tube voltage for coronary CT angiography. *AJR Am J Roentgenol* 2011;196(4):801–806. doi:10.2214/AJR.10.5786.

12a   **Answer D.** The image shows delayed enhancement along the left anterior descending coronary artery territory from an acute myocardial infarction with microvascular obstruction and no myocardial thinning indicating an acute infarction. Myocardial infarction and delayed enhancement are associated with wall motion abnormalities and decreased ventricular function.

References: Boagert J, et al. Remote myocardial dysfunction after acute anterior myocardial infarction: impact of left ventricular shape on regional function: a magnetic resonance myocardial tagging study. *J Am Coll Cardiol* 2000;35(6):1525–1534. doi:10.1016/S0735-1097(00)00601-X.

Marra MP, Lima JAC, Iliceto S. MRI in acute myocardial infarction. *Eur Heart J* 2011;32(3):284–293. doi:10.1093/eurheartj/ehq409.

12b   **Answer E.** A severely decreased ejection measures <35%. Patients with severely decreased ejection fractions are at higher risk for arrhythmia and may require device placements (AICDs).

13   **Answer C.** During isovolumetric contraction of the ventricles, the pressure within the ventricle rises; however, the volume within the ventricle does not change. During isovolumetric contraction, the tricuspid and mitral valves are closed. The pressure in the ventricles, however, is not yet greater than the systemic pressure, and as a result, the aortic and pulmonic valves are closed.

References: http://www.cvphysiology.com/Heart%20Disease/HD002b.htm

http://www.austincc.edu/emeyerth/isovolum.htm

14a   **Answer C.** The three-chamber image shows narrowing along the left ventricular outflow tract. There is also dephasing artifact along the left ventricular outflow tract indicating turbulent flow and velocity elevation in this patient with a diagnosis of hypertrophic cardiomyopathy.

References: Bogaert J, Olivotto I. MR imaging in hypertrophic cardiomyopathy: from magnet to bedside. *Radiology* 2014;273(2):329–348. doi:10.1148/radiol.14131626.

Chun EJ, et al. Hypertrophic cardiomyopathy: assessment with MR imaging and multidetector CT. *Radiographics* 2010;30(5):1309–1328. doi:10.1148/rg.305095074.

14b   **Answer B.** Patients with hypertrophic cardiomyopathy have an increased myocardial mass, an elongated mitral valve leaflet, and decreased left ventricular compliance. The increased mass makes it difficult for blood to fill the left ventricle during diastole and leads to diastolic dysfunction. Patients with diastolic dysfunction have an increased left atrial pressure and an increased left atrial kick in an attempt to further fill the left ventricle.

References: Bogaert J, Olivotto I. MR imaging in hypertrophic cardiomyopathy: from magnet to bedside. *Radiology* 2014;273(2):329–348. doi:10.1148/radiol.14131626.

Chun EJ, et al. Hypertrophic cardiomyopathy: assessment with MR imaging and multidetector CT. *Radiographics* 2010;30(5):1309–1328. doi:10.1148/rg.305095074.

15 **Answer C.** Preload is altered by the volume of blood within the ventricle. Factors that increase central venous return will increase blood in the ventricle and thereby increase the preload. A noncompliant ventricle will cause less blood to be in the ventricle. An elevated heart rate will afford less time and less blood to fill the ventricle. Ligating a fistula will decrease venous return, thereby decreasing blood volume and preload. Reduced atrial pressure and decreased atrial contraction will result in less blood filling the ventricles and a reduced preload.

References: Suzanne C, O'Connell S, Bare BG, et al. *Brunner & Suddarth's textbook of medical-surgical nursing*, Volume 1. Philadelphia, PA: Wolters Kluwer Health/Lippincott Williams & Wilkins, 2010:824.

http://cvphysiology.com/Cardiac%20Function/CF007.htm

16 **Answer C.** During a phase-contrast acquisition, the VENC should be set at a value greater than the maximum expected velocity. Once the sequence is started, protons in the blood will experience a phase shift proportional to their velocity, while nonmoving objects have no phase shift in response to the pulses. If the velocity of blood is higher than the VENC, the phase shift will be >180 degrees and aliasing will occur. As long as the VENC is larger than the fastest velocity of blood, no aliasing will occur.

References: Ferreira PF, et al. Cardiovascular magnetic resonance artefacts. *J Cardiovas Magn Reson* 2013;15:41. doi:10.1186/1532-429X-15-41.

Lee VS. *Cardiovascular MR: physical principles to practical protocols*. Philadelphia, PA: Lippincott Williams & Wilkins, 2006:206.

17 **Answer D.** Metoprolol is a type of beta-blocker that can be administered orally or intravenously to patients undergoing cardiac CTA. Metoprolol acts by selectively blocking the beta-1 receptor. As a result, the heart rate and blood pressure will decrease and it will have a net negative ionotropic effect on the heart.

References: Marx JA. *"Cardiovascular drugs". Rosen's emergency medicine: concepts and clinical practice*, 8th ed. Philadelphia, PA: Elsevier/Saunders, 2014. Chapter 152. ISBN 1455706051.

http://www.nlm.nih.gov/medlineplus/druginfo/meds/a682864.html

18a **Answer C.** The image shows a tricuspid aortic valve at end-ventricular systole in a patient with severe aortic stenosis. The valve leaflets are thickened and calcified with only a small open valve area. Severe aortic stenosis is diagnosed with a valve area measuring <1.0 cm^2 (by valve planimetry). Other values characteristic of aortic stenosis can be quantified by cardiac MRI and include a velocity gradient >40 mm Hg or a velocity jet >4.0 m/sec.

References: Feuchtner G. Imaging of cardiac valves by computed tomography. *Scientifica* 2013;2013:13. Article ID 270579. doi:10.1155/2013/270579.

John AS. Magnetic resonance to assess the aortic valve area in aortic stenosis: how does it compare to current diagnostic standards? *J Am Coll Cardiol* 2003;42(3):519–526. doi:10.1016/S0735-1097(03)00707-1.

18b **Answer D.** The pressure gradient can be calculated using the modified Bernoulli equation (pressure gradient (mm Hg) = 4 Vmax^2) where the maximum velocity (Vmax) is reported in meters per second

Using the above equation and values: 150 cm/sec = 1.5 m/sec
Pressure gradient = 4 (1.5 m/sec)^2
Pressure gradient = 9 mm Hg

References: Feuchtner G. Imaging of cardiac valves by computed tomography. *Scientifica* 2013;2013:13. Article ID 270579. doi:10.1155/2013/270579.

John AS. Magnetic resonance to assess the aortic valve area in aortic stenosis: how does it compare to current diagnostic standards? *J Am Coll Cardiol* 2003;42(3):519–526. doi:10.1016/S0735-1097(03)00707-1.

19a **Answer C.** The image shows an aortic valve in diastole. At this moment, the aortic valve should be fully closed (complete coaptation); however, centrally, the valve is open. Incomplete coaptation of the valve is a sign of aortic insufficiency. Aortic insufficiency will result in an increased end-diastolic volume and ventricular dilation secondary to backflow of blood from the aorta into the ventricle. The severity of aortic insufficiency can be quantified by cardiac MRI using a phase-contrast sequence.

References: Cawley PJ, et al. Valvular heart disease: changing concepts in disease management cardiovascular magnetic resonance imaging for valvular heart disease technique and validation. *Circulation* 2009;119:468–478. doi:10.1161/CIRCULATIONAHA.107.742486.

Feuchtner G. Imaging of cardiac valves by computed tomography. *Scientifica* 2013;2013:13. Article ID 270579. doi:10.1155/2013/270579.

19b **Answer C.** Aortic insufficiency can be graded from mild to severe. Severe aortic insufficiency can be diagnosed by a regurgitant volume >60 mL/beat or a regurgitant fraction >50%. Other features associated with aortic insufficiency include holodiastolic flow reversal in the descending aorta, incomplete leaflet coaptation, increased end-diastolic volume, and ventricular dilation.

References: Cawley PJ, et al. Valvular heart disease: changing concepts in disease management cardiovascular magnetic resonance imaging for valvular heart disease technique and validation. *Circulation* 2009;119:468–478. doi:10.1161/CIRCULATIONAHA.107.742486.

Maurer G. Aortic regurgitation. *Heart* 2006;92(7):994–1000. doi:10.1136/hrt.2004.042614.

20a **Answer B.** The image is from a phase-contrast cardiac MRI acquisition. The sequence produces two data sets (magnitude image and phase velocity maps). When acquiring the data set, the user sets the VENC (encoding velocity range measured by the sequence). The VENC should be set at a value greater than the maximum expected velocity. If the actual velocity is greater than the VENC, aliasing will occur (the abnormality seen in this image). This can be solved by repeating the sequence with a higher VENC.

References: Ferreira PF, et al. Cardiovascular magnetic resonance artefacts. *J Cardiovas Magn Reson* 2013;15:41. doi:10.1186/1532-429X-15-41.

Lee VS. *Cardiovascular MR: physical principles to practical protocols*. Lippincott Williams & Wilkins, 2006:206.

20b **Answer A.** The phase-contrast cardiac MRI acquisition produces two data sets (magnitude image and phase velocity maps). The images are viewed, and the vessel of interest is evaluated with contour lines placed over the area of interest.

References: Ferreira PF, et al. Cardiovascular magnetic resonance artefacts. *J Cardiovas Magn Reson* 2013;15:41. doi:10.1186/1532-429X-15-41.

Lee VS. *Cardiovascular MR: physical Principles to practical protocols*. Lippincott Williams & Wilkins, Philadelphia, PA: 2006:206.

21 **Answer B.** Beta-blockers are negative inotropic agents. As a result, once beta-blockers are administered, they will decrease myocardial contractility. The Frank-Starling curve is a graphical tool that shows how cardiac output changes in response to changes in heart rate or stroke volume. The administration of beta-blockers will reduce contractility and heart rate resulting in a shift of the curve down and to the right. A positive inotrope would shift the curve up and to the left.

References: Marx JA. *"Cardiovascular drugs". Rosen's emergency medicine: concepts and clinical practice*, 8th ed. Philadelphia, PA: Elsevier/Saunders, 2014. Chapter 152. ISBN 1455706051.

http://www.nlm.nih.gov/medlineplus/druginfo/meds/a682864.html

http://www.cvphysiology.com/Cardiac%20Function/CF003.htm

22a **Answer A.** The image shows an unroofed coronary sinus with abnormal connection between the left atrium and the coronary sinus. This results in a left to right shunt with a connection between the left and right atrium via the coronary sinus defect. An unroofed coronary sinus can be associated with a left SVC.

References: Kim H, Choe YH, Park SW, et al. Partially unroofed coronary sinus: MDCT and MRI findings. *AJR Am J Roentgenol* 2010;195(5):W331–W336. doi:10.2214/AJR.09.3689.

Ootaki Y, et al. Unroofed coronary sinus syndrome: diagnosis, classification and surgical treatment. *J Thorac Cardiovas Surg* 2003;126(5):1655–1656.

22b **Answer A.** The Qp/Qs is the ratio of the flow in the pulmonary circulation to the flow in the systemic circulation. It is obtained by using phase-contrast sequence to measure the flow in the pulmonary artery and the aorta. A Qp/Qs value of 1.5 or greater suggests that the shunt is significant and may trigger an intervention.

References: Kim H, Choe YH, Park SW, et al. Partially unroofed coronary sinus: MDCT and MRI findings. *AJR Am J Roentgenol* 2010;195(5):W331–W336. doi:10.2214/AJR.09.3689.

Ootaki Y, et al. Unroofed coronary sinus syndrome: diagnosis, classification and surgical treatment. *J Thorac Cardiovas Surg* 2003;126(5):1655–1656.

Rajiah P, Kanne JP. Cardiac MRI: Part 1, cardiovascular shunts. *AJR Am J Roentgenol* 2011;197(4):W603–W620. doi:10.2214/AJR.10.7257.

23 **Answer C.** The patient has a prior cardiac stent in the right coronary artery. The left main coronary artery contains noncalcified plaque, which narrows the lumen by 50%. Stenosis of 50% or greater in the left main coronary artery or of either coronary ostia will cause a significant reduction in flow (significant stenosis). The left main coronary artery gives rise to the left anterior descending and left circumflex coronary arteries. Given that the stenosis is proximal to these vessels, these territories will have perfusion defects.

References: Fathala A. Myocardial perfusion scintigraphy: techniques, interpretation, indications and reporting. *Ann Saudi Med* 2011;31(6):625–634. doi:10.4103/0256-4947.87101.

Kinis S, et al. Normal and variant coronary arterial and venous anatomy on high-resolution CT angiography. *AJR Am J Roentgenol* 2007;188:1665–1674.

24a **Answer D.** The image shows noncalcified plaque in the proximal right coronary artery. The plaque causes more than 70% narrowing of the proximal right coronary artery indicating a significant stenosis and the territory likely to contain a perfusion defect when further investigated by stress testing.

References: Fathala A. Myocardial perfusion scintigraphy: techniques, interpretation, indications and reporting. *Ann Saudi Med* 2011;31(6):625–634. doi:10.4103/0256-4947.87101.

Kinis S, et al. Normal and variant coronary arterial and venous anatomy on high-resolution CT angiography. *AJR Am J Roentgenol* 2007;188:1665–1674.

24b **Answer D.** A flow-limiting stenosis by CTA that does not involve the ostium or left main correlates with stenosis >70%. Plaque causing 70% on CCTA are likely to cause compromised flow when evaluated by invasive coronary angiography.

References: Kinis S, et al. Normal and variant coronary arterial and venous anatomy on high-resolution CT angiography. *AJR Am J Roentgenol* 2007;188:1665–1674.

http://www.scct.org/advocacy/coverage/PubGuidelines.pdf

25 **Answer B.** Sublingual nitroglycerin is given to dilate the coronary arteries thereby improving their visualization. In particular, sublingual nitroglycerin helps improve the visualization of the distal divisions of the coronary arteries. Beta-blockers are given to decrease motion of the coronary arteries. No medication is routinely given to improve ventricular function or decrease radiation dose.

References: Chun EJ, et al. Effects of nitroglycerin on the diagnostic accuracy of electrocardiogram-gated coronary computed tomography angiography. *J Comput Assist Tomogr* 2008;32(1):86–92. doi:10.1097/rct.0b013e318059befa.

Decramer I, et al. Effects of sublingual nitroglycerin on coronary lumen diameter and number of visualized septal branches on 64-MDCT angiography. *Am J Roentgenol* 2008;190:219–225.

26 **Answer A.** Sublingual nitroglycerin should not be administered to a patient who has taken sildenafil within 24 hours secondary to the risk of severe hypotension. Sublingual nitroglycerin dilates the coronary arteries and improves their visualization. If a patient has taken tadalafil, sublingual nitroglycerin should be administered for at least 48 hours due to the longer half-life of the drug and the risk of hypotension.

References: Cheitlin MD, Hutter AM, Brindis RG, et al. ACC/AHA Expert Consensus Document. Use of sildenafil (Viagra) in patients with cardiovascular disease. *Circulation* 1999;99:168–177. doi:10.1161/01.CIR.99.1.168.

Kloner RA, et al. Time course of the interaction between tadalafil and nitrates. *J Am Coll Cardiol* 2003;42(10):1855–1860.

27 **Answer C.** The ejection fraction is calculated by the following formula:

$$\left[\left(\text{End Diastolic Volume} - \text{End Diastolic Volume}\right)/\text{End Diastolic Volume}\right] \times 100$$
$$\text{EF} = \left(100 - 40\right)/100 \times 100$$
$$\text{EF} = 60\%$$

At end diastole, the ventricular volume will be at its maximum, while at end systole, the ventricular volume will be at its minimum. The difference between these entities is the stroke volume. A normal ejection fraction measures 55%. A diminished ejection fraction can be associated with reduced mortality and an increased of developing ventricular thrombus or arrhythmia.

Reference: Guyton AC, Hall JE. *Textbook of medical physiology*, 11th ed. Princeton, NJ: Elsevier Saunders, 2006:108. ISBN 0-7216-0240-1.

28 **Answer D.** Atrial fibrillation is the most common sustained arrhythmia, and its incidence is increasing with the progressively aging population. Atrial fibrillation can be associated with stroke, and up to 20% to 25% of strokes are caused by atrial fibrillation. In atrial fibrillation, the atria are constantly being activated in a chaotic manner by arrhythmogenic foci at the pulmonary vein ostia, the coronary sinus, or along the atria. The electrical impulses bypass the normal electrical coordinated conduction process that begins in the SA node. This results in too many signals reaching the AV node and ventricles resulting in the ventricles beating too fast (>100 beats/min).

References: Schotten U, et al. Pathophysiological mechanisms of atrial fibrillation: a translational appraisal. *Am Physiol Soc* 2011;91(1):265–325. doi:10.1152/physrev.00031.2009.

Waktare J. Cardiology patient page: atrial fibrillation. *Circulation* 2002;106:14–16. doi:10.1161/01.CIR.0000022730.66617.D9.

29 **Answer A.** Cardiac MRI (CMRI) can be used to calculate myocardial mass by calculating the difference between epicardial and endocardial volumes and multiplying the value by the specific density of the myocardium (1.05 g/mL). Because of the high spatial resolution of CMR and the volumetric acquisition of the entire heart, myocardial mass can be determined with excellent accuracy and reproducibility.

References: Bezante GP, et al. Left ventricular myocardial mass determination by contrast enhanced colour Doppler compared with magnetic resonance imaging. *Heart* 2005;91(1): 38–43. doi:10.1136/hrt.2003.023234.

Higgins CB, Sakuma H. Heart disease: functional evaluation with MR imaging. *Radiology* 1996;199:307–315.

30 **Answer B.** Diastolic dysfunction occurs when the left ventricle cannot fill with blood during ventricular diastole secondary to ventricular stiffness or impaired ventricular relaxation. As a result, the stroke volume and end-diastolic volume are reduced, and patients have heart failure with a normal ejection fraction. The left atrium will progressively enlarge during the course of diastolic dysfunction.

References: European Study Group on Diastolic Heart Failure. How to diagnose diastolic heart failure. *Eur Heart J* 1998;19:990–1003.

Zile MR, Brutsaert DL. Clinical cardiology: new frontiers new concepts in diastolic dysfunction and diastolic heart failure: part I diagnosis, prognosis, and measurements of diastolic function. *Circulation* 2002;105:1387–1393. doi:10.1161/hc1102.105289.

31 **Answer C.** A chamber measuring >5.5 cm is considered dilated. Dilated cardiomyopathy (DCM) can also manifest with heterogeneous wall thickness, wall thinning, preserved right ventricular mass, and late gadolinium enhancement. Three patterns of late gadolinium enhancement can occur and include mid wall late gadolinium enhancement, subendocardial delayed enhancement, or no late gadolinium enhancement.

References: Francone M. Role of cardiac magnetic resonance in the evaluation of dilated cardiomyopathy: diagnostic contribution and prognostic significance. *ISRN Radiol* 2014;2014:16. Article ID 365404. doi:10.1155/2014/365404.

McCrohon JA, Moon JCC, Prasad SK, et al. Differentiation of heart failure related to dilated cardiomyopathy and coronary artery disease using gadolinium-enhanced cardiovascular magnetic resonance. *Circulation* 2003;108(1):54–59.

32 **Answer B.** Aortic insufficiency will result in an increased stroke volume, increased preload (due to the volume from the regurgitant fraction), progressive dilation of the left ventricular cavity (from the regurgitant volume), increased afterload (initially due to the increased pressure needed by the myocardium to eject the increased blood volume), and loss of an isovolumetric relaxation phase since blood is continuously entering the ventricle.

Reference: Bekeredjian R, Grayburn PA. Contemporary reviews in cardiovascular medicine valvular heart disease aortic regurgitation. *Circulation* 2005;112:125–134. doi:10.1161/CIRCULATIONAHA.104.488825.

33a **Answer B.** The image shows a myxoma adjacent to the inflow of the left inferior pulmonary vein partially blocking its inflow to the left atrium. The most common location for a cardiac myxoma is the left atrium, and while it can be attached to the interatrial septum via a broad base, it can prolapse through the mitral valve, embolize, or obstruct the pulmonary veins.

References: Grebenec ML, et al. Cardiac myxoma: imaging features in 83 patients. *Radiographics* 2002;22(3):673–689.

Stevens LH, et al. Left atrial myxoma: pulmonary infarction caused by pulmonary venous occlusion. *Ann Thorac Surg* 1987;43(2):215–217.

33b **Answer A.** Hemodynamics are an essential part of cardiac physiology. Normal values for the heart include the following:

RA, 1–8 mm Hg; LA, 4–12 mm Hg
RV, 15–30/1–8 mm Hg; LV, 100–140/4–12 mm Hg
PA, 15–30/4–12 mm Hg; Ao, 100–140/60–80 mm Hg

When the pulmonary capillary wedge pressure, which is usually similar to the left atrial pressure, approaches 20 mm, the patient will develop interstitial edema, and when the value is >20 mm Hg, the patient will have alveolar edema.

Reference: Grossman W (ed.). *Cardiac catheterization and angiography*, 3rd ed. Philadelphia, PA: Lea & Febiger, 1986. http://www.uptodate.com/contents/cardiac-catheterization-techniques-normal-hemodynamics

34 **Answer B.** The heart of competitive athletes can undergo a series of changes secondary to the cardiovascular activity. In most cases, the left atrium, left ventricle, and right ventricle will dilate and the myocardial mass will increase.

Reference: Maron BJ, Pelliccia A. Contemporary reviews in cardiovascular medicine the heart of trained athletes cardiac remodeling and the risks of sports, including sudden death. *Circulation* 2006;114:1633–1644. doi:10.1161/CIRCULATIONAHA.106.613562.

4 Ischemic Heart Disease

Brian Pogatchnik, MD • Amar B. Shah, MD, MPA • Sachin Malik, MD

QUESTIONS

1 In the below images, the abnormality of the right coronary artery (RCA) is most closely associated with which of the following in this patient with chest pain but no EKG changes?

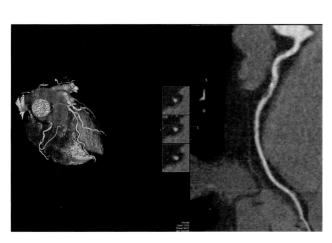 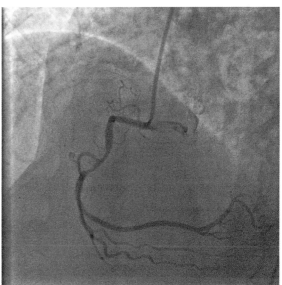

    A. Lateral wall hypokinesis
    B. Significant restriction of blood flow to the inferior wall
    C. RCA occlusion
    D. ST-elevation myocardial infarction (STEMI)

2 In addition to hypotension and severe aortic stenosis, use of which of the following drugs precludes the use of sublingual nitroglycerin for cardiac CTA?

    A. Metformin
    B. Sildenafil
    C. Diltiazem
    D. Atorvastatin

3a A 67-year-old male was brought emergently to the cath lab for an ST-elevation myocardial infarction (STEMI). The patient was found to have single-vessel disease and underwent percutaneous coronary intervention (PCI). Based on the images shown, which of the following coronary arteries was intervened upon?

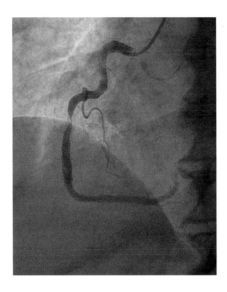 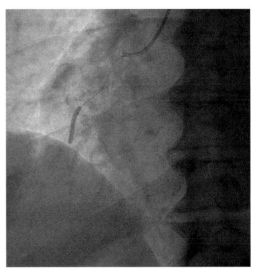

A. Left main artery (LM)
B. Left anterior descending artery (LAD)
C. Left circumflex artery (LCx)
D. Right coronary artery (RCA)

3b On hospital day 3, the patient underwent cardiac magnetic resonance imaging (CMR). Late gadolinium enhancement (LGE) short-axis basal (left), mid (middle), and apical (right) images are shown below. According to the American Heart Association's (AHA) 17-segment model, how many segments of the RCA territory are viable?

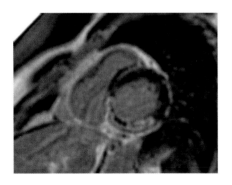 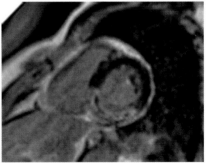 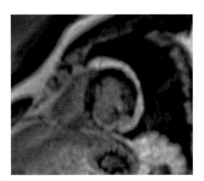

A. Zero
B. One
C. Two
D. Three

4 An otherwise healthy 60-year-old male presents to the emergency department with chest pain, and the initial troponin was negative. A coronary CTA was performed and a stenosis was seen in the proximal to mid LAD measuring approximately 70%. According to CAD-RADS, what additional modifier should be added to this CAD-RADS 4A lesion?

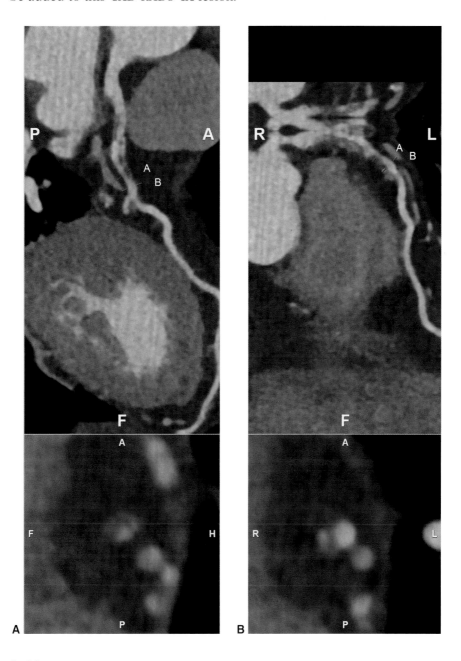

A. N
B. S
C. G
D. V

5 Which statement is correct regarding the patency of left internal mammary artery (LIMA) and saphenous vein bypass grafts (SVG) at 10 years?

A. LIMA > SVG
B. LIMA < SVG
C. LIMA = SVG
D. Indeterminate

6   A coronary CTA is ordered for a 72-year-old patient with shortness of breath. As part of the examination, a calcium score is performed and the below image is obtained. (Total calcium score is calculated at 2,286 Agatston units.) Which of the following conclusions is accurate?

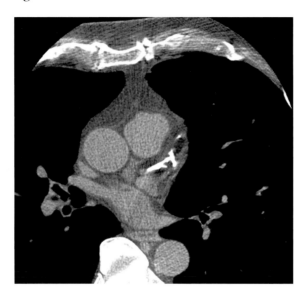

A. The patient has atherosclerotic plaque.
B. High-grade stenosis is likely.
C. The patient is at low risk for a coronary event.
D. Aortic stenosis is likely.

7   The following scan parameters were used to obtain the image in a patient with a heart rate of 60 beats/min: kVp = 120; mA = 700; gantry rotation speed = 320 msec; contrast volume = 80 mL; contrast rate = 6.5 mL/sec; and slice thickness = 0.625 mm. The poor image quality in this case is most likely from?

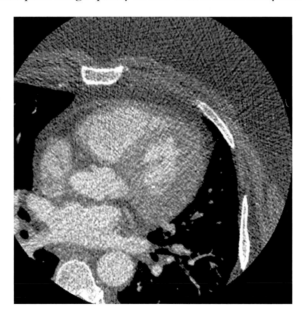

A. Poor temporal resolution
B. Elevated body mass index
C. Incorrect contrast timing
D. Too high spatial resolution

8   A 66-year-old patient is status post myocardial infarction 2 days ago. Which of the following conclusions can be made?

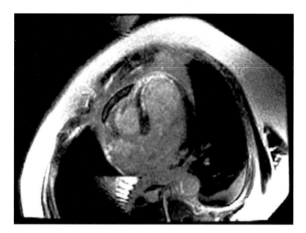

A. There is thrombus at the apex.
B. The septal myocardium is viable.
C. The lesion was most likely in the left circumflex coronary artery.
D. The septum is normokinetic.

9   Which of the following sequelae of prior LAD territory myocardial infarct is shown?

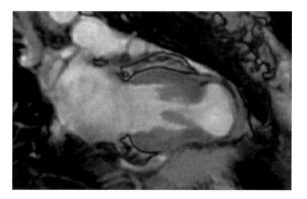

A. Pseudoaneurysm
B. Interventricular septal rupture
C. Pericarditis
D. Aneurysm

10 Which of the following clinical scenarios is an appropriate indication for coronary CTA based on current appropriate use criteria?

A. Acute ST-elevation myocardial infarction
B. Acute non–ST-elevation myocardial infarction
C. Stable anginal symptoms with a normal ECG stress test
D. Coronary CTA in a patient with a known 2.0-mm stent in the LAD to assess disease

11 Which of the following statements is correct regarding the area of low signal in the anterior wall on this delayed enhancement sequence?

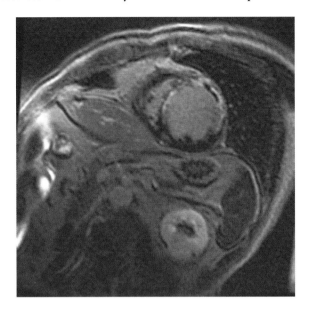

A. It is an area of normal nulled myocardium.
B. It represents an area without reflow and carries a less favorable prognosis.
C. It represents hibernating myocardium.
D. It indicates that a suboptimal inversion time was used during acquisition.

12 A patient undergoes coronary CTA with CT-derived fractional flow reserve (FFR$_{CT}$) analysis and the following report is generated. How many major coronary vessels likely have hemodynamically significant stenoses?

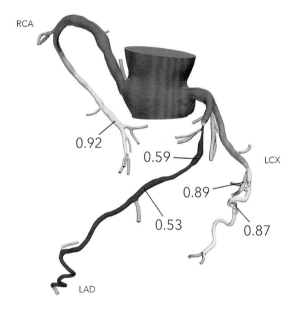

A. One
B. Two
C. Three
D. Four

13 A 40-year-old female patient presents to the ER with chest pain, negative cardiac enzyme tests, and a normal EKG. A review of the medical record reveals she presented 2 months prior with similar symptoms. At that time, she underwent a coronary CTA, which was normal. What is the next step?

A. Repeat coronary CTA.
B. Admission and stress test
C. Catheter angiography
D. Evaluate for possible noncardiac causes of chest pain.

14 A 39-year-old male with no past medical history presents to the ER with chest pain. The workup reveals a normal ECG and negative cardiac enzymes. He undergoes a coronary CTA angiogram (shown below). Based on the images and clinical trials, which of the following is a reasonable plan of disposition?

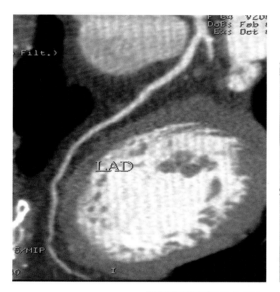

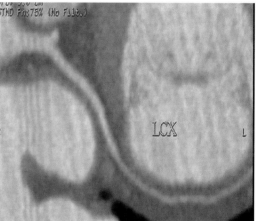

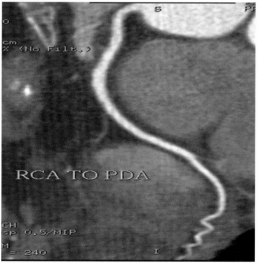

A. Discharge to home
B. Admit to telemetry
C. Stress test
D. Cardiology consult for possible catheterization

15 In adults, what is the most common cause of the abnormality seen here?

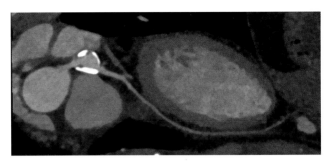

    A. Kawasaki disease

    B. Spontaneous coronary artery dissection

    C. Atherosclerosis

    D. Marfan syndrome

16 As time from injection of gadolinium increases during a delayed enhancement sequence, what adjustment, if any, must be made to the inversion time to preserve quality of myocardial nulling?

    A. Increase the inversion time.

    B. Decrease the inversion time.

    C. No change necessary

17 The images below are taken from the same patient. The findings should be reported as

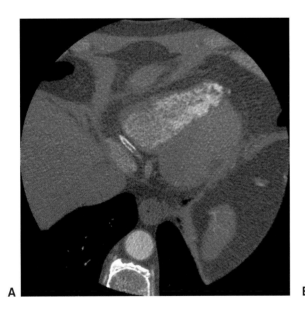

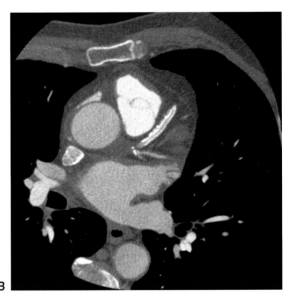

    A. Patent LAD stent and RCA stent

    B. Occluded LAD and RCA stent

    C. Patent LAD stent and occluded RCA stent

    D. Occluded LAD stent and patent RCA stent

18 A patient presents for cardiac MRI 3 days following myocardial infarction. On admission, catheterization reveals severe stenosis in the left anterior descending and right coronary arteries. On admission day 2, new-onset mitral regurgitation is discovered, and the patient develops right upper lobe pulmonary edema. What complication of infarction should be considered?

A. Aneurysm formation
B. Thrombus formation
C. Papillary muscle infarction
D. Pericardial effusion

19 Stent thrombosis after percutaneous intervention can be due to the failure to comply with which of the following prescribed regimen?

A. Statin therapy
B. Inotropic therapy
C. Beta-blocker therapy
D. Dual antiplatelet therapy

20a A 101-year-old female presented to the emergency department with left arm pain. A retrospectively gated coronary CTA was obtained. Based on the images shown, which of the following coronary arteries most likely contains the culprit lesion that would explain the patient's acute presentation?

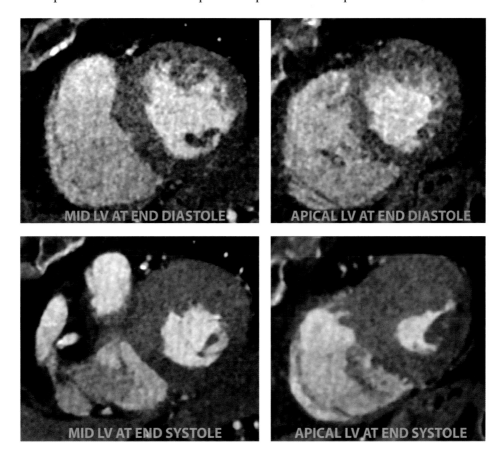

A. Left main artery (LM)
B. Left anterior descending artery (LAD)
C. Left circumflex artery (LCx)
D. Right coronary artery (RCA)

20b Based on the images shown, what would be the most appropriate CAD-RADS score for this patient?

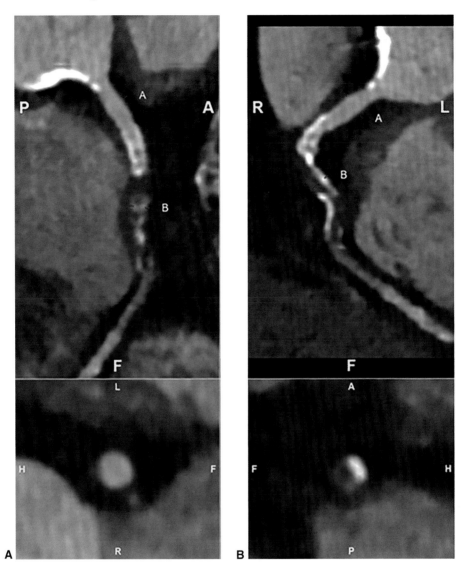

A. CAD-RADS 1
B. CAD-RADS 2
C. CAD-RADS 3
D. CAD-RADS 5

21 An 80-year-old male with a history of coronary artery bypass grafts (left internal mammary artery to the LAD and vein graft to the RCA) has noted new exertional chest pain. The referring provider is concerned for potential bypass graft failure. Given the patient's frailty and extensive comorbidities, the referring provider would like an initial noninvasive approach to evaluate for graft patency and requests a coronary CTA. What change to the usual protocol used in patients without bypass grafts must be made to best evaluate the grafts in this patient?

A. Extend scan range superiorly to top of the aortic arch.
B. Extend scan range superiorly through clavicles.
C. Extend scan range inferiorly through the renal arteries.
D. No change in scan range

22 The placement of the cardiac support devices in the chest radiograph is most often associated with which clinical parameters?

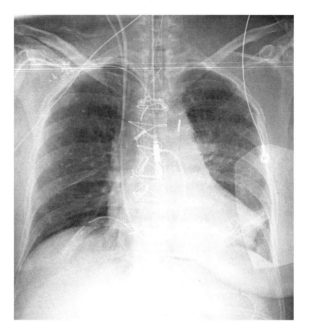

A. Atrial fibrillation
B. Isolated left bundle-branch block
C. Acute myocardial infarction with cardiogenic shock
D. Placement of a stent in a patient with stable angina

23 What is the dose of adenosine typically given for adenosine stress perfusion MRI?

A. 25 µg/kg/min
B. 50 µg/kg/min
C. 100 µg/kg/min
D. 140 µg/kg/min

24 Percutaneous coronary intervention (PCI) in symptomatic patients with stable coronary artery disease receiving optimal medical therapy has which of the following benefit?

A. Improved survival
B. Decreased risk of future major adverse cardiac events
C. Decreased angina
D. Decreased survival

25 Which of the following patients is best suited for coronary CTA?

A. A 35-year-old female with atypical chest pain during emotional stress
B. A 47-year-old male with a history of smoking, family history of CAD, and atypical chest pain
C. A 55-year-old female with a history of smoking, atrial fibrillation, and atypical chest pain
D. A 76-year-old male with a history of smoking and angina

26 A 74-year-old male with a heart rate of 51 underwent a retrospectively gated coronary CTA with tube current modulation to evaluate coronary anatomy and left ventricular function. The following ECG tracing was created by the CT scanner when making a diagnostic reconstruction of the best diastolic phase. What do the thick white horizontal lines (arrows) under the ECG tracing represent?

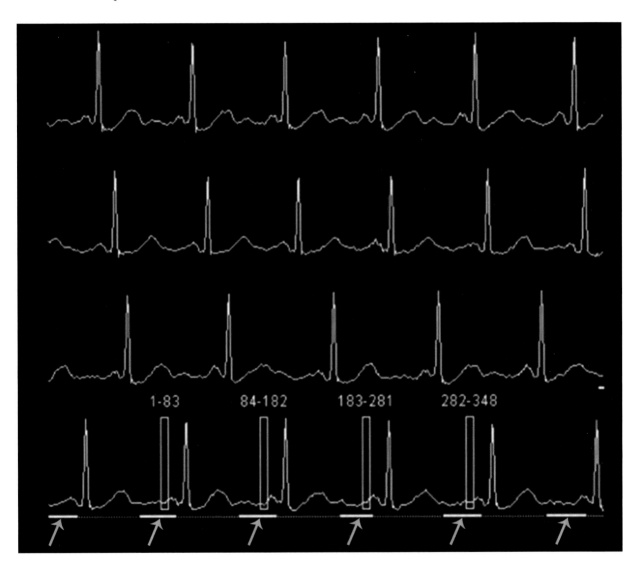

A. Increased tube current used to scan during this phase
B. Reduced tube current used to scan during this phase
C. No tube current used to scan during this phase
D. Reconstruction artifact

27 A 50% stenosis in which of the following coronary arteries typically carries the worst prognosis?

A. Right coronary artery (RCA)
B. Left main artery (LM)
C. Left anterior descending artery (LAD)
D. Left circumflex artery (LCx)

28a A 47-year-old female presents with chest pain and no prior cardiac history. Labs show elevated troponin. What is the most likely diagnosis?

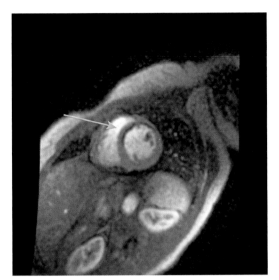
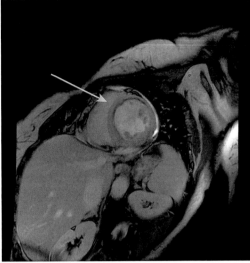
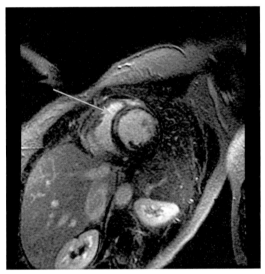

    A. Myocarditis
    B. Acute myocardial infarction
    C. Old myocardial infarction
    D. Sarcoidosis

28b What coronary artery territory does this abnormality involve?

    A. LAD
    B. LCX
    C. PDA
    D. RCA

28c Compared to infarct without microvascular obstruction, what is the prognosis of infarct with microvascular obstruction?

    A. Worse
    B. Better
    C. Same

29   A 57-year-old male presents for a cardiac MRI to assess myocardial viability several weeks after an acute myocardial infarction. On coronary catheterization, the patient was noted to have severe three-vessel disease. A follow-up echocardiogram demonstrated a left ventricular ejection fraction of 25% and severe hypokinesis of the anterior wall. Based on the clinical history and image shown, which of the following most accurately describes the anterior wall of the left ventricle?

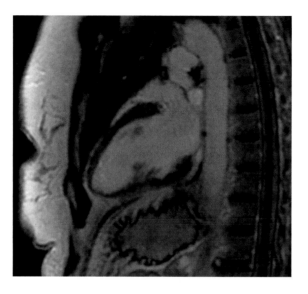

A. Normal myocardium
B. Nonviable myocardium
C. Stunned myocardium
D. Hibernating myocardium

30   A 65-year-old male with a past medical history of hyperlipidemia undergoes an adenosine stress cardiac MRI to evaluate intermittent anginal symptoms. What is the most likely diagnosis?

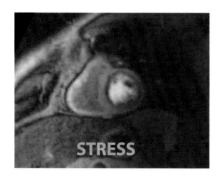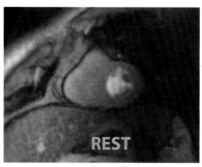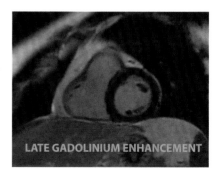

A. Myocarditis
B. Sarcoidosis
C. Dark rim artifact
D. Three-vessel ischemia

ANSWERS AND EXPLANATIONS

1 **Answer B.** The curved multiplanar reformat of the RCA (right-dominant system) demonstrates mixed plaque within the proximal vessel resulting in severe (roughly 80%) stenosis. A more proximal lesion consisting of noncalcified plaque causes 40% to 50% stenosis. A lesion is considered hemodynamically significant if it causes >70% stenosis. This is based on myocardial blood flow studies. The lateral wall is perfused by the circumflex, not the RCA. Contrast is noted throughout the lumen indicating partial patency. STEMI is caused by acute plaque rupture and acute total occlusion.

Reference: Uren NG, Melin JA, De Bruyne B, et al. Relation between myocardial blood flow and severity of coronary-artery stenosis. *N Engl J Med* 1994;330(25):1782–1788.

2 **Answer B.** During coronary CTA, sublingual nitroglycerin (SL NTG) is given for coronary artery dilation. Patients who have taken a phosphodiesterase inhibitor (i.e., sildenafil) should not take oral nitrates until 48 hours after the last dose due to the risk of hypotension and syncope. Similarly, hypotension is a contraindication for nitroglycerin due to the blood pressure effects caused by nitroglycerin. Patients with hypertrophic obstructive cardiomyopathy and severe aortic stenosis can be detrimental from reduced preload caused by the nitroglycerin. A review of the patient's medication list is mandatory prior to performing coronary CTA.

References: Amsterdam EA, Wenger NK, Brindis RG, et al. 2014 AHA/ACC guideline for the management of patients with non-ST-elevation acute coronary syndromes: a report of the American College of Cardiology/American Heart Association Task Force on Practice Guidelines. *Circulation* 2014;130(25):e344–e426.

Kloner RA, Hutter AM, Emmick JT, et al. Time course of the interaction between tadalafil and nitrates. *J Am Coll Cardiol* 2003;42(10):1855–1860.

3a **Answer D.** Knowing the angiographic views of the coronary arteries greatly augments one's ability to interpret other cardiac imaging modalities. These coronary angiographic images were obtained in the left anterior oblique (LAO) position, which best demonstrates the course of the RCA prior to diverging into the posterior lateral (PL) and posterior descending (PDA) branches (assuming right dominance). In the LAO view, the RCA typically forms the letter "C" as it wraps around in the right atrioventricular groove. LAO images can be differentiated from the right anterior oblique (RAO) views used to evaluate the LM, LAD, and LCx by which side of the screen the spine is on. The spine is on the right side of the image if the position is LAO and vice versa.

The image on the left shows injection of contrast into the RCA via a catheter parked in its ostium. A single stenosis is seen measuring approximately 90% in the mid RCA just distal to a prominent acute marginal branch. The image on the right shows the deployment of a stent at the location that was previously stenotic.

Reference: Aquilina O, Grech V, Felice H, et al. Normal adult coronary angiography. *Images Paediatr Cardiol* 2006;8(2):1–16.

3b **Answer A.** In order to standardize nomenclature across different imaging modalities (echocardiography, MRI, etc.), the AHA adopted a 17-segment model to describe the vascular territories of the left ventricular myocardium. The basal and mid segments are divided into six 60-degree territories, the apical segments are divided into four 90-degree segments, and the apex is a segment of its own. According to this model, five myocardial segments are assigned to the RCA territory: namely, the basal inferoseptal, basal inferior, mid inferoseptal, mid inferior, and apical inferior segments.

Although this model matches the vascular distribution in the majority of patients, there is considerable variability in vascular territories of the coronary arteries, and none of these segments are 100% specific to the RCA itself. Care must be given to evaluation of the overall distribution of pathology on CMR and comparison made with prior imaging that may show coronary anatomy before assigning a lesion on CMR to a specific vascular territory.

The CMR images in this patient demonstrate transmural LGE in the basal inferoseptal, basal inferior, basal inferolateral, mid inferoseptal, mid inferior, and apical inferior segments with scattered areas of microvascular obstruction (MVO). MVO is identified as areas of hypointensity within the infarcted myocardium. These regions are consistent with an acute myocardial infarction given the MVO and normal wall thickness of the affected territories. Since the LGE affects more than 50% of the myocardial thickness, these regions are considered nonviable. Therefore, none of the six segments would be considered viable.

References: Cerqueira MD, Weissman NJ, Dilsizian V, et al. Standardized myocardial segmentation and nomenclature for tomographic imaging of the heart. A statement for healthcare professionals from the Cardiac Imaging Committee of the Council on Clinical Cardiology of the American Heart Association. *Circulation* 2002;105(4):539–542.

Ortiz-pérez JT, Rodríguez J, Meyers SN, et al. Correspondence between the 17-segment model and coronary arterial anatomy using contrast-enhanced cardiac magnetic resonance imaging. *JACC Cardiovasc Imaging* 2008;1(3):282–293.

4 **Answer D.** According to the Coronary Artery Disease—Reporting and Data System (CAD-RADS), there are four modifiers that can be added to a classification. These are N (nondiagnostic), S (stent), G (graft), and V (vulnerability). Vulnerability can be reported if a vessel has two of the four following features at the site of stenosis: positive remodeling, low attenuation plaque, spotty calcifications, and the napkin ring sign.

In positive remodeling, the outer diameter of the coronary artery expands greater than the diameter of normal adjacent vessel (as seen in this case). Specifically, this is defined as the ratio of outer vessel diameter at the site of plaque divided by the average outer diameter of the vessel proximal and distal to the plaque >1.1. Low attenuation plaque typically describes a vulnerable lipid-rich core of an atheroma with a region containing plaque measuring <30 Hounsfield units (HU). Although not discreetly measured on these images, the plaque measured >30 HU in this case. Spotty calcifications are defined as calcifications <3 mm measuring >130 HU surrounded by noncalcified plaque (not seen in this case). Finally, the napkin ring sign is defined as a peripheral rim of higher attenuation with lower central attenuation in a plaque (present in this case).

Thus, the correct answer would be V as the plaque exhibits both positive remodeling and a napkin ring sign. Multiple studies have demonstrated these features to indicate an increased likelihood of plaque rupture, thereby resulting in a myocardial infarction. As such, vulnerable plaque is important to note as it can warrant more aggressive management.

This patient's study is clearly diagnostic, so N would not be the correct choice. Similarly, no graft or stent is seen in these images; therefore, a G and S would be incorrect as well.

References: Cury RC, Abbara S, Achenbach S, et al. CAD-RADS™: coronary artery disease—reporting and data system: an expert consensus document of the Society of Cardiovascular

Computed Tomography (SCCT), the American College of Radiology (ACR) and the North American Society for Cardiovascular Imaging (NASCI). Endorsed by the American College of Cardiology. *J Am Coll Radiol* 2016;13(12 Pt A):1458–1466.e9.

Kolossváry M, Szilveszter B, Merkely B, et al. Plaque imaging with CT-a comprehensive review on coronary CT angiography based risk assessment. *Cardiovasc Diagn Ther* 2017;7(5):489–506. doi:10.21037/cdt.2016.11.06.

5   **Answer A.** Graft patency at 10 years was 61% for saphenous vein grafts compared with 85% for left internal mammary artery grafts ($p < 0.001$).

Reference: Goldman S, et al. Long-term patency of saphenous vein and left internal mammary artery grafts after coronary artery bypass surgery: results from a Department of Veterans Affairs Cooperative Study. *J Am Coll Cardiol* 2004;44(11):2149–2156.

6   **Answer A.** Coronary artery calcification occurs in proportion to underlying plaque burden but not degree of stenosis. While it has been shown that a calcium score of >100 AU carries a 5× increased risk of a coronary event than a score <100, the presence of high-grade stenosis cannot be accurately determined on a calcium score image alone, as this does not account for occult noncalcified plaque. Additionally, it is possible that calcium is mostly intramural and does not cause significant luminal narrowing.

References: Guerci AD, et al. Relation of coronary calcium score by electron beam computed tomography to arteriographic findings in asymptomatic and symptomatic adults. *Am J Cardiol* 1997;79:128–133.

Yadon A, et al. Coronary calcification, coronary disease risk factors, C-reactive protein, and atherosclerotic cardiovascular disease events: the St. Francis Heart Study. *J Am Coll Cardiol* 2005;46(1):158–165.

7   **Answer B.** All scan parameters listed above are within reasonable protocol limits. The body habitus in this patient, however, is causing significant attenuation of the x-ray and increased image noise. BMI > 39 can potentially lead to nondiagnostic studies and is a relative contraindication.

Reference: Raff GL, et al. SCCT guidelines on the use of coronary computed tomographic angiography for patients presenting with acute chest pain to the emergency department: a report of the Society of Cardiovascular Computed Tomography Guidelines Committee. *J Cardiovas Comput Tomogr* 2014;8:254-271.

8   **Answer B.** Infarcted tissue demonstrates subendocardial enhancement or (when extensive) transmural enhancement. If <50% of the affected wall demonstrates scarring/enhancement, it is deemed viable, and revascularization has been shown to improve postinfarction ejection fraction and clinical outcome.

References: Cummings KW, et al. A pattern based approach to assessment of delayed enhancement in nonischemic cardiomyopathy at MR imaging. *Radiographics* 2009;29:89–103.

Kim R, et al. The use of contrast enhanced magnetic resonance imaging to identify reversible myocardial dysfunction. *N Engl J Med* 2000;343(2):1445–1453.

9   **Answer D.** Two-chamber bright blood image of the heart from a cardiac MRI demonstrates severe left ventricular apical thinning and a wide-mouthed apical outpouching most compatible with an aneurysm. Ventricular aneurysms are typically defined as severely thinned myocardium replaced by fibrous/scar tissue and surrounded by epicardium and endocardium. These are usually the result of prior myocardial infarction. These can be seen in as many as 8% to 15% of patients with Q-wave myocardial infarctions. The vast majority of these (as high as 85%) involve the left ventricular apex and/or apical anterior segments. Typically, true aneurysms are wide-mouthed (neck-to-mouth ratio of 0.9 to 1.1), dyskinetic, and demonstrate subendocardial or transmural enhancement. Associated mural thrombus is common and typically warrants anticoagulation.

Clot formation is augmented by stasis of flow in the aneurysm. The scar tissue itself may also act as a procoagulant. Aneurysms frequently cause ventricular arrhythmias. However, unlike pseudoaneurysms of the left ventricle, true aneurysms rarely rupture. Aneurysms may be surgically repaired in cases of intractable arrhythmias or heart failure failing to respond to medical therapy.

Ventricular pseudoaneurysms form when there is rupture of the myocardium and the leak is contained by pericardial adhesions or scar tissue. The majority are caused by transmural myocardial infarctions. These are usually seen with inferior wall infarcts. Some other potential etiologies include surgery, trauma, and infection. When caused by myocardial infarctions, they tend to happen 3 to 7 days after the infarct. Typically, pseudoaneurysms are narrow-mouthed (neck-to-mouth ratio of 0.25 to 0.5) and dyskinetic or akinetic. These may have associated pericardial enhancement and thickening thought to be a result of irritation from the acute bleed at the time of rupture. Without surgical treatment, mortality can be as high as 50%.

In practice, there is often overlap of imaging features between aneurysms and pseudoaneurysms. Surgery may be the only way to obtain a definitive diagnosis.

Interventricular septal rupture is not seen and could not be evaluated with only a two-chamber view of the heart. The given image does not clearly demonstrate pericardial thickening to suggest pericarditis. In addition, double inversion recovery dark blood and late gadolinium enhancement images would better evaluate for pericardial thickening and enhancement. Pericarditis that occurs in the context of injury to the heart such as infarct is referred to as Dressler syndrome.

References: Antman EM, Anbe DT, Armstrong PW, et al. ACC/AHA guidelines for the management of patients with ST-elevation myocardial infarction. *Circulation* 2004;110(5):588–636. www.acc.org/qualityandscience/clinical/statements.htm. Accessed on August 24, 2006.

Glower DG, Lowe EL. Left ventricular aneurysm. In: Edmunds LH (ed.). *Cardiac surgery in the adult*. New York: McGraw-Hill, 1997:677.

Nagle RE, Williams DO. Natural history of ventricular aneurysm without surgical treatment. *Br Heart J* 1974;36(10):1037.

Rao G, Zikria EA, Miller WH, et al. Experience with sixty consecutive ventricular aneurysm resections. *Circulation* 1974;50(2 Suppl):II149.

Reeder GS, Lengyel M, Tajik AJ, et al. Mural thrombus in left ventricular aneurysm: incidence, role of angiography, and relation between anticoagulation and embolization. *Mayo Clin Proc* 1981;56(2):77–81.

10 **Answer C.** Coronary CTA has a negative predictive value >95% and is an excellent test to exclude coronary artery disease. In particular, it has been shown to be of value when evaluating low-risk patients with atypical chest pain, low-risk patients with negative or equivocal stress testing, and in the emergency room setting to evaluate patients with acute chest pain who are of low to medium risk (shown in ACRIN-PA and ROMICAT-II clinical trials).

Reference: Taylor AJ, et al. ACCF/SCCT/ACR/AHA/ASE/ASNC/NASCI/SCAI/SCMR 2010 appropriate use criteria for cardiac computed tomography. Evaluation of graft patency after CABG has an appropriateness score of 8/9 in a symptomatic patient. *Circulation* 2010;122:e525–e555.

11 **Answer B.** Microvascular obstruction (MVO), also known as no-reflow phenomenon is a focus of infracted myocardium where obstruction of the microvasculature does not allow contrast to perfuse the tissue. Following infarction, administered contrast resides in the interstitium and creates the scar seen on delayed enhancement images. In areas where the microvasculature is obstructed, the contrast never reaches the interstitium, and this tissue appears as very dark signal surrounded by an enhancing scar on both sides. MVO is recognized as a poor prognostic indicator and marker of subsequent adverse LV remodeling.

Reference: Wu K. CMR of microvascular obstruction and hemorrhage in myocardial infarction. *J Cardiovasc Magn Reson* 2012;14:68.

12 **Answer A.** FFR_{CT} uses computational fluid dynamics to estimate the hemodynamic significance of a stenosis. The added value of FFR_{CT} is particularly noticeable in long segment stenoses or serial stenoses, as the additive effects of these lesions may be underestimated by a single 2D measurement. Studies have shown that combined with standard coronary CTA measurements, it can result in fewer unnecessary invasive angiographic studies without harm to the patient. Measurements are made 2 cm from identified sites of stenosis in vessels >1.8 mm in diameter. An $FFR_{CT} > 0.8$ indicates a high likelihood of the stenosis being nonobstructive, values from 0.76 to 0.80 are indeterminate, and values ≤ 0.75 indicates a high likelihood the stenosis is hemodynamically significant. In this example, only the LAD contains FFR_{CT} values below 0.75, suggesting only one vessel has hemodynamically significant disease.

Reference: Lu MT, Ferencik M, Roberts RS, et al. Noninvasive FFR derived from coronary CT angiography: management and outcomes in the PROMISE trial. *JACC Cardiovasc Imaging* 2017;10(11):1350–1358.

13 **Answer D.** Long-term data are now available for patients who underwent coronary CTA in the emergency room. Current data suggest that a normal CTA in a low-risk patient presenting to the ER has a "warranty period" of up to 2 years meaning a rescan is not necessary as there has been no recorded incident of ACS within 2 years in this population.

Reference: Schlett CL, et al. Prognostic value of CT angiography for major adverse cardiac events in patients with acute chest pain from the emergency department. *JACC Cardiovas Imaging* 2011;4(5):481–491.

14 **Answer A.** Several clinical trials such as ACRIN-PA, CT-STAT, and ROMICAT have demonstrated the utility of coronary CTA for low-risk emergency room patients presenting with chest pain. Current data support the position that a CCTA-based strategy for low- to intermediate-risk patients presenting with a possible acute coronary syndrome allows for the safe, expedited discharge home rather than admission and continued monitoring.

Reference: Litt HI, et al. CT angiography for safe discharge of patients with possible acute coronary syndromes. *N Engl J Med* 2012;366:1393–1403.

15 **Answer C.** Curved multiplanar reformation of the left anterior descending artery from a coronary CTA shows a peripherally calcified aneurysm involving the distal left main and proximal left anterior descending arteries (arrow). The most common cause of coronary artery aneurysms in an adult is atherosclerosis.

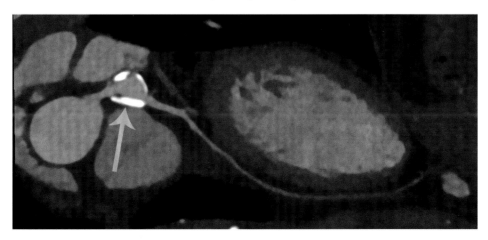

Coronary artery aneurysms are rare, seen in about 1% of all patients. Predisposing factors include entities such as atherosclerosis (most common in adults), Kawasaki disease, congenital factors, Marfan syndrome, and prior surgical/interventional procedures. Like many other arteries in the human body, coronary artery aneurysms are defined as focal dilation at least 1.5 times the caliber of the adjacent normal vessel. On the other hand, coronary artery ectasia is defined as a diffuse dilation at least 1.5 times the caliber of a normal vessel. When identified on coronary imaging, it is important to note the size, morphology (saccular vs. fusiform), the presence of branch vessels, and the presence of mural thrombus.

References: Cohen P, O'gara PT. Coronary artery aneurysms: a review of the natural history, pathophysiology, and management. *Cardiol Rev* 2008;16(6):301–304.

Kawsara A, Núñez Gil IJ, Alqahtani F, et al. Management of coronary artery aneurysms. *JACC Cardiovasc Interv* 2018;11(13):1211–1223.

16 **Answer A.** Selecting the appropriate TI or inversion time is extremely important for obtaining accurate imaging results. The TI is chosen to "null" normal myocardium (normal myocardium will not retain gadolinium, whereas injured myocardium will retain gadolinium). In principle, the optimal TI at which normal myocardium is nulled (black) must be determined by imaging iteratively with different inversion times. As time progresses after gadolinium administration, normal myocardium will have increased signal and a longer inversion time must be chosen to null its signal.

Reference: Kim R, et al. How we perform delayed enhancement imaging. *J Cardiovas Magnet Reson* 2003;5(3):505–514.

17 **Answer C.** Image A shows low attenuation within the distal RCA stent placed remotely. The low attenuation material is secondary to thrombus, which has developed over time. Image B shows two patent stents in the LAD. In general, stents >3.0 mm in size are readily evaluable, while stents measuring <2.5 mm can be difficult to evaluate.

References: Hong C, Chrysant GS, Woodard PK, et al. Coronary artery stent patency assessed with in-stent contrast enhancement measured at multi-detector row CT angiography: initial experience. *Radiology* 2004;233(1):286–291.

Martine R-J, Rémy J. *Integrated cardiothoracic imaging with MDCT*. Berlin, Germany: Springer Verlag, 2009.

18 **Answer C.** Myocardial infarction carries many associated complications that include apical aneurysm formation, decreased ejection fraction, ventriculoseptal defect formation, and papillary muscle infarction.

In one study, the incidence of rupture of the papillary muscle was found to be 0.9%. The clinical features usually occur during the first week after infarction. More common is slight mitral regurgitation without pulmonary edema from papillary muscle dysfunction.

Reference: Clements SD Jr, et al. Ruptured papillary muscle, a complication of myocardial infarction: clinical presentation, diagnosis, and treatment. *Clin Cardiol* 1985;8:93–103.

19 **Answer D.** After a successful procedure, coronary stents can fail to maintain vessel patency due to stent thrombosis or in-stent restenosis. Stent thrombosis can occur early, late, or very late following stent placement and is more common with bare metal stent placement. The incidence of thrombosis has decreased following the development and use of drug-eluting stents and anticoagulation therapy. Current guidelines for bare-metal stents require dual antiplatelet therapy for 1 month and for 1 year following placement of a drug-eluting stent.

References: Mahnken AH. CT imaging of coronary stents: past present and future. *ISRN Cardiol* 2012;2012(1):286–291. Article ID 139823.

Maluenda G, Ben-dor I, Gaglia MA, et al. Clinical outcomes and treatment after drug-eluting stent failure: the absence of traditional risk factors for in-stent restenosis. *Circ Cardiovasc Interv* 2012;5(1):12–19.

20a Answer D. Mid and basal apical short-axis images of the heart at end-diastole and end-systole demonstrate hypoenhancement and severe hypokinesis of the mid inferior, mid inferoseptal, and apical inferior walls compatible with myocardial infarction. These segments are most commonly supplied by the right coronary artery in a right dominant system. A notable exception would be in a patient with left dominant coronary circulation. This happens when the posterior descending artery arises from the left circumflex artery and is seen in approximately 9% of patients. The mid anterior, mid anteroseptal, apical septal, and apical anterior segments are typically supplied by the left anterior descending artery. The mid anterolateral and inferolateral segments are supplied by the left circumflex coronary artery.

In patients with acute myocardial infarction, the myocardium loses its ability to contract initially from decreased aerobic metabolism by the cardiomyocytes due to decreased blood flow from the coronary stenosis or occlusion. After approximately 20 minutes of ischemic time, the myocardium begins to undergo necrosis beginning along the subendocardial surface, extending to the subepicardial surface over time. This has been described as the "wavefront phenomenon" and is an important concept to understand as many imaging features used to detect ischemic heart disease rely on this phenomenon.

References: Knaapen M, Koch AH, Koch C, et al. Prevalence of left and balanced coronary arterial dominance decreases with increasing age of patients at autopsy. A postmortem coronary angiograms study. *Cardiovasc Pathol* 2013;22(1):49–53.

Reimer KA, Lowe JE, Rasmussen MM, et al. The wavefront phenomenon of ischemic cell death. 1. Myocardial infarct size vs duration of coronary occlusion in dogs. *Circulation* 1977;56(5):786–794.

20b Answer D. Curved multiplanar reformation and short-axis views of the right coronary artery demonstrate a long segment occlusion of the mid RCA. According to the Coronary Artery Disease—Reporting and Data System (CAD-RADS), the degree of coronary stenosis is graded from 0 to 5, in roughly 25% increments. The scores are as follows: 0 (0% stenosis), 1 (1% to 24% stenosis), 2 (25% to 49% stenosis), 3 (50% to 69% stenosis), 4A (70% to 99% stenosis), 4B (left main >50% stenosis or 70% to 99% stenosis in all three coronary arteries), and 5 (100% total occlusion). Generally, CAD-RADS scores from 0 to 2 are considered "negative," and nonatherosclerotic causes of chest pain should be considered. On the other hand, scores of CAD-RADS 3 to 5 are considered "positive" for potential hemodynamically significant coronary artery atherosclerosis and warrant further testing. A score of CAD-RADS 3 typically should receive functional testing to determine the clinical significance of the stenosis. Scores of 4 to 5 usually undergo invasive coronary angiograms, although functional or viability testing may be performed in certain scenarios. Multiple large randomized control trials have demonstrated that a negative coronary CTA effectively rules out coronary atherosclerosis as a cause of acute chest pain and can spare the patient unnecessary admissions and additional testing.

Reference: Cury RC, Abbara S, Achenbach S, et al. CAD-RADS™: coronary artery disease—reporting and data system: an expert consensus document of the Society of Cardiovascular Computed Tomography (SCCT), the American College of Radiology (ACR) and the North American Society for Cardiovascular Imaging (NASCI). Endorsed by the American College of Cardiology. *J Am Coll Radiol* 2016;13(12 Pt A):1458–1466.e9.

21 **Answer B.** The two most common vessels used for coronary artery bypass grafting are the greater saphenous vein and the left internal mammary artery. Saphenous vein grafts (SVG) are typically used given their size and ease of harvesting. SVGs are typically anastomosed to the ascending aorta and distal to the target lesion in the coronary artery of interest. Primary reasons for using the left internal mammary artery are its proximity to the heart, relatively good long-term patency rates, and need for only single (distal) anastomosis. The origin of the left internal mammary artery is most commonly from the left subclavian artery. The most common variant anatomy is an origin from the left thyrocervical trunk. Therefore, in order to investigate graft patency in this patient, the scan range would need to extend from the clavicles through the base of the heart.

Extending the range to the top of the aortic arch may miss the left internal mammary artery origin from the proximal left subclavian artery. Extending the scan range inferiorly to the renal arteries will not help evaluate graft patency. Not changing the scan range at all would not fully visualize the bypass grafts.

Reference: Shahoud JS, Burns B. Anatomy, thorax, internal mammary (internal thoracic) arteries. [Updated 2019 Jan 4]. In: *StatPearls* [Internet]. Treasure Island, FL: StatPearls Publishing, 2020. https://www.ncbi.nlm.nih.gov/books/NBK537337/

22 **Answer C.** The image demonstrates an endotracheal tube and nasogastric tube and bilateral chest tubes. An intra-aortic balloon pump is noted along with a percutaneous left ventricular assist device. These circulatory support devices are placed in the setting of acute myocardial infarction with shock requiring hemodynamic support.

References: Delgado D, et al. Mechanical circulatory assistance state of the art. *Circulation* 2002;106:2046–2050.

Naidu SS. Novel percutaneous cardiac assist devices: the science of and indications for hemodynamic support. *Circulation* 2011;123(5):533–543. doi: 10.1161/CIRCULATIONAHA. 110.945055.

23 **Answer D.** Advances in cardiac MRI allow for stress perfusion imaging in addition to delayed enhancement imaging for scar. Stress perfusion imaging has the added advantage of detecting inducible subendocardial hypoperfusion. Intravenous adenosine is typically given at a dose of 140 µg/kg/min during stress perfusion imaging.

References: Kramer C, et al. Standardized cardiovascular magnetic resonance imaging (CMR) protocols, society for cardiovascular magnetic resonance: board of trustees task force on standardized protocols. *J Cardiovas Magn Reson* 2008;10:35.

Vogel-Claussen J, et al. Comprehensive adenosine stress perfusion MRI defines the etiology of chest pain in the emergency room: comparison with nuclear stress test. *J Magn Reson Imaging* 2009;30(4):753–762.

24 **Answer C.** Percutaneous coronary intervention (PCI) in symptomatic patients with stable ischemic heart disease receiving optimal medical therapy has only been shown to improve angina. It has not been proven to improve survival nor decrease future myocardial infarctions. PCI in patients with stable CAD is only recommended if patients have unacceptable symptoms or cannot tolerate optimal medical therapy.

References: Kureshi F, Jones PG, Buchanan DM, et al. Variation in patients' perceptions of elective percutaneous coronary intervention in stable coronary artery disease: cross sectional study. *BMJ* 2014;349:g5309. doi:10.1136/bmj.g5309.

Sedlis SP, Hartigan PM, Teo KK, et al. Effect of PCI on long-term survival in patients with stable ischemic heart disease. *N Engl J Med* 2015;373(20):1937–1946. doi:10.1056/NEJMoa1505532.

25 **Answer B.** Coronary CTA should ideally be done in patients with low to moderate pretest probability for coronary artery disease. Of the choices given, the 47-year-old male with a smoking and family history of coronary artery disease best fits this category. The 35-year-old female would have very low probability for coronary artery disease and other etiologies for her chest pain should be considered. The 55-year-old female could potentially be a good candidate but has atrial fibrillation, which is not ideal for coronary CTA due to ECG gating difficulties. A 76-year-old with angina has high probability of coronary artery disease so would ideally undergo invasive coronary catheterization.

Reference: American College of Cardiology Foundation Task Force on Expert Consensus Documents; Mark DB, Berman DS, Budoff MJ, et al. ACCF/ACR/AHA/NASCI/SAIP/SCAI/SCCT 2010 expert consensus document on coronary computed tomographic angiography: a report of the American College of Cardiology Foundation Task Force on Expert Consensus Documents. *Circulation* 2010;121(22):2509–2543. doi:10.1161/CIR.0b013e3181d4b618.

26 **Answer A.** The solid and dotted white lines represent the portion of the ECG tracing during which the image was being acquired. The solid line represents increased tube current and the dotted line represents reduced tube current. Given the low heart rate of the patient, diagnostic coronary artery images could be obtained using only diastole, which is typically around 70% of the R–R interval. Therefore, increased tube current was only used during this time to acquire the images with the least amount of noise. In this case, since left ventricular function was also being evaluated, images were acquired during the rest of the cardiac cycle, but at a lower tube current to reduce dose (dotted white line) since function can usually still be evaluated in noisy images. Note that in practice, there is a short ramp up and ramp down of tube current since the scanner is not able to instantaneously switch between maximum and minimum tube currents.

Reference: Litmanovich DE, Tack DM, Shahrzad M, et al. Dose reduction in cardiothoracic CT: review of currently available methods. *Radiographics* 2014;34(6):1469–1489.

27 **Answer B.** In any vascular stenosis, the more proximal the lesion, the larger the territory affected by the stenosis. This is no different in the heart. Typically, the LAD perfuses a little over one-third of the left ventricular myocardium. The RCA and LCx both perfuse just under one-third each (assuming right dominant anatomy). Therefore, the LM will typically supply over two-thirds of the left ventricular myocardium since it bifurcates into the LAD and LCx. In the case of left dominant circulation, the entire left ventricular myocardium is supplied via the LM. Consequently, atherosclerotic lesions in the LM carry the highest risk of any coronary artery, and studies have found that lesions as low as 50% can carry significant risks. As such, the American College of Cardiology/American Heart Association and the European Society of Cardiology all recommend revascularization in patients with at least 50% stenosis in the LM regardless of symptoms.

Reference: Ramadan R, Boden WE, Kinlay S. Management of left main coronary artery disease. *J Am Heart Assoc* 2018;7(7):e008151. doi:10.1161/JAHA.117.008151.

28a **Answer B.** Perfusion image shows subendocardial perfusion abnormality in the anteroseptal region. On the b-SSFP image, there is persistent hypointensity in the anterior septal endocardium. On the late gadolinium enhancement image, there is evidence for microvascular obstruction (MVO) (subendocardial area of nonenhancement due to inability for blood to flow into the microvasculature), normal myocardial thickness, and enhancement of the infarct in the mid wall indicating an acute myocardial infarction.

MVO is an important feature to note on imaging for a multitude of reasons, one of these is that it can help elucidate the chronicity of the infarction. MVO is most pronounced in the acute setting and will slowly resolve in the subacute phase and should be absent when the infarction is chronic. The majority of MVO will resolve within 4 to 6 weeks.

Myocarditis and sarcoidosis typically cause mid myocardial or subepicardial delayed enhancement, whereas the vast majority of subendocardial delayed enhancement will be secondary to myocardial infarctions.

Reference: Abbas A, Matthews GH, Brown IW, et al. Cardiac MR assessment of microvascular obstruction. *Br J Radiol* 2015;88(1047):20140470. doi:10.1259/bjr.20140470.

28b **Answer A.** The anteroseptal myocardial segment is almost always supplied by the left anterior descending coronary artery (LAD).

28c **Answer A.** Infarcts with microvascular obstruction have worse prognosis than infarcts without microvascular obstruction. It is associated with adverse left ventricular remodeling, persistent LV dysfunction with worsened ejection fraction, and increased likelihood of future major adverse cardiac events.

Reference: Hamirani YS, Wong A, Kramer CM, et al. Effect of microvascular obstruction and intramyocardial hemorrhage by CMR on LV remodeling and outcomes after myocardial infarction: a systematic review and meta-analysis. *JACC Cardiovas Imaging* 2014;7(9):940–952. doi:10.1016/j.jcmg.2014.06.012.

29 **Answer D.** Two-chamber late gadolinium enhancement image of the heart does not demonstrate any abnormal late gadolinium enhancement. The abnormal contractility precludes a diagnosis of normal myocardium. No fibrosis is seen to suggest nonviable myocardium. That leaves two potential etiologies for the viable myocardium in this case: stunned or hibernating. Stunned myocardium refers to dysfunctional myocardium in the setting of recent ischemia (typically <15 minutes or infarction would occur). This typically resolves within weeks of the inciting event. Hibernating myocardium refers to chronic myocardial dysfunction from persistently reduced perfusion by the coronary arteries. Both can result in reduced contractility without abnormal late gadolinium enhancement. Stunned myocardium will usually have a normal resting perfusion on first-pass perfusion sequences (not shown in this case), while hibernating myocardium will demonstrate reduced flow in the affected regions. In this case, the history gives us the answer. The patient had presented with an acute event several weeks prior. At this point, any stunned myocardium should have resolved or potentially become hibernating. Hibernating myocardium is especially important to recognize as these areas often exhibit vastly improved contractility after coronary revascularization.

Reference: Souto ALM, Souto RM, Teixeira ICR, et al. Myocardial viability on cardiac magnetic resonance. *Arq Bras Cardiol* 2017;108(5):458–469. doi:10.5935/abc.20170056.

30 **Answer D.** Adenosine stress cardiac MRI is commonly used to assess for hemodynamically significant epicardial coronary artery disease. It works based on the idea that the epicardial coronary arteries and arterioles will dilate in response to increased oxygen demands by cardiomyocytes during stress. In regions of significant stenosis, these arteries and arterioles cannot dilate to keep up with the perfusion demands of the myocardium during stress and a relative perfusion defect becomes apparent on first-pass perfusion imaging. The typical vasodilator stress protocol involves first-pass perfusion imaging under stress, at rest, and late gadolinium enhancement imaging. If a stress perfusion defect resolves on rest images and there is no late gadolinium enhancement, then inducible hypoperfusion is present. If a stress perfusion defect persists on rest images and there is no late gadolinium enhancement, then it is most likely dark rim artifact. Rarely, resting ischemia has been reported. If a stress perfusion defect resolves on rest images and there is late gadolinium enhancement, then an infarct is present. Peri-infarct ischemia is seen when the size of the stress perfusion defect is greater than the area of late gadolinium enhancement. When an infarct is present, the perfusion defect appears to resolve on rest images because they are acquired after stress images, so the infarcted myocardium is now enhancing and no longer distinguishable as a perfusion defect. Note that stress cardiac MRI can also be performed with dobutamine looking at function, perfusion, or both.

In this patient, the stress images demonstrate a circumferential subendocardial hypointense ring that resolves on the rest images. No late gadolinium enhancement is seen, excluding scar. These findings are consistent with inducible ischemia, though since it is circumferential, all three vascular territories would be involved. This was later confirmed by catheter angiography.

The dark rim artifact is commonly seen on perfusion images, though typically is present for the first few frames after the contrast enters the myocardium and will quickly resolve. Initially, this was felt to possibly represent microvascular disease, but now, it is agreed upon to be an artifact. The etiology of the artifact is not entirely clear but may be related to Gibbs ringing, susceptibility artifact, or volume averaging. Recently, some studies have shown that quantitative perfusion stress MRI may be able to help distinguish between dark rim artifact and microvascular disease (also microvascular angina or cardiac syndrome X). Dark rim artifact causes a decrease in signal intensity in a subendocardial distribution, whereas microvascular disease does not have a change in signal intensity—rather only the relative appearance of decreased signal intensity due to the increased signal of the surrounding "normally" perfusing myocardium. Finally, there are no findings to suggest myocarditis on these images.

References: Di Bella EV, Parker DL, Sinusas AJ. On the dark rim artifact in dynamic contrast-enhanced MRI myocardial perfusion studies. *Magn Reson Med* 2005;54(5):1295–1299.

Lipinski MJ, McVey CM, Berger JS, et al. Prognostic value of stress cardiac magnetic resonance imaging in patients with known or suspected coronary artery disease: a systematic review and meta-analysis. *J Am Coll Cardiol* 2013;62(9):826–838.

Cardiomyopathy

Jean Jeudy, MD • Sachin Malik, MD

QUESTIONS

1a A 21-year-old male with a history of palpitations and dizziness while playing basketball undergoes a cardiac MRI for further workup. Which of the following best describes the abnormality identified by the arrows in the images below?

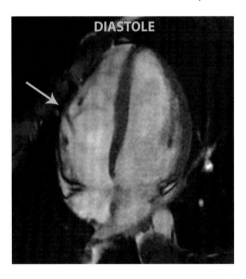
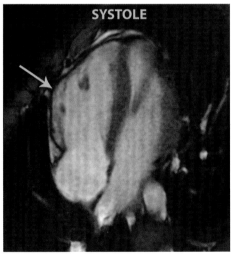

A. Right ventricular dyskinesia
B. Right ventricular thrombus
C. Right ventricular fat deposition
D. Right ventricular late gadolinium enhancement

1b Functional analysis of the cardiac MRI revealed a left ventricular ejection fraction of 56% and a right ventricular ejection fraction of 36%. In this patient, these findings could suggest which of the following diagnoses?

A. Hypertrophic cardiomyopathy
B. Restrictive cardiomyopathy
C. Arrhythmogenic right ventricular dysplasia
D. Constrictive pericarditis

2 A short axis late gadolinium enhancement image at the level of the mid left ventricle is shown. The pattern of fibrosis shown has been commonly associated with which of the following?

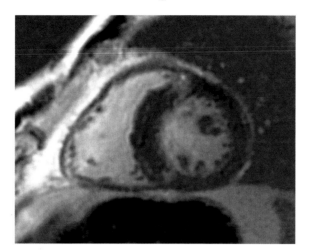

    A. Pulmonary hypertension
    B. Myocardial infarction
    C. Constrictive pericarditis
    D. Anderson-Fabry disease

3 Which process best characterizes the imaging findings?

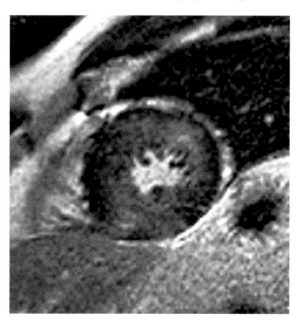

    A. Myocardial infarction
    B. Hypertrophic cardiomyopathy
    C. Myocarditis
    D. Arrhythmogenic right ventricular dysplasia

4   A 27-year-old male presented after an episode of syncope while playing soccer. Based on the abnormality seen in the images below from his cardiac MRI, what is the most likely diagnosis?

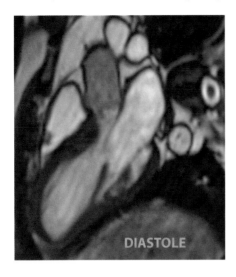
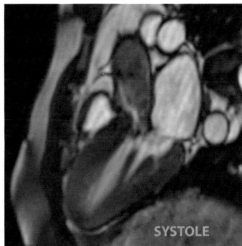

A. Sarcoidosis

B. Amyloidosis

C. Arrhythmogenic right ventricular dysplasia

D. Hypertrophic cardiomyopathy

5   The patient is a 26-year-old with worsening heart failure. Given the imaging findings, what is the most likely explanation for the patient's condition?

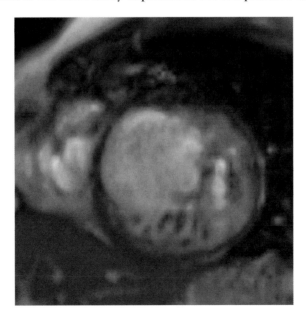

A. Restrictive cardiomyopathy

B. Constrictive pericarditis

C. Hypertrophic cardiomyopathy

D. Left ventricular noncompaction

6 Patient is referred for atypical chest pain and exercise intolerance over the last few months. No personal or family history of cardiac disease is otherwise noted. Given the imaging findings, what is the most likely etiology of the patient's condition?

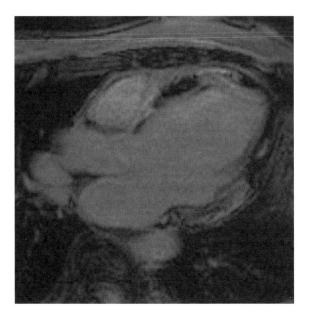

A. Myocardial infarction
B. Hypertrophic cardiomyopathy
C. Myocarditis
D. Arrhythmogenic right ventricular dysplasia

7 A 36-year-old woman without significant past medical history presents with acute chest pain while attending a funeral. She was found to have elevated troponins and taken for emergent cardiac catheterization. No obstructive coronary artery disease was found. Apical four-chamber images during diastole and systole from a transthoracic echocardiogram are shown below. Which of the following is the most likely etiology?

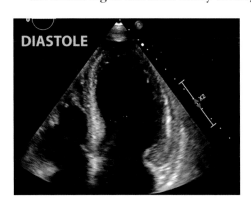
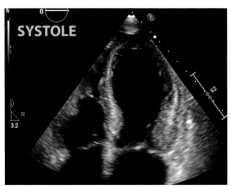

A. Dilated cardiomyopathy
B. Hypertrophic cardiomyopathy
C. Stress-induced cardiomyopathy
D. Ischemic cardiomyopathy

8   A 16-year-old male with a history of thalassemia major is referred for cardiac MR due to worsening shortness of breath and decreased systolic function on echocardiography. The examination was performed on a 1.5T scanner. As part of the examination, a T2* of the myocardium is obtained which was calculated at 12.9 msec. Additional images from the examination are shown below. What is the most likely cause of the patient's condition?

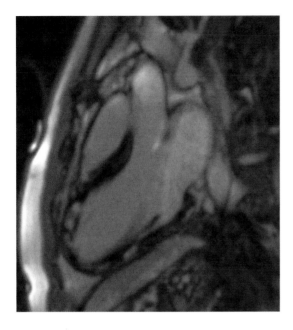 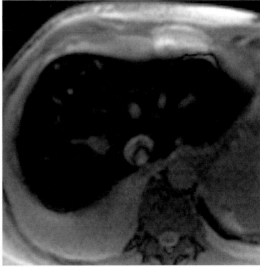

A. Myocardial infarction
B. Hypertrophic cardiomyopathy
C. Arrhythmogenic right ventricular dysplasia
D. Hemochromatosis

9   Which of the following could explain the abnormality in the image shown below?

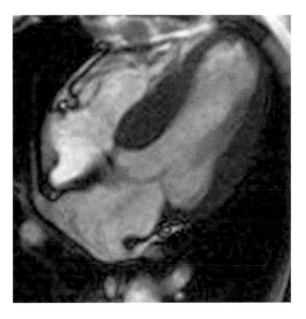

A. Ventricular noncompaction
B. Severe aortic stenosis
C. Uhl anomaly
D. Annuloaortic ectasia

10 A 27-year-old male has a syncopal episode while playing soccer. He was resuscitated by medical personnel in the field and brought to the emergency department. On review of family history, he notes that he had an uncle who unexpectedly died at the same age playing basketball. Cardiac MR demonstrates the following:

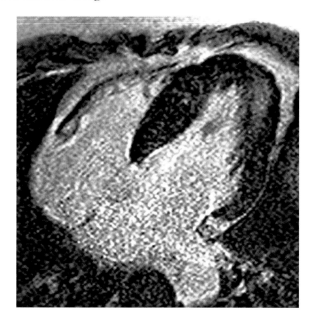

Given the clinical presentation and the imaging findings, what treatment recommendation would you suggest?

A. Beta-blockers
B. ICD
C. ACE inhibitors
D. Steroid therapy

11 A patient with cardiomyopathy and peripheral eosinophilia presents with the following imaging findings:

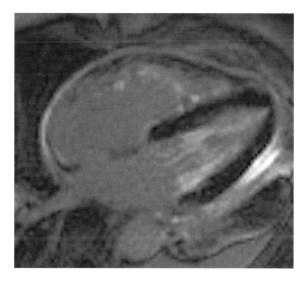

Which abnormality most likely reflects the underlying cardiomyopathy?

A. Loeffler endocarditis
B. Myocardial infarction
C. Cardiac sarcoidosis
D. Amyloidosis

12 A 33-year-old male with progressive shortness of breath presented to the emergency room where he was found to have second-degree heart block. Echocardiography showed normal systolic dysfunction, but moderate diastolic dysfunction. Based on the history and images from his cardiac MR shown below, which of the following is the most likely diagnosis?

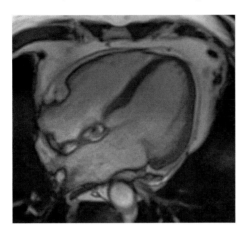 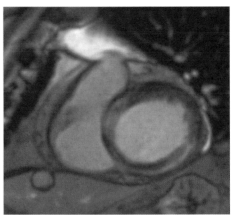

A. Restrictive cardiomyopathy
B. Ischemic cardiomyopathy
C. Hypertrophic cardiomyopathy
D. Constrictive pericarditis

13 A 47-year-old patient with worsening heart failure presents for evaluation by cardiac MR. A representative image is noted below. Which of the following is most closely associated with the MR finding?

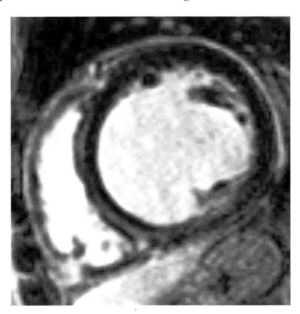

A. Nonischemic dilated cardiomyopathy
B. Sarcoid cardiomyopathy
C. Arrhythmogenic right ventricular cardiomyopathy
D. Ischemic cardiomyopathy with septal infarct

14 A 77-year-old male with multiple myeloma has worsening dyspnea with global ventricular hypertrophy and decreased left ventricular function by echocardiography. Cardiac MR was ordered for further evaluation.

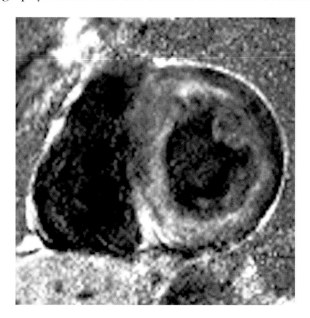

Given the clinical history and imaging findings, which of the following diagnoses best characterize the underlying cardiomyopathy?

A. Amyloidosis
B. Dilated cardiomyopathy
C. Hypertrophic cardiomyopathy
D. Iron overload cardiomyopathy

15a A 19-year-old male presents with palpitations and syncope while working out at the gym. He undergoes a cardiac MRI for further evaluation. In the images below, what is the best explanation for the finding identified by the arrow?

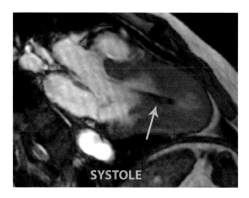
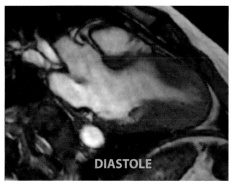

A. Turbulent flow
B. Calcification
C. Mitral regurgitation
D. Thrombus

15b Additional images from his cardiac MRI examination are shown. Given the clinical presentation and imaging findings, what is the most likely diagnosis?

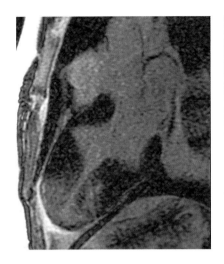 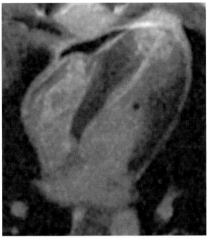 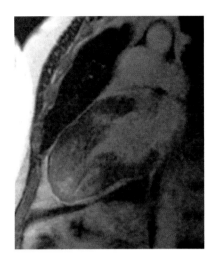

    A. Dilated cardiomyopathy
    B. Hypertrophic cardiomyopathy
    C. Iron overload cardiomyopathy
    D. Stress-induced cardiomyopathy

16 A 27-year-old male presents with 2 days of atypical chest pain. History reveals a recent upper respiratory tract infection. Examination shows a low-grade fever. Echocardiography notes a small pericardial effusion, but normal systolic function and left ventricular wall motion. He is referred for a cardiac MRI for further evaluation. Based on the information provided and MR images below, what is the most likely diagnosis?

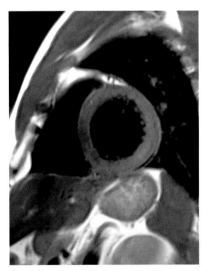 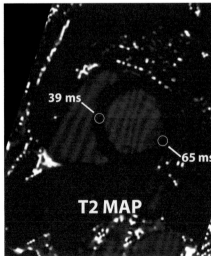 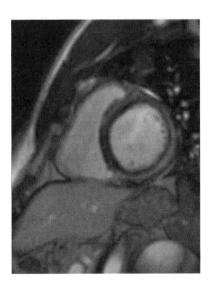

    A. Myocardial infarction
    B. Myocarditis
    C. Hypertrophic cardiomyopathy
    D. Constrictive pericarditis

17a A 27-year-old male without any prior medical history presents to his primary physician with progressive dyspnea and difficulty with exercise over the last couple of months. A cardiac MR reveals decreased left ventricular function and the following imaging findings:

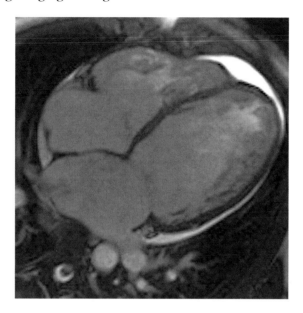

Given the clinical history and imaging, which of the following best characterizes the patient's cardiomyopathy?

A. Dilated cardiomyopathy
B. Inflammatory cardiomyopathy (myocarditis)
C. Ventricular noncompaction
D. Chronic hypertensive changes

17b Which of the following is a complication of the previous abnormality?

A. Conduction abnormalities
B. Left ventricular hypertrophy
C. Ventricular aneurysms
D. Valvular stenosis

18 A 67-year-old male with end stage renal disease on dialysis was recently found to have new severe left ventricular hypertrophy and a reduced left ventricular ejection fraction of 41%. Images from a 99m-Technetium pyrophosphate SPECT examination are shown. In this patient, which of the following abnormalities may be seen on cardiac MRI?

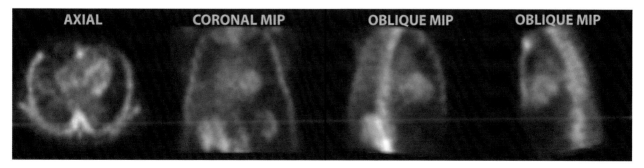

A. Difficulty nulling the myocardium
B. Right ventricular outflow tract aneurysm
C. Pericardial thickening and enhancement
D. Systolic anterior motion of the anterior mitral valve leaflet

19 What other abnormality may be associated with the finding highlighted by the arrows in the images below?

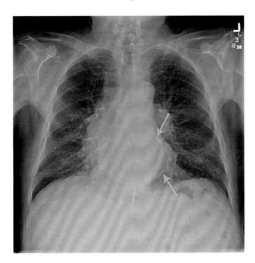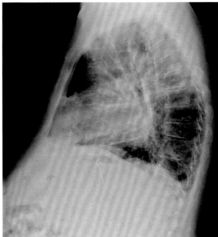

A. Difficulty nulling the myocardium
B. Turbulent flow across the mid LV cavity
C. Noncompacted to compacted LV myocardium ratio of 3.2 at end-diastole
D. Ventricular interdependence

20a A 28-year-old male presents with progressive muscle loss and muscle weakness. History reveals that he had an older sibling with similar symptoms who died of sudden cardiac death at the age of 30. Based on the cardiac MR images shown, what best explains the abnormality identified by the arrows?

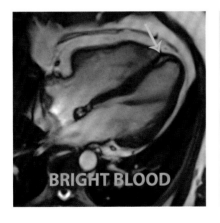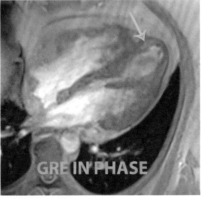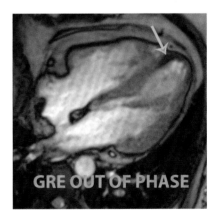

A. Intramyocardial microvascular obstruction
B. Intramyocardial edema
C. Intramyocardial fat
D. Intramyocardial hemorrhage

20b A short axis phase reconstruction late gadolinium enhancement image through the mid left ventricle is shown in the same patient. Given the clinical presentation and imaging findings. What is the most likely diagnosis?

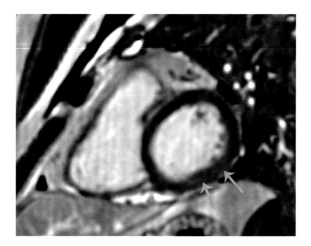

    A. Ischemic cardiomyopathy
    B. Endomyocardial fibrosis
    C. Acute myocarditis
    D. Myotonic dystrophy

21a A 67-year-old female presents with a several month history of exertional dyspnea and fatigue. History reveals a remote history of mediastinal radiation for lymphoma. On examination, she is found to have elevated jugular venous distension, ascites, and lower extremity edema. Cardiac MR is performed for further evaluation. Based on the clinical history and images shown, which of the following would this patient also be expected to have?

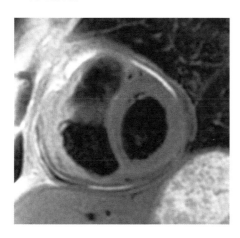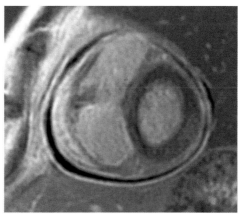

    A. Descending thoracic aortic diastolic flow reversal
    B. Ventricular interdependence
    C. Microvascular obstruction
    D. First pass subendocardial hypoperfusion

21b Additional MR images are shown from the same examination. The abnormality highlighted by the arrows suggests the presence of which of the following?

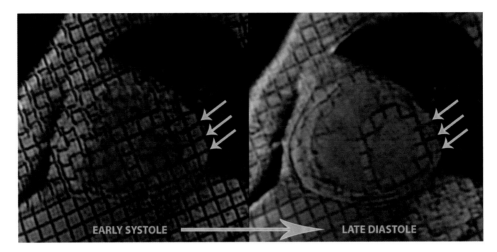

A. Myocyte necrosis
B. Right ventricular dyskinesia
C. Left ventricular hypertrophy
D. Myocardial–pericardial adhesions

22 In restrictive cardiomyopathy, what is the relationship of ventricular compliance and diastolic volume?

A. Increased ventricular compliance with reduced diastolic volume
B. Decreased ventricular compliance with increased diastolic volume
C. Increased ventricular compliance with increased diastolic volume
D. Decreased ventricular compliance and reduced diastolic volume

23 Which MR sequence quantifies the severity of iron deposition in iron overload cardiomyopathies?

A. T2*
B. Late gadolinium enhancement
C. Chemical shift imaging
D. T1

24 A 27-year-old woman presents with dyspnea, edema, and palpitations. She has no prior medical history and gave birth to a healthy newborn child 2 months ago, but still complains of progressive symptoms. An echocardiogram was performed and reports a dilated left ventricle with an EF of 35% and no other wall motion abnormalities. Which form of cardiomyopathy is most likely?

A. Postpartum
B. Amyloidosis
C. Hypertrophic
D. ARVD

25 A 55-year-old male with a history of syncope while jogging was found to have frequent episodes of nonsustained ventricular tachycardia. He was referred for a cardiac MRI for further evaluation, which was performed on a 3T scanner. Based on the images shown what is the best explanation for the increase in extracellular volume (ECV)?

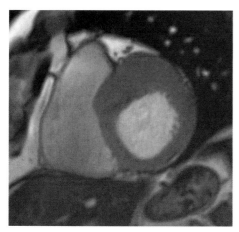
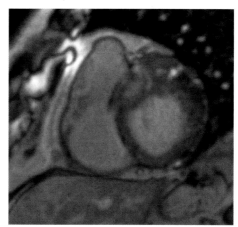

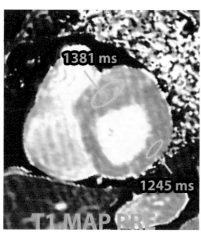
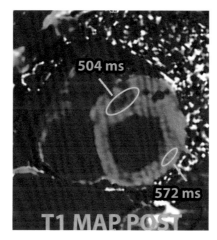
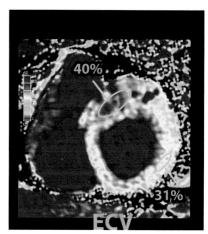

A. Interstitial fibrosis
B. Hemorrhage
C. Iron overload
D. Fat deposition

26a A 37-year-old female with a history of pulmonary sarcoidosis presented with worsening shortness of breath and syncope. Workup revealed third-degree heart block and a reduced left ventricular ejection fraction of 34%. FDG-PET CT was obtained. How would you best describe the cardiac findings?

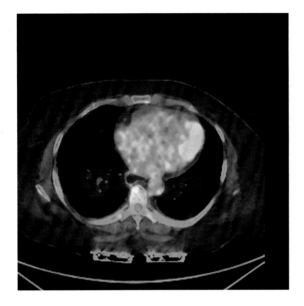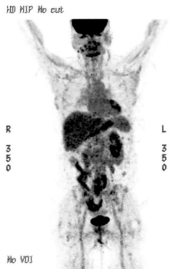

A. No uptake
B. Diffuse uptake
C. Focal uptake

26b What is the most likely diagnosis?

A. Cardiac sarcoidosis
B. Noncompaction cardiomyopathy
C. Hemochromatosis
D. Constrictive pericarditis

26c When performing FDG-PET CT to evaluate for cardiac sarcoidosis patients are instructed to switch to a high-fat, low-carbohydrate diet. What is the goal of this preparation?

A. Decrease glucose uptake by infarcted myocardium.
B. Increase glucose uptake by infarcted myocardium.
C. Decrease glucose uptake by normal myocardium.
D. Increase glucose uptake by normal myocardium.

27 A 57-year-old male with multiple myeloma presents with progressive heart failure symptoms. He is referred for CMR to rule out amyloidosis. Which of the following MR findings would be consistent with the diagnosis?

A. Dilated thin walled ventricles on precontrast GRE sequences
B. Asymmetric septal hypertrophy on postcontrast T1 sequences
C. Dyskinetic right ventricular wall motion on cine SSFP sequences
D. Difficulty nulling the myocardium on postcontrast inversion recovery sequences

28 A 54-year-old female presents with premature ventricular complexes (PVCs). Study was done to assess for ARVD. Images below are in end diastole and end systole. The bulge seen in systole in the RV wall near the apex represents what?

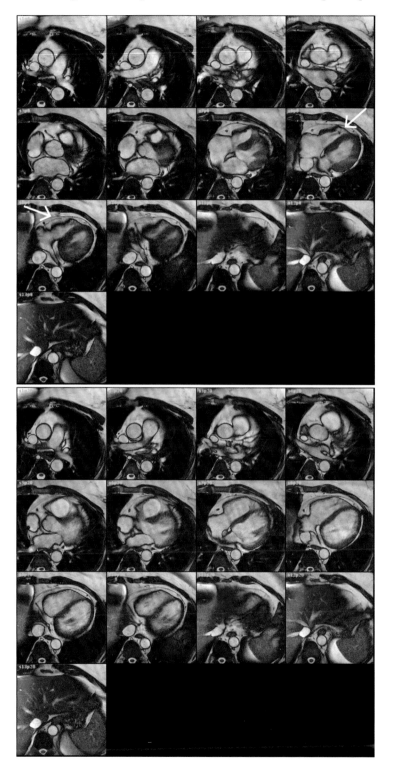

    A. Normal finding in isolation of other RV wall motion abnormalities
    B. Abnormal finding consistent with minor criterion for ARVD
    C. Abnormal finding consistent with major criterion for ARVD

ANSWERS AND EXPLANATIONS

1a **Answer A.** Images from a four-chamber view of the heart during systole and diastole are shown. The arrow highlights an area of the lateral right ventricular wall, which bulges outward during systole compatible with dyskinesia. No mass is seen to suggest thrombus. Fat deposition and late gadolinium enhancement cannot be fully assessed with the images provided.

1b **Answer C.** Arrhythmogenic right ventricular dysplasia (ARVD) is a genetic cardiomyopathy with an incidence of the familial form of ARVD that is estimated between 15% and 50%. The diagnosis is based on clinical and nonclinical criteria, including family history, which are subdivided into major and minor criteria. A "definite" diagnosis consists of two major criteria or one major and two minor criteria, or four minor criteria. A "borderline" diagnosis consists of one major and one minor criterion or three minor criteria. Finally, a "possible" diagnosis consists of one major or two minor criteria.

The original criteria were revised in 2010 to include specific abnormalities that may be detected on MRI and echocardiography. Primary imaging criteria on MRI include a combination of

a. Regional RV akinesia, dyskinesia, or dyssynchronous RV contraction
b. Findings of right ventricular dysfunction, of which severity determines whether a major or minor criteria is reached:
   i. RV end-diastolic volume index $\geq$110 mL/m^2 (male) or $\geq$100 mL/m^2 (female)
   Or RV ejection fraction $\leq$40%, which in combination with (a) would fulfill a Major criteria
   ii. RV end-diastolic volume index 100 to 109 mL/m^2 (male) or 90 to 99 mL/m^2 (female)
   Or RV ejection fraction 40% to 44%, which in combination with (a) would fulfill a Major criteria

Other morphologic abnormalities such as fat infiltration and delayed enhancement images are detectable by MRI but have not been considered sensitive enough to be in the diagnostic criteria. Fat deposition has also been reported on CT, including reports of left ventricular intramyocardial fat deposition. However, note that fat in the LV in a subendocardial or transmural distribution is much more commonly related to prior myocardial infarction.

This patient has a major criteria for ARVD due to the RV dyskinesia and RV ejection fraction <40%.

References: Marcus FI, McKenna WJ, Sherrill D, et al. Diagnosis of arrhythmogenic right ventricular cardiomyopathy/dysplasia proposed modification of the task force criteria. *Circulation* 2010;121(13):1533–1541.

Tavano A, Maurel B, Gaubert J-Y, et al. MR imaging of arrhythmogenic right ventricular dysplasia: what the radiologist needs to know. *Diagn Interv Imaging* 2015;96(5):449–460.

2 **Answer A.** The image shows anterior and posterior interventricular hinge point enhancement (arrows).

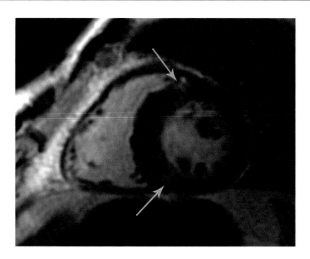

This pattern of fibrosis has been associated with pulmonary hypertension, right ventricular volume and pressure overload states, hypertrophic cardiomyopathy, and less commonly nonischemic dilated cardiomyopathies. Myocardial infarction would have subendocardial or transmural fibrosis in a coronary artery distribution. Constrictive pericarditis does not classically have myocardial fibrosis unless from another concurrent process. Anderson-Fabry disease has been associated with mesocardial or epicardial fibrosis in the basal to mid inferolateral left ventricular wall. Knowing the typical patterns of fibrosis are very high yield for the CORE examination.

Select high yield associations and patterns to know include the following:

Infarct: subendocardial or transmural in a *coronary artery distribution*

Amyloidosis: global subendocardial, global patchy subendocardial/mesocardial, and basal inferolateral wall

Nonischemic dilated cardiomyopathy: mesocardial septum

Hypertrophic cardiomyopathy: mesocardial particularly in areas of hypertrophy, hinge points

Systemic sclerosis: mesocardial septal, patchy mesocardial

Myocarditis: *mesocardial/epicardial lateral wall*, patchy mesocardial/epicardial, may also see pericardial enhancement (i.e., myopericarditis)

Anderson-Fabry, Myotonic Dystrophy, Chagas disease: mesocardial/epicardial of basal to mid inferolateral wall

Sarcoidosis: basal and mid septal, patchy throughout

ARVD: RV wall

Endomyocardial fibrosis: diffuse subendocardial

Hypertensive cardiomyopathy: diffuse patchy mesocardial

Post cardiac transplantation: diffuse subendocardial

References: Cummings KW, et al. A pattern-based approach to assessment of delayed enhancement in nonischemic cardiomyopathy at MR imaging. *Radiographics* 2009;29:89–103.

Lamacie MM, et al. The added value of cardiac magnetic resonance in muscular dystrophies. *J Neuromuscul Dis* 2019;6(4):389–399.

3   **Answer B.** Short-axis view of the heart demonstrating marked hypertrophy of the left ventricle. The MR sequence is an inversion recovery technique with an inversion time to null the myocardium and assess for late gadolinium enhancement. In this case, there is patchy enhancement within the midmyocardium with more focal fibrosis in anterolateral and inferoseptal segments. Findings are consistent with hypertrophic cardiomyopathy.

The pattern of enhancement is atypical for infarction, which should primarily be subendocardial. Left ventricular hypertrophy and patchy enhancement can be seen with amyloidosis. However, the nulling of the myocardium is characteristically difficult because of the T1 properties of the amyloid protein and diffusely increased extracellular volume.

Hypertrophic cardiomyopathy (HCM) is a genetic disorder characterized by left ventricular hypertrophy (wall thickness >12 to 15 mm) but is also heterogeneous in presentation, prognosis, and treatment strategies. Pathologic hallmarks of HCM include myocyte disarray and interstitial fibrosis.

Several imaging phenotypes are recognized (e.g., asymmetric [septal] HCM, apical HCM, symmetric HCM [concentric HCM], and midventricular HCM). In addition, RV hypertrophy may be seen in isolation or in conjunction with LV hypertrophy. Increased LV wall thickness may result in narrowing of the left ventricular outflow tract (LVOT). Systolic anterior motion of the anterior mitral leaflet may also be observed, which can increase LVOT obstruction and decrease coronary and systemic outflow.

LV wall thickness, presence of underlying perfusion abnormalities, and fibrosis as evidenced by late gadolinium enhancement are important imaging markers pointing to increased risk for sudden death in HCM patients.

References: Hoey ETD, Teoh JK, Das I, et al. The emerging role of cardiovascular MRI for risk stratification in hypertrophic cardiomyopathy. *Clin Radiol* 2014;69(3):221–230.

Maron BJ. Hypertrophic cardiomyopathy: a systematic review. *JAMA* 2002;287(10):1308–1320.

4 **Answer D.** Three-chamber view bright blood images of the heart during diastole and systole show turbulent flow across the left ventricular outflow tract due to systolic anterior motion of the anterior mitral valve leaflet consistent with hypertrophic cardiomyopathy. The blue dots (image below) show the position of the anterior mitral valve leaflet.

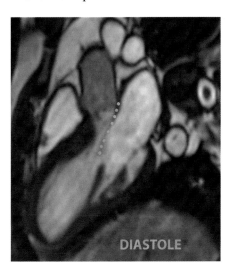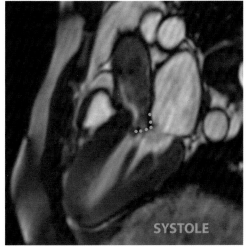

During ventricular systole, the mitral valve should be closed but is pulled forward into the left ventricular outflow tract with resultant turbulent flow as seen by the dephasing of the flow jets. The mechanism is thought to be one or both of the following: venturi effect, decrease in LVOT diameter results in increased velocity and reduced pressure which then pulls the anterior mitral leaflet forward; or, an anatomic abnormality of a more anterior and inward location of the papillary muscles which results in a pushing of the mitral valve toward the septum during early systole.

Systolic anterior motion of the anterior mitral valve leaflet is not commonly associated with any of the other answer choices.

Reference: Walker CM, et al. Systolic anterior motion of the mitral valve. *J Thorac Imaging* 2012;27(4):W87.

5   **Answer D.** Midventricular short-axis SSFP image of the heart demonstrates significantly increased trabeculation of the left ventricular cavity relative to normal compacted myocardium. This appearance is compatible with left ventricular noncompaction (VNC). Note that the papillary muscles are often not well formed in the setting of VNC.

Left ventricular noncompaction, also known as spongiform cardiomyopathy, is a congenital myocardial abnormality that can present in either childhood or adulthood. VNC occurs due to persistence of noncompacted endocardium characteristic of the early fetal period before myocardial compaction is complete. The left ventricle is usually affected, and it may be either dilated or hypertrophied.

Echocardiography or MRI is the diagnostic method of choice for detecting VNC cardiomyopathy and is characterized by prominent trabeculations associated with deep intertrabecular recesses. Diagnostic clues include ≥3 trabeculations in one imaging plane located apically from the insertion of the papillary muscles and a ratio of noncompacted myocardium to compacted myocardium of more than 2.3:1 (sensitivity, 86%; specificity, 99%).

Patients with VNC have high morbidity and mortality as a result of heart failure, ventricular arrhythmias, and systemic embolism. Sudden death by arrhythmia is most often the cause of death. Unfortunately, there is no specific therapy for VNC with the only definitive treatment being cardiac transplant.

References: Petersen SE, Selvanayagam JB, Wiesmann F, et al. Left ventricular noncompaction: insights from cardiovascular magnetic resonance imaging. *J Am Coll Cardiol* 2005;46(1):101–105.

Zenooz NA, Zahka KG, Siwik ES, et al. Noncompaction syndrome of the myocardium: pathophysiology and imaging pearls. *J Thorac Imaging* 2010;25(4):326–332.

6   **Answer C.** Inversion recovery sequence demonstrating nulling of the myocardium and multifocal areas of late gadolinium enhancement in mid- and epicardial distribution. The findings are most compatible with myocarditis. The epicardial distribution is not compatible with infarction. Hypertrophic cardiomyopathy typically has asymmetric thickening and a familial association. Arrhythmogenic right ventricular cardiomyopathy typically demonstrates abnormalities in right ventricular motion and increased right ventricular size.

Myocarditis (inflammatory cardiomyopathy) is inflammation of the heart caused by a variety of pathogens and triggers (e.g., viral, bacterial, fungal infections, drug toxicity, or postradiation). Despite the etiology, the inflammation culminates in leukocytic cell infiltration, nonischemic degeneration, myocyte necrosis, and cardiac dysfunction. Presence of late gadolinium enhancement (LGE) is an indication of irreversible myocardial necrosis and fibrosis.

The "Lake Louise Criteria" is a consensus criteria used to determine the likelihood of myocarditis by cardiac MRI. These were updated in 2018 to now define two main criteria to support the diagnosis which include a T2-based criterion and a T1-based criterion. T2-based criterion identifies myocardial edema and includes an increase in myocardial signal intensity on T2-weighted images and myocardial T2 prolongation on T2 maps. T1-based criterion identifies nonischemic myocardial injury and include an increase in myocardial T1 on T1 maps, an increase in extracellular volume, and nonischemic pattern of late gadolinium enhancement. Supportive criteria include imaging findings of pericarditis and reduced left ventricular systolic function.

References: Ferreira VM, Schulz-Menger J, Holmvang G, et al. Cardiovascular magnetic resonance in nonischemic myocardial inflammation: expert recommendations. *J Am Coll Cardiol* 2018;72(24):3158–3176.

Friedrich MG, Sechtem U, Schulz-Menger J, et al. Cardiovascular magnetic resonance in myocarditis: a JACC white paper. *J Am Coll Cardiol* 2009;53(17):1475–1487.

Yilmaz A, Ferreira V, Klingel K, et al. Role of cardiovascular magnetic resonance imaging (CMR) in the diagnosis of acute and chronic myocarditis. *Heart Fail Rev* 2013;18(6):747–760.

7 **Answer C.** The apical four-chamber images of the heart demonstrate expected thickening of the basal walls (arrows) during systole, but no substantial thickening or contraction of the mid to apical left ventricular septal and lateral walls.

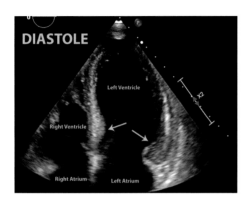 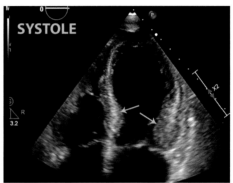

Given the symptoms of chest pain and elevated troponins, the primary concern would be the presence of an obstructive coronary lesion and need for immediate coronary intervention. The absence of coronary disease and the characteristic appearance of apical dilation on the echocardiogram are compatible with stress-induced cardiomyopathy, also called Takotsubo cardiomyopathy.

Takotsubo cardiomyopathy (TTC) is a rapidly reversible form of acute heart failure reported to be triggered by stressful events and associated with a distinctive left ventricular (LV) contraction pattern. TTC mimics acute coronary syndrome in clinical presentation in the absence of angiographically significant coronary artery stenosis.

Variants of TTC include apical, midventricular, basal, or biventricular "ballooning." The most common form is severe apical akinesis and hypercontractility of the basal segments ("apical ballooning"). Typically, cardiac MR does not show any late gadolinium enhancement which helps differentiate Takotsubo cardiomyopathy from anterior myocardial infarction.

Many studies report a good long-term prognosis. However, the acute phase of TTC can be life threatening. Complications, which may occur in the acute setting, include heart failure, arrhythmia, cardiogenic shock, LVOT obstruction, mitral regurgitation, ventricular thrombus, and cardiac rupture.

Treatment of TTC during the acute phase is mainly symptomatic treatment. Patients with TTC usually have a good prognosis and almost complete recovery is seen in 96% of cases.

References: Eitel I, Schuler G, Gutberlet M, et al. Biventricular stress-induced (takotsubo) cardiomyopathy with left midventricular and right apical ballooning. *Int J Cardiol* 2011;151(2):e63–e64.

Virani SS, Khan AN, Mendoza CE, et al. Takotsubo cardiomyopathy, or broken-heart syndrome. *Tex Heart Inst J* 2007;34(1):76–79.

8 **Answer D.** The first image on the left is a three-chamber view from a late gadolinium enhancement sequence which demonstrates patchy mesocardial and epicardial fibrosis throughout the left ventricle. Axial SSFP image on the right shows dark appearance of the liver compatible with iron deposition and signal loss due to susceptibility. Myocardial T2* of 12.9 msec is low and compatible with iron deposition. Taken together, these findings are most compatible with hemochromatosis.

Iron overload cardiomyopathy (IOC) is a secondary form of cardiomyopathy resulting from the accumulation of iron in the myocardium. IOC may result from hereditary disorders of iron metabolism (e.g., cardiomyopathy in hemochromatosis, thalassemia) or may be secondary due to multiple transfusions or abnormalities of hemoglobin synthesis leading to aberrant erythropoiesis.

Two main imaging phenotypes are generally noted—infiltration of the ventricular myocardium resulting in a restrictive cardiomyopathy, common in primary hemochromatosis, and a dilated cardiomyopathy with severe diastolic dysfunction in the early stages of secondary hemochromatosis. Echocardiography may not be able to distinguish IOC from idiopathic dilated cardiomyopathy. Deposition of iron in the myocardium causes a decrease in T2* relaxation time, which can be detected by multiecho gradient sequences on cardiac MRI. T2* values associated with IOC are typically <20 msec. The iron load is considered severe if the value is <10 msec. Varying amounts of delayed enhancement may also be observed depending on the severity of fibrosis.

References: Anderson L. Cardiovascular T2-star (T2*) magnetic resonance for the early diagnosis of myocardial iron overload. *Eur Heart J* 2001;22(23):2171–2179.

Kremastinos DT, Farmakis D. Iron overload cardiomyopathy in clinical practice. *Circulation* 2011;124(20):2253–2263.

9 **Answer B.** The four-chamber bright blood image of the heart shows severe basal septal hypertrophy (BSH). Although commonly seen in the setting of hypertrophic cardiomyopathy, BSH can also be seen with severe aortic stenosis. Based on autopsy series and echocardiographic data, about 10% of patients with hemodynamically significant AS show asymmetric thickening of the septum. Recent studies have demonstrated that hypertrophic heart disease from valvular aortic stenosis implicates a poor prognosis early and late after aortic valve replacement.

Noncompaction cardiomyopathy is characterized by prominent endocardial trabeculations in the left ventricle. Uhl anomaly is a rare cardiac disorder in which there is partial or complete absence of the right ventricular myocardium. Annuloaortic ectasia refers to enlargement of the aortic root and proximal ascending aorta. This is associated with connective tissue disorders such as Marfan syndrome and Ehlers-Danlos syndrome.

References: Di Tommaso L, Stassano P, Mannacio V, et al. Asymmetric septal hypertrophy in patients with severe aortic stenosis: the usefulness of associated septal myectomy. *J Thorac Cardiovasc Surg* 2013;145(1):171–175.

Diaz T, Pencina MJ, Benjamin EJ, et al. Prevalence, clinical correlates, and prognosis of discrete upper septal thickening on echocardiography: the Framingham Heart Study. *Echocardiography* 2009;26(3):247–253.

Kelshiker MA, Mayet J, Unsworth B, et al. Basal septal hypertrophy. *Curr Cardiol Rev* 2013;9(4):316–324.

10 **Answer B.** Horizontal long axis image of the heart demonstrates marked left ventricular thickening with mild asymmetric thickening of the septum, consistent with hypertrophic cardiomyopathy (HCM). Patchy late gadolinium enhancement is also observed near the left ventricular (LV) apex, compatible with areas of myocardial fibrosis.

HCM is a clinically and genetically heterogeneous disorder, characterized most commonly by left ventricular hypertrophy. HCM has a range of potential outcomes including heart failure and sudden cardiac death, but also survival to normal life expectancy.

The estimated prevalence of HCM of 1 in 500 is based on data originally collected almost 20 years ago. However, advances in HCM, including enhanced understanding of the underlying molecular and genetic substrate, contemporary family screening, and more sensitive diagnostic cardiac imaging, suggest that the prevalence of HCM may be underestimated. Although many patients remain asymptomatic with a benign natural history, sudden death (SD) can occur as the initial manifestation of the disease in otherwise asymptomatic or mildly symptomatic young (<25 years of age) patients.

Conventional risk factors for SD in HCM include family history HCM-related sudden death; one of more episodes of unexplained recent syncope; LV hypertrophy >30 mm; nonsustained ventricular tachycardia on 24-hour electrocardiography; and hypotensive blood pressure response to exercise. Cardiac magnetic resonance (CMR) imaging has emerged as a precise diagnostic tool and powerful adjunct in assessing risk of SD with HCM. CMR provides characterization of morphologic phenotypes of LV wall thickening, often not reliably visualized with standard echocardiographic cross-sectional planes. The presence of late gadolinium enhancement (LGE) in HCM patients has been shown to have a sevenfold increased risk for potential lethal ventricular tachyarrhythmias compared with those without LGE. Although large prospective studies validating its utility are still emerging, many experts consider the presence of LGE as influential in the decision of placing an ICD in HCM patients currently classified as intermediate risk.

References: Efthimiadis GK, Pagourelias ED, Gossios T, et al. Hypertrophic cardiomyopathy in 2013: current speculations and future perspectives. *World J Cardiol* 2014;6(2):26–37.

Hoey ETD, Teoh JK, Das I, et al. The emerging role of cardiovascular MRI for risk stratification in hypertrophic cardiomyopathy. *Clin Radiol* 2014;69(3):221–230.

Semsarian C, Ingles J, Maron MS, et al. New perspectives on the prevalence of hypertrophic cardiomyopathy. *J Am Coll Cardiol* 2015;65(12):1249–1254.

11 **Answer A.** Horizontal long axis image of the heart demonstrates subendocardial late gadolinium enhancement involving both ventricles. The remaining myocardium nulls appropriately. Although infarction is classically subendocardial, the distribution of the abnormality does not follow a vascular distribution. The unremarkable nulling of the remaining myocardium is atypical in amyloid. Cardiac sarcoidosis is usually mid- to epicardial in its involvement.

Eosinophil-mediated myocarditis can occur in association with parasitic infection (tropical endomyocardial fibrosis) or Churg-Strauss syndrome (a necrotizing small vessel vasculitis) or can occur as an idiopathic entity (termed Loeffler endocarditis or hypereosinophilic syndrome). Classically, three clinicohistologic stages have been described:

1. Acute necrotic stage—characterized by subendocardial necrosis as well as constitutional symptoms, pulmonary infiltrates, atrioventricular valve regurgitation, and biventricular failure

2. Subacute thrombotic stage—characterized by thrombosis, splinter hemorrhages, and more severely resulting in cerebral, splenic, renal, and coronary infarctions

3. Late fibrotic stage—characterized by late-stage fibrosis of the endomyocardial surface of either or both left and right ventricles

Cardiac MR is instrumental in identifying markers of eosinophilic involvement including myocardial inflammation, mural thrombi, and endocardial fibrosis. The use of first-pass perfusion MRI allows differentiation of perfused and enhancing myocardium from poorly vascularized and hypoenhancing thrombus or eosinophilic infiltrate. Late gadolinium enhancement images typically show intense global subendocardial enhancement that is not limited to a vascular territory. Nonenhancing thrombi may also be observed in left and right ventricular apices.

Endomyocardial fibrosis and especially cardiac thromboembolic events originating from mural thrombus may cause potentially fatal complications or irreversible neurologic defects if not appropriately treated without delay. Follow-up MRI can help document therapeutic improvement with reduction of left ventricular mass and improved contractile function along with simultaneous improvement of clinical symptoms.

References: Kleinfeldt T, Ince H, Nienaber CA. Hypereosinophilic syndrome: a rare case of Loeffler's endocarditis documented in cardiac MRI. *Int J Cardiol* 2011;149(1):e30–e32.

Mannelli L, Cherian V, Nayar A, et al. Loeffler's endocarditis in hypereosinophilic syndrome. *Curr Probl Diagn Radiol* 2012;41(4):146–148.

Perazzolo Marra M, Thiene G, Rizzo S, et al. Cardiac magnetic resonance features of biopsy-proven endomyocardial diseases. *JACC Cardiovasc Imaging* 2014;7(3):309–312.

12 Answer A. The four-chamber bright blood image of the heart from a cardiac MRI (left image) shows normal biatrial size, normal biventricular size, normal LV wall thickness, and normal pericardial thickness. The short axis late gadolinium enhancement image at the base of the LV from a cardiac MRI (right image) demonstrates mesocardial and epicardial fibrosis throughout the lateral, inferior, and septal walls. Note absence of pericardial thickening, pericardial effusion, and pericardial enhancement. This patient has a restrictive cardiomyopathy and was subsequently diagnosed with cardiac sarcoidosis.

Restrictive cardiomyopathy (CMP) refers to a group of primary or secondary infiltrative disorders characterized by normal left ventricular cavity size and systolic function but with increased myocardial stiffness and decreased ventricular compliance. Primary restrictive cardiomyopathies include endomyocardial fibrosis, Loeffler endomyocarditis, and idiopathic primary restrictive CMP. Secondary types of restrictive CMP are more common and are typically due to conditions where the heart is affected as part of a multisystem disorder such as in amyloidosis, sarcoidosis, or hemochromatosis. The morphologic appearance in restrictive CMP can demonstrate atrial enlargement and left ventricular hypertrophy. The presence of myocardial late gadolinium enhancement is a key distinguisher that strongly favors restrictive cardiomyopathy over constrictive pericarditis.

Ischemic cardiomyopathy would be expected to have fibrosis in a coronary artery distribution compatible with prior myocardial infarct. Hypertrophic cardiomyopathy would be expected to have left ventricular hypertrophy and primarily mesocardial fibrosis. Constrictive pericarditis may have a constellation of findings including pericardial effusion, pericardial thickening, pericardial enhancement, ventricular interdependence, and myocardial–pericardial adhesions.

References: Belloni E, De Cobelli F, Esposito A, et al. MRI of cardiomyopathy. *Am J Roentgenol* 2008;191(6):1702–1710.

Gupta A, Singh Gulati G, Seth S, et al. Cardiac MRI in restrictive cardiomyopathy. *Clin Radiol* 2012;67(2):95–105.

Hughes S. Cardiomyopathies. In: Suvarna SK (ed.). *Cardiac pathology*. London: Springer, 2013:183–200.

13 **Answer A.** Short-axis inversion recovery sequence after contrast demonstrates linear late gadolinium enhancement in the midwall of the interventricular septum.

A linear midwall septal stripe of late gadolinium enhancement has been described in approximately 30% of patients with nonischemic dilated cardiomyopathies. The location of the stripe does not follow a pattern consistent with ischemic disease. The abnormality is thought to develop secondary to replacement fibrosis, which has been reported in pathologic samples and may be related to subclinical foci of myocardial ischemia. This linear abnormality has been suggested as a marker for increased risk of sudden cardiac death, since the fibrosis may predispose to electrical instability.

Reference: Cummings KW, Bhalla S, Javidan-Nejad C, et al. A pattern-based approach to assessment of delayed enhancement in nonischemic cardiomyopathy at MR imaging. *Radiographics* 2009;29(1):89–103.

14 **Answer A.** Short-axis image of the left ventricle demonstrates diffusely abnormal nulling of the myocardium on inversion recovery sequences. Classically, with the blood pool containing the largest concentration of gadolinium, the inversion time of the blood pool occurs before nulling of the myocardium. In this case, subendocardial myocardium has traversed its null point before the blood pool, and the remaining myocardium reaches its null point near the same time as the blood pool. This gross aberration of late gadolinium enhancement is almost exclusively seen in the setting of amyloid deposition.

Cardiac amyloidosis is the most common infiltrative type of secondary restrictive cardiomyopathies and is caused by the deposition of insoluble amyloid protein fibrils in the interstitium of the myocardium. Cardiac amyloidosis may be classified according to the type of amyloid fibril protein deposited. The most common type of amyloidosis to affect the heart is AL amyloidosis due to the deposition of amyloid fibrils complexed with monoclonal kappa and lambda immunoglobulin light chains. AL amyloidosis is principally associated with plasma cell dyscrasias (e.g., B-cell lymphoma, Waldenstrom macroglobulinemia, multiple myeloma). Mutations in the gene for transthyretin predominantly result in neurologic and heart disease, and with some mutations, amyloid deposits are exclusive to the myocardium. Fragments of serum amyloid A protein are responsible for AA (secondary) amyloidosis, which is associated with a variety of chronic inflammatory disorders, but rarely associated with cardiac involvement.

No single noninvasive test or abnormality is pathognomonic of cardiac amyloid; diagnosis of cardiac amyloid has usually relied on (1) echocardiographic assessment, especially measurement of LV wall thickness, subjective assessment of myocardial appearance, and evaluation of diastolic function/restrictive physiology, and (2) histopathologic findings of amyloid deposition on endomyocardial biopsy.

The high spatial resolution and signal-to-noise ratio of cardiac MR permit reproducible measurement of cardiac chamber volumes and mass, as well as LV and atrial septal wall thickness. The main feature of cardiac amyloidosis is diffuse myocardial thickening including the atria and valves. Biatrial dilation and restriction of diastolic filling may also be seen associated with depressed systolic ventricular function and reduced wall compliance, which in later stages can evolve to overt restrictive CMP.

Tissue characterization with LGE provides unique clinical value in further assessment of amyloid infiltration. The pattern of late gadolinium enhancement is characterized by a diffuse, heterogeneous subendocardial distribution that may resemble an incorrect myocardial signal suppression due to an inappropriate choice of inversion time.

References: Maceira AM. Cardiovascular magnetic resonance in cardiac amyloidosis. *Circulation* 2005;111(2):186–193.

Selvanayagam JB, Leong DP. MR imaging and cardiac amyloidosis: where to go from here? *JACC Cardiovasc Imaging* 2010;3(2):165–167.

15a **Answer A.** Three-chamber bright blood images of the heart during diastole and systole demonstrate midventricular hypertrophy and a linear band of hypointensity in the mid cavity seen only during systole. This is most compatible with artifact from turbulent flow. The severe mid and apical left ventricular hypertrophy causes severe narrowing versus obliteration of the mid LV cavity at systole. This results in turbulent flow and increased velocities across the mid LV cavity. Calcification and thrombus would persist during diastole. Mitral regurgitation would be seen across the mitral valve with the jet extending into the left atrium.

15b **Answer B.** Three-chamber (left), four-chamber (middle), and two-chamber (right) late gadolinium enhancement images of the heart show mesocardial fibrosis throughout the hypertrophied mid and apical left ventricular wall. In combination with the history and flow acceleration across the mid-LV cavity findings are most compatible with hypertrophic cardiomyopathy. Dilated, iron overload, and stress-induced cardiomyopathy would not be expected to have flow acceleration and systolic cavity narrowing/obliteration. Stress-induced cardiomyopathy rarely shows late gadolinium enhancement and is characterized by apical hypokinesis and ballooning.

References: Amano Y, et al. Cardiac MR imaging of hypertrophic cardiomyopathy: techniques, findings, and clinical relevance. *Magn Reson Med Sci* 2018;17(2):120–131.

Hoey ETD, Teoh JK, Das I, et al. The emerging role of cardiovascular MRI for risk stratification in hypertrophic cardiomyopathy. *Clin Radiol* 2014;69(3):221–230.

16 **Answer B.** Short-axis T2 dark blood (left), T2 map (middle), and late gadolinium enhancement images (right) through the mid left ventricle are shown. The T2 dark blood image demonstrates increased signal intensity through the lateral wall, inferior wall, anterior wall, and portions of the anteroseptal wall compatible with edema. The T2 map confirms this finding by demonstrating corresponding areas of T2 prolongation compatible with myocardial edema. The parametric T2 map is a technique used to quantify T2-values throughout the myocardium allowing for evaluation of focal and diffuse disease. T2 maps may also be advantageous to T2 dark blood images which may suffer from susceptibility artifact, slow flow artifact, and incomplete spectral fat saturation. Normal values can be variable and are dependent on MR field strength and acquisition technique. In the images shown there is clearly T2 prolongation in the lateral wall (65 msec) compared to the septum (39 msec). The late gadolinium enhancement images demonstrated epicardial fibrosis throughout nearly the entire LV with some sparing of the septum. This patient meets the Lake Louise consensus criteria for acute myocarditis by demonstrating a T1-based criterion (fibrosis) and a T2-based criterion (myocardial edema, T2 prolongation). Please see the answer to Question 6 for more discussion of this criteria.

Myocarditis (inflammatory cardiomyopathy) is defined as an inflammatory disorder of the myocardium, characterized by leukocytic cell infiltration, nonischemic degeneration, myocyte necrosis, and cardiac dysfunction. Clinical presentation is variable in severity, ranging from asymptomatic to cardiogenic shock. Myocarditis is typically associated with other viral symptoms 7 to 10 days after the onset of the systemic illness. Young adults are most commonly affected. The mean age of patients with giant-cell myocarditis is 42 years, whereas the mean age of adult patients with other forms of myocarditis has been reported to range from 20 to 51 years. Most patients respond well to standard heart failure therapy. However, in severe cases, mechanical circulatory support or heart transplantation may be indicated. More than 75% of patients with acute myocarditis gain spontaneous recovery, except in patients with giant-cell myocarditis.

Myocardial infarction would have a pattern of fibrosis that follows a coronary artery distribution. Hypertrophic cardiomyopathy typically has left ventricular hypertrophy and mesocardial fibrosis. Constrictive pericarditis typically has a constellation of findings including pericardial thickening, pericardial effusion, pericardial enhancement, ventricular interdependence, and myocardial–pericardial adhesions.

References: Cooper LT Jr. Myocarditis. *N Engl J Med* 2009;360(15):1526–1538.

Maisch B, Pankuweit S. Current treatment options in (peri)myocarditis and inflammatory cardiomyopathy. *Herz* 2012;37(6):644–656.

17a **Answer C.** SSFP, horizontal long-axis image demonstrates biventricular dilation and notable trabeculation involving both chambers, consistent with ventricular noncompaction. Also noted is the absence of well-formed papillary muscles.

Ventricular noncompaction (VNC), also known as spongiform cardiomyopathy, is a congenital myocardial abnormality that can present in either childhood or adulthood. VNC occurs due to persistence of noncompacted endocardium characteristic of the early fetal period before myocardial compaction is complete.

Echocardiography is usually the first modality obtained for the assessment of VNC cardiomyopathy and characteristically demonstrates prominent trabeculations associated with deep intertrabecular recesses. Noncompacted segments are usually hypokinetic, and global ventricular function is commonly decreased. RV involvement has been described but rarely in isolation.

With the advent of ECG gating, computed tomography has expanded its role in identification of the disorder. It has better spatial resolution, allows for better visualization of trabeculations than echo, and is not limited by acoustic windows. Cardiac MR is the most robust modality with the capability of multiplanar imaging of the heart, evaluation of ventricular function, and tissue characterization of the myocardium.

References: Petersen SE, Selvanayagam JB, Wiesmann F, et al. Left ventricular non-compaction: insights from cardiovascular magnetic resonance imaging. *J Am Coll Cardiol* 2005;46(1):101–105.

Zenooz NA, Zahka KG, Siwik ES, et al. Noncompaction syndrome of the myocardium: pathophysiology and imaging pearls. *J Thorac Imaging* 2010;25(4):326–332.

17b **Answer A.** The triad of heart failure symptoms, conduction abnormalities, and embolic events is the major clinical manifestation in patients with left ventricular noncompaction (VNC). A substantial percentage of these patients have a dilated left ventricle with systolic dysfunction, mimicking dilated cardiomyopathy. Criteria suggesting the diagnosis of VNC include ≥3 trabeculations in one imaging plane and a ratio of noncompacted myocardium to compacted myocardium of more than 2.3:1.

In adults, various forms of congenital heart disease are associated with left VNC, particularly stenotic lesions of the left ventricular outflow tract, Ebstein's anomaly, and tetralogy of Fallot. VNC is rarely associated with muscular dystrophies, unclassified myopathies, or neuropathies. One particular association, Barth syndrome, is an X-linked recessive disorder that is typically characterized by cardiomyopathy, skeletal myopathy, growth retardation, and neutropenia.

There is no specific therapy for VNC. Because of a high incidence of thromboembolic events, all patients should receive systemic anticoagulation. Heart failure is treated with conventional therapies. Since the main causes of death are arrhythmias, antiarrhythmic medications should be considered for all VNC patients, whether symptomatic or not. Also, in some patients, implantation of a defibrillator may be necessary.

References: Jefferies JL, Towbin JA. Dilated cardiomyopathy. *Lancet* 2010;375(9716):752–762.

Stähli BE, Gebhard C, Biaggi P, et al. Left ventricular non-compaction: prevalence in congenital heart disease. *Int J Cardiol* 2013;167(6):2477–2481.

Udeoji DU, Philip KJ, Morrissey RP, et al. Left ventricular noncompaction cardiomyopathy: updated review. *Ther Adv Cardiovasc Dis* 2013;7(5):260–273.

Zenooz NA, Zahka KG, Siwik ES, et al. Noncompaction syndrome of the myocardium: pathophysiology and imaging pearls. *J Thorac Imaging* 2010;25(4):326–332.

18   **Answer A.** This patient has cardiac amyloidosis. There are two types of cardiac amyloidosis: AL type (acquired) and transthyretin-related (TTR). TTR has two subtypes: hereditary (ATTR) and nonhereditary (senile systemic amyloidosis, SSA). The images shown demonstrate almost diffuse uptake of radiotracer throughout the left ventricle compatible with amyloidosis. Normally, there should not be any myocardial uptake on this examination. PET and SPECT imaging can be used to image cardiac amyloid. Cardiac amyloid-specific PET radiotracers are generally under investigation, not well validated, or not available in the United States. SPECT bone imaging radiotracers (99m-Technetium DPD and PYP) have a high specificity for ATTR amyloidosis but show little to no uptake in AL amyloidosis.

Difficulty nulling the myocardium is a finding seen in cardiac amyloidosis on cardiac MRI. This is due to altered contrast kinetics related to rapid washout of contrast from the blood pool into the increased extracellular space. Normally, blood nulls before myocardium since the gadolinium in the blood pool results in T1 shortening. With altered contrast kinetics, the myocardium nulls before the blood pool. Other cardiac MRI findings of amyloid include late gadolinium enhancement of the atrial walls, left ventricular hypertrophy, biatrial enlargement, pleural effusions, increased T1 values when using T1 parametric mapping, and increased extracellular volume (calculated with hematocrit level, precontrast T1 mapping, and postcontrast T1 mapping).

Right ventricular outflow tract aneurysm would be associated with arrhythmogenic right ventricular dysplasia. Pericardial thickening and enhancement could be seen with acute or constrictive pericarditis. Systolic anterior motion of the anterior mitral valve leaflet would be seen with left ventricular outflow tract obstruction in a patient with hypertrophic cardiomyopathy.

Reference: Falk RH, et al. How to image cardiac amyloidosis: a focused practical review. *Circ Cardiovasc Imaging* 2014;7(3):552–562.

19 **Answer D.** The arrows in the two-view chest x-ray identify pericardial calcifications. This finding would support a clinical diagnosis of constrictive pericarditis. Ventricular interdependence can be seen with constrictive pericarditis. Since the pericardium is scarred or calcified, it is no longer compliant and does not allow the ventricles to fully increase in size when blood is flowing in from the atria during diastole. During early diastole at inspiration, there is an inflow of blood into the right ventricle resulting in flattening or bulging of the interventricular septum toward the left ventricle. This is also called the septal bounce sign. Difficulty nulling the myocardium is seen with cardiac amyloid. Turbulent flow across the mid LV cavity is seen with the mid-ventricular form of hypertrophic cardiomyopathy. A noncompacted to compacted LV myocardium ratio of >2.3 at end-diastole supports a diagnosis of noncompaction cardiomyopathy.

Reference: Bogaert J, Francone M. Pericardial disease: value of CT and MR imaging. *Radiology* 2013;267(2):340–356.

20a **Answer C.** The abnormality in the apical septal wall is centrally hyperintense with a hypointense rim on bright blood images and demonstrates some signal drop out from in phase to out of phase images. Signal characteristics are most compatible with intramyocardial fat. Microvascular obstruction typically occurs within a myocardial infarct in the acute setting. This would not be expected to have intravoxel fat. Edema and hemorrhage also would not be expected to have intravoxel fat.

20b **Answer D.** The arrows in the short axis phase reconstruction late gadolinium enhancement image through the mid left ventricle highlight mesocardial fibrosis in the mid inferolateral wall. In conjunction with the history and intramyocardial fat seen in the apical septal wall, this patient most likely has myotonic dystrophy. Myotonic dystrophy is an autosomal dominant disorder characterized by progressive muscle loss and weakness. Histologically, fibrosis and fat deposition can be seen in the skeletal muscles. Myotonic dystrophy type 2 usually has an onset of symptoms in the 20s and 30s. Reported cardiac MR abnormalities include mesocardial fibrosis of the basal to mid inferolateral wall, intramyocardial fat deposition, prolonged native T1 values, and increased extracellular volumes in patients with fibrosis.

Ischemic cardiomyopathy is unlikely given the patient's relatively young age and lack of subendocardial fibrosis in a coronary artery distribution to indicate myocardial infarct. While old myocardial infarcts can develop areas of fibrofatty infiltration, these are usually subendocardial to transmural in a coronary artery distribution rather than intramyocardial.

Findings of endomyocardial fibrosis include diffuse subendocardial fibrosis, LV apical thrombi, and atrial enlargement. In the acute phase, these patients present with a febrile illness. In the chronic phase, these patients present with symptoms of restrictive physiology including ascites and hepatosplenomegaly. In acute myocarditis, patients typically present with atypical chest pain, diffuse ST elevations on EKG, troponin elevation, and recent history of upper respiratory tract infection. On MR, they may have patchy mesocardial and epicardial areas of fibrosis. In the acute phase, myocardial edema may also be seen.

References: Schmacht L, et al. Cardiac involvement in myotonic dystrophy type 2 patients with preserved ejection fraction: detection by cardiovascular magnetic resonance. *Circ Cardiovasc Imaging* 2016;9:e004615.

Turkbey EB, et al. Assessment of cardiac involvement in myotonic muscular dystrophy by T1 mapping on magnetic resonance imaging. *Heart Rhythm* 2012;9(10):1691–1697.

21a **Answer B.** T2-weighted dark blood (left) and phase reconstruction from late gadolinium enhancement (right) short-axis images through the left ventricle demonstrate near circumferential pericardial thickening, pericardial enhancement, and a small pericardial effusion. Based on the history, the patient most likely has constrictive pericarditis and would also be expected to have ventricular interdependence. Since the pericardium is scarred or calcified, it is no longer compliant and does not allow the ventricles to fully increase in size when blood is flowing in from the atria during diastole. During early diastole at inspiration, there is an inflow of blood into the right ventricle resulting in flattening or bulging of the interventricular septum toward the left ventricle. This is called ventricular interdependence (also septal bounce sign).

Descending thoracic aortic diastolic flow reversal is seen in severe aortic regurgitation. Microvascular obstruction is a poor prognostic sign seen in acute myocardial infarcts. First pass subendocardial hypoperfusion (during stress such as from adenosine, regadenoson, or dobutamine) would be indicative of ischemia if no corresponding late gadolinium enhancement or infarct if with corresponding late gadolinium enhancement.

21b **Answer D.** The images shown are from a sequence called spatial modulation of magnetization (SPAMM), or myocardial "tagging." Tagging is a robust, noninvasive technique that provides evaluation of myocardial contractility, strain, and torsion. Saturation bands, or tags, are created by perturbations of the magnetization field perpendicular to the imaging plane. This can be done with a grid or lines. The resulting tags follow myocardial motion during the cardiac cycle, thus reflecting the underlying myocardial deformation.

The myocardial tagging images shown suggest myocardial–pericardial adhesions along the lateral wall of the left ventricle. When going from systole to diastole, the tags (grid lines in this case) deform and lose signal intensity with LV contraction and pericardial motion. There are three grid lines that do not deform or break from early systole to end diastole (dotted lines). The grid line running perpendicular to the dotted lines is roughly at the demarcation point between the left ventricle and pericardium. Also note the almost complete disappearance of the grid lines in the stomach (asterisk) due to motion of the air and food products in this area. Extensive myocardial–pericardial adhesions were confirmed during surgical pericardial stripping.

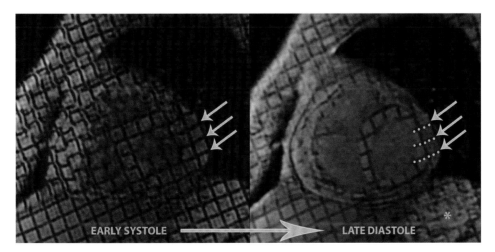

Reference: Shehata ML, Cheng S, Osman NF, et al. Myocardial tissue tagging with cardiovascular magnetic resonance. *J Cardiovasc Magn Reson* 2009;11(1):55.

22 **Answer D.** Both restrictive and constrictive diseases exhibit an abrupt reduction in filling, increased backpressure, and impaired stroke volume. Restrictive cardiomyopathy is characterized by normal left ventricular cavity size and systolic function but with decreased diastolic volume and ventricular compliance. Imaging often reveals thickening of the ventricles with biatrial enlargement secondary to a differential of intracardiac chamber pressures.

Constrictive pericarditis is characterized by fibrous or calcific thickening of the pericardium, which leads to discordance in normal diastolic filling of the heart—reduced left ventricular filling, which corresponds to increased right ventricular filling. This manifests as a variance in the septal curvature during diastolic filling and characteristic "septal bounce." Intracardiac pressures are typically equal throughout the cardiac chambers.

While constrictive pericarditis is an extracardiac constraint, restrictive cardiomyopathy is an intrinsic myocardial disease of the ventricle. Respiratory variation of ventricular filling and ejection velocities may be modestly present in constriction but is absent in restrictive right ventricular disease.

It is important to distinguish between constrictive pericarditis and restrictive cardiomyopathy because treatment for the former condition is surgical and treatment for the latter is medical.

References: Henein MY, Sheppard M. Restrictive cardiomyopathy. In: Henein MY (ed.). *Clinical echocardiography*. London, UK: Springer, 2012:203–212.

Henein MY, Sheppard M. Pericardial disease. In: Henein MY (ed.). *Clinical echocardiography*. London, UK: Springer, 2012:251–266.

23 **Answer A.** Iron overload cardiomyopathy can occur either as a result of inappropriate excess iron absorption, as in the case of hemochromatosis or thalassemia major, or due to multiple transfusions. Myocardial iron content cannot be predicted from serum ferritin or liver iron, and conventional assessments of cardiac function can only detect those with advanced disease.

The measurement of T2* relaxation by cardiac MR is the most widely used technique for the direct assessment of myocardial iron because it is fast and robust, is reproducible, and is sensitive to iron deposition. T2* relaxation is the combined effect of T2 relaxation and the effect of magnetic field nonuniformities. Excess iron in the tissues induces a significant loss of signal due to changes in magnetic susceptibility, causing a shortening of T2* values. As iron accumulates in the normal storage form in the heart, the T2* falls, but there is minimal effect on cardiac function until a threshold is reached where the iron storage capacity is exhausted. Once this critical level is reached, rapid deterioration of cardiac function occurs. Thus, cardiac T2* is a powerful predictor of the subsequent development of heart failure. Iron clears more slowly from the heart than the liver, which may contribute to the high mortality of patients with established cardiomyopathy despite intensive chelation.

LGE is widely used to detect macroscopic fibrosis in a range of nonischemic cardiomyopathies, and the presence of LGE is associated with the development of cardiac events, including heart failure. LGE, however, is not specific for iron deposition. Additionally, macroscopic fibrosis, which is commonly identified in other pathologies, is less common in iron overload cardiomyopathies, particularly at early stages. Newer developing techniques such as T1 mapping may play a more critical role in the evaluation of early microscopic changes in the future.

References: Kirk P, Carpenter JP, Tanner MA, et al. Low prevalence of fibrosis in thalassemia major assessed by late gadolinium enhancement cardiovascular magnetic resonance. *J Cardiovas Magn Reson* 2011;13(1):8.

Kirk P, Roughton M, Porter JB, et al. Cardiac T2* magnetic resonance for prediction of cardiac complications in thalassemia major. *Circulation* 2009;120(20):1961–1968.

24 **Answer A.** Peripartum/postpartum cardiomyopathy (PPCM) is a disorder associated with pregnancy distinguished by ventricular dilation and decreased systolic function, leading to symptoms of heart failure. PPCM is diagnosed when the following three criteria are met:

1. Heart failure develops in the last month of pregnancy or within 5 months of delivery.
2. Reduced systolic function, with an ejection fraction (EF) <45%
3. No other cause for heart failure with reduced EF can be found.

Most patients (80%) present within 3 months of delivery, with the minority presenting in the last month of pregnancy (10%) or 4 to 5 months postpartum (10%). Because there is a significant overlap between symptoms related to pregnancy, especially toward the end of the third trimester or after delivery, and heart failure, the diagnosis may be initially missed or delayed.

Reference: Givertz MM. Peripartum cardiomyopathy. *Circulation* 2013;127(20):e622–e626.

25 **Answer A.** Short-axis bright blood (top left) and late gadolinium enhancement images (top right) demonstrate severe anterior/anteroseptal LV wall hypertrophy and corresponding patchy mesocardial fibrosis. This patient has septal variant hypertrophic cardiomyopathy. Using the lateral wall as an internal reference, in the area of LV hypertrophy and mesocardial fibrosis, the precontrast T1 maps (bottom left) demonstrate relative T1 prolongation, the postcontrast T1 maps (bottom middle) demonstrate greater relative T1 shortening, and the ECV maps (bottom right) demonstrate a relative increase in ECV.

Parametric T1 mapping is an MR technique that allows for the quantification of the intrinsic T1 values of individual pixels. This can be used for the evaluation of focal and diffuse myocardial disease. After contrast administration T1 values are expected to decrease as gadolinium spreads into the intravascular and interstitial space. More gadolinium leads to shorter T1 times. The ECV reflects the amount of volume not taken up by the cells. For example, after an infarct, there is myocardial necrosis which leads to less volume taken up by myocytes and hence an increase in ECV. ECV can be calculated by using precontrast T1 maps, postcontrast T1 maps, and correcting for hemoglobin. In this case, the best explanation for the increase in ECV is interstitial fibrosis in this patient with hypertrophic cardiomyopathy. Hemorrhage, iron overload, and fat deposition would all be expected to have shortened precontrast T1 values, which are not seen in this patient. Note that reference T1 values are highly variable and depend on multiple factors including magnetic field strength.

Reference: Roy C, Slimani A, de Meester C, et al. Age and sex corrected normal reference values of T1, T2, T2* and ECV in healthy subjects at 3T CMR. *J Cardiovasc Magn Reson* 2017;19:72.

26a **Answer C.** Axial fused FDG-PET CT at the level of the heart (left) and a maximum intensity projection from a whole-body FDG-PET (right) demonstrate focal uptake in the mid to apical lateral wall of the left ventricle (arrows).

Although not histologically validated, one proposed method of interpretation of FDG-PET CT for cardiac sarcoidosis is using the descriptors of no uptake, diffuse uptake, focal uptake, and focal on diffuse uptake. Other proposed methods use both the resting perfusion and FDG-PET images to attempt to describe the stage of disease. The spectrum of findings ranges from normal perfusion and no FDG uptake (normal), mild to severe perfusion abnormality and FDG uptake (active), to severe perfusion abnormality and no or low FDG uptake (fibrosis).

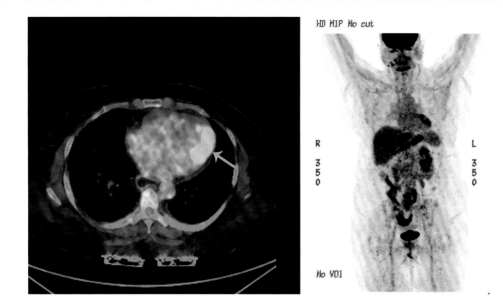

26b **Answer A.** A clinical and histologic diagnosis of cardiac sarcoidosis can be made using the Japanese Ministry Guidelines for the diagnosis of cardiac sarcoidosis. A histologic diagnosis can be made when myocardial biopsy demonstrates noncaseating granulomas. A clinical diagnosis can be made when there is a confirmed diagnosis of extracardiac sarcoidosis in conjunction with 2+ of 4 major criteria or 1 of 4 major criteria and 2+ of 5 minor criteria. Major criteria include atrioventricular block, basal thinning of the interventricular septum, 67-gallium uptake in the heart, and LV ejection fraction <50%. Minor criteria include abnormal EKG findings, abnormal echocardiography findings, perfusion defect on 201-thallium or 99m-technetium myocardial scintigraphy, myocardial delayed enhancement on cardiac MRI, and myocardial biopsy showing interstitial fibrosis or monocyte infiltration.

26c **Answer C.** FDG-PET uptake assesses active inflammation, which is characterized by increased glucose metabolism, particularly by activated macrophages. PET scanning protocols for cardiac sarcoidosis aim to suppress the physiologic uptake of FDG by the myocardium by switching to free fatty acid metabolism. Suppressing physiologic glucose metabolism of the myocardium increases the specificity for active inflammation in areas of increased FDG uptake. Patterns suggestive of active cardiac sarcoidosis are mainly focal areas of FDG uptake and focal on top of diffuse uptake. FDG-PET CT may be used to guide and monitor steroid dosage and duration since steroid treatment has been shown to decrease the size and intensity of myocardial FDG uptake. Non-viable infarcted myocardium would not be expected to have any FDG uptake regardless of the patient's diet.

Reference: Skali H, Schulman AR, Dorbala S. 18F-FDG PET/CT for the assessment of myocardial sarcoidosis. *Curr Cardiol Reports* 2013;15(4):352.

27 **Answer D.** Amyloidosis causes accumulation of an abnormal interstitial protein and expansion of extracellular space within the myocardium. As a consequence, suppression of myocardial signal using inversion recovery sequences becomes difficult due to the global abnormality of the myocardium. Diffuse subendocardial or transmural enhancement of the myocardium may be observed in a noncoronary distribution.

Reference: Pandey T, Jambhekar K, Shaikh R, et al. Utility of the inversion scout sequence (TI scout) in diagnosing myocardial amyloid infiltration. *Int J Cardiovasc Imaging* 2013;29(1):103–112.

28 Answer A. This bulge along the RV wall has been described as "apicolateral bulge" and is considered a benign variant in the absence of other RV wall motion abnormalities. This would not give any imaging criterion for the diagnosis of ARVD. Note the normal RV size in this patient.

Reference: Rastegar N, Burt JR, Corona-Villalobos CP, et al. Cardiac MR findings and potential diagnostic pitfalls in patients evaluated for arrhythmogenic right ventricular cardiomyopathy. *Radiographics* 2014;34(6):1553–1570.

6 Cardiac Masses

Joe Y. Hsu, MD • Jean Jeudy, MD

QUESTIONS

1 Primary cardiac lymphoma can be characterized by which of the following features?

A. Uncommon in immunocompetent patients
B. Histologically different from thoracic lymphoma
C. May present with large pericardial effusion
D. Most commonly of T-cell origin

2 Patient with breast cancer status post chemotherapy. One year after therapy, echocardiography reveals a decrease of left ventricular ejection fraction from 55% at baseline to a 40% currently. The patient is asymptomatic. Which MR parameter would be most helpful in revealing underlying myocardial injury?

A. End-diastolic volume
B. T1 mapping
C. Phase-contrast imaging
D. SSFP imaging

3 Which MR characteristic would be most helpful in determining thrombus versus mass?

A. Enhancement with gadolinium
B. Low signal on T2-weighted images
C. Intrinsic signal on SSFP sequences
D. Extended TI on delayed enhancement

4 A patient presents with hepatic PEComa with metastases to the liver and heart. Which best describes the type of involvement?

A. Direct extension
B. Hematogenous
C. Lymphatic
D. Transvenous

5 The patient has imaging reports from two different facilities, one describing a cardiac lipoma and the other describing lipomatous hypertrophy of the interatrial septum. The best parameter to discriminate the two would be

A. Attenuation value on computed tomography
B. Saturation of signal on fat-saturation MR techniques
C. Absence of FDG avidity on PET imaging
D. High signal on conventional T1-weighted images

6 Which of the following diagnoses best characterize the imaging findings?

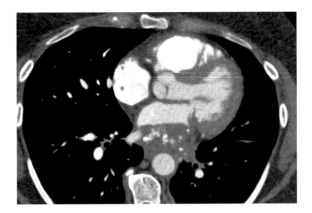

    A. Thrombus
    B. Myxoma
    C. LA osteosarcoma
    D. Lymphoma

7 After an abnormality is observed on preoperative echo, follow up ECG gated CT was performed. Which of the following is the best diagnosis?

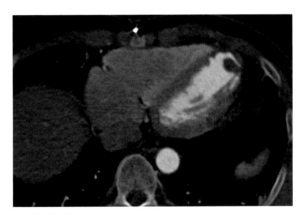

    A. Thrombus
    B. Myxoma
    C. Papillary fibroelastoma
    D. Intracardiac metastases

8 You have an infant who has been diagnosed with multiple cardiac rhabdomyomas. What else should you look for?
    A. Renal cysts
    B. Renal angiomyolipomas
    C. Hepatic adenomas
    D. Atrial myxomas

9   A 25-year-old patient with increasing shortness of breath is found to have
    a large cardiac mass diagnosed by transthoracic echocardiography. A
    multimodality workup confirms the extent of the mass, and eventual biopsy
    reveals a primary pericardial mesothelioma (PPM). Which of the following
    statements best characterizes the disorder?

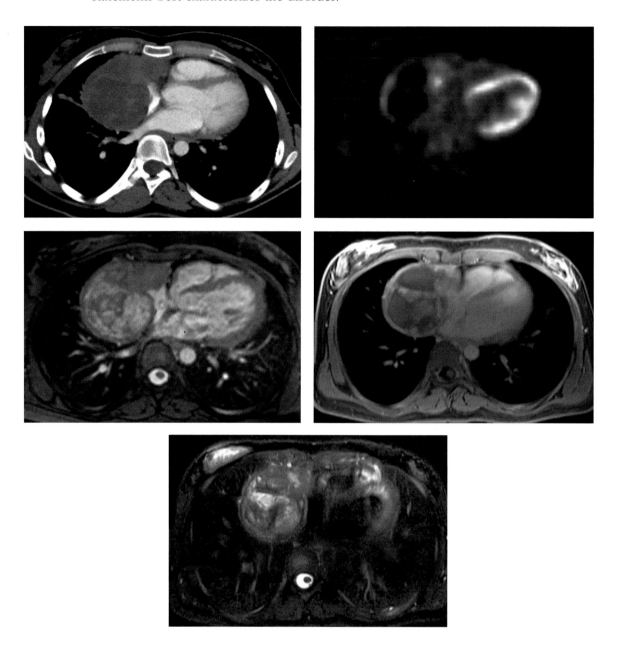

A. Strong association with calcified pleural plaques
B. Benign course with good prognosis despite aggressive features
C. Constrictive pericarditis is a common clinical presentation.
D. PPM is histologically distinct from pleural mesothelioma.

10 Which of the following diagnoses best characterize the imaging findings?

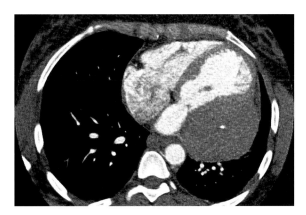

A. Fibroma
B. Myxoma
C. Angiosarcoma
D. Papillary fibroelastoma

11 Which of the following diagnoses best correlate with the imaging findings?

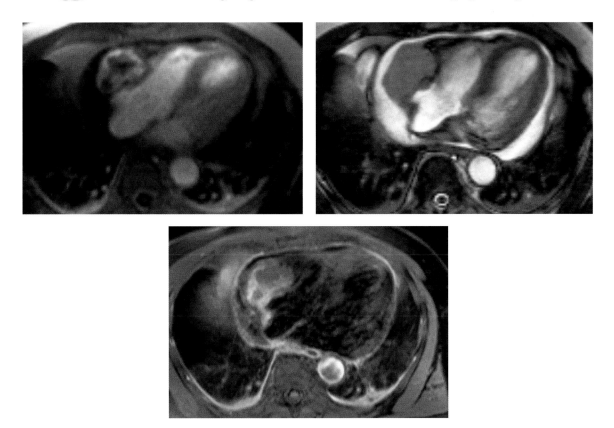

A. Lymphoma
B. Thrombus
C. Angiosarcoma
D. Rhabdomyoma

12a The abnormality is in

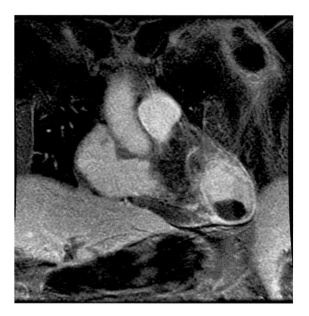

    A. The left atrium
    B. The left ventricle
    C. The right atrium
    D. The right ventricular outflow tract (RVOT)
    E. The aorta

12b What is the best treatment for this lesion?
    A. Surgical resection
    B. Chemotherapy
    C. No treatment
    D. Anticoagulation

12c What is the most common type of mass seen in the heart?
    A. Myxoma
    B. Angiosarcoma
    C. Thrombus
    D. Rhabdomyoma
    E. Melanoma

13 Metastatic tumors to the heart most often involve
    A. Myocardium
    B. Pericardium
    C. Endocardium

14a Where is the abnormality?

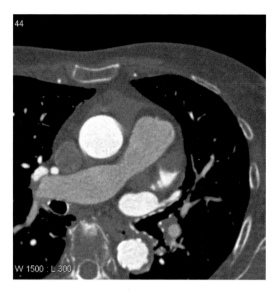

    A. Aorta
    B. Pulmonary artery
    C. Pulmonary vein
    D. Left atrium
    E. Left atrial appendage

14b This image was obtained immediately after the first image. What happened to the abnormality?

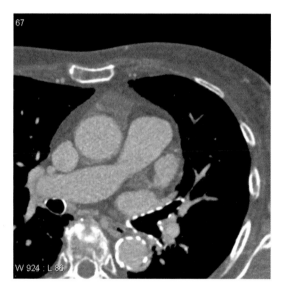

    A. It is still there.
    B. There is no abnormality.
    C. The abnormality embolized.

14c What modality is most often used to evaluate for left atrial appendage thrombus?

    A. CTA
    B. MRI
    C. Transesophageal echocardiogram
    D. Transthoracic echocardiogram

15 This mass is most likely due to

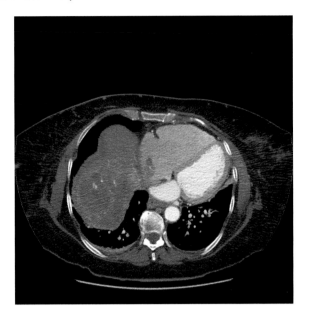

A. Thrombus
B. Metastasis
C. Myxoma
D. Infection
E. Lymphoma

16 An 18-year-old male presents with chest pain and history of febrile illness. No other cardiac history documented, but chart notes history of similar chest pain, fever, and rash at age 4. What is the next step?

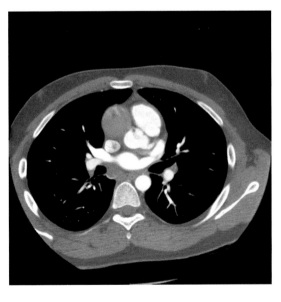 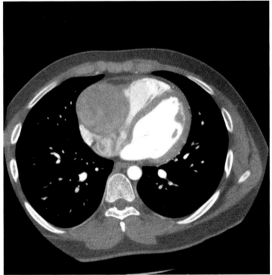

A. Catheter angiography
B. CT-guided biopsy
C. Chemotherapy
D. Cardiac MRI

17a A 50-year-old male presents with a history of chest pain. Where is the abnormality?

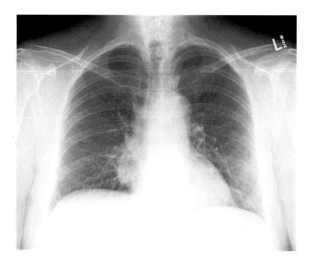

    A. No abnormality
    B. Right lower lobe
    C. Ascending aorta
    D. Right heart border
    E. Left atrium

17b What is the treatment for this lesion?

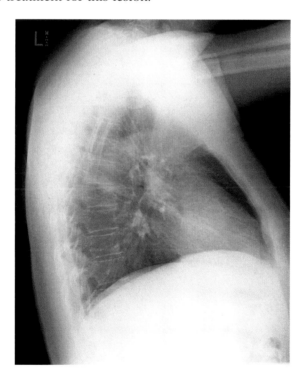

    A. No treatment
    B. Surgical resection
    C. Serial MRI
    D. Chemotherapy

18 What is the treatment for this patient?

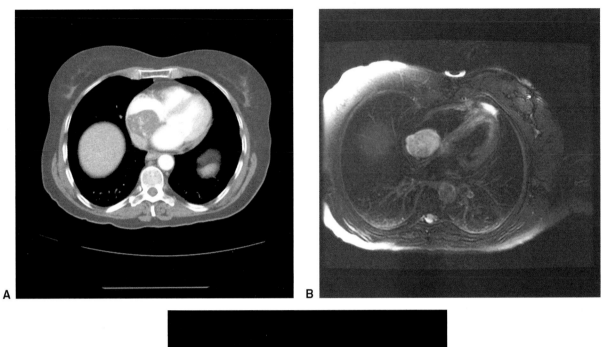

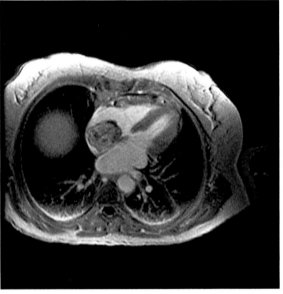

A. Anticoagulation
B. Chemotherapy
C. Surgery
D. Endovascular thrombolysis

19 What feature most suggests a benign lesion?

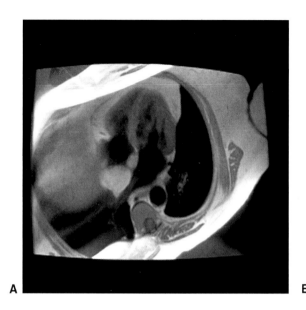

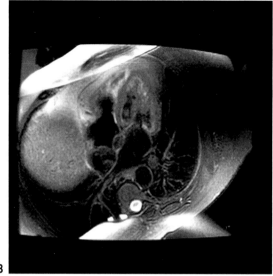

A   B

    A. Right atrial location
    B. Sparing of fossa ovalis
    C. Fluid suppression
    D. Lack of enhancement

20a What is the treatment for this lesion?

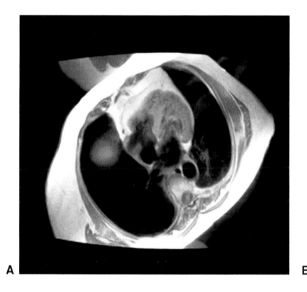

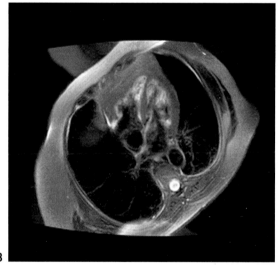

A   B

    A. Surgery
    B. Anticoagulation
    C. Chemotherapy
    D. No treatment is necessary.

20b What is an advantage of inversion recovery fat suppression over chemical fat suppression?

A. It is specific for fat.
B. It does not suppress contrast enhancement.
C. It does not require high field strength.
D. It is inherently high in signal.

21a Which chamber of the heart is abnormal based on this radiograph in a 3-year-old boy?

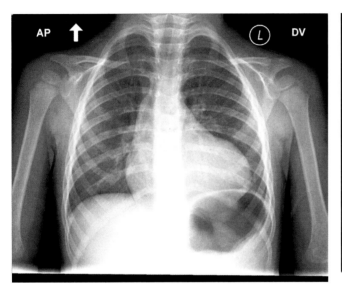 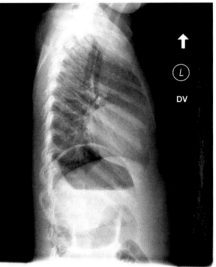

A. Left atrium
B. Left ventricle
C. Right atrium
D. Right ventricle

21b What is the most common type of primary cardiac tumor in a 3-year-old boy?

A. Rhabdomyoma
B. Myxoma
C. Fibroma
D. Teratoma

21c What is the best treatment for this tumor?

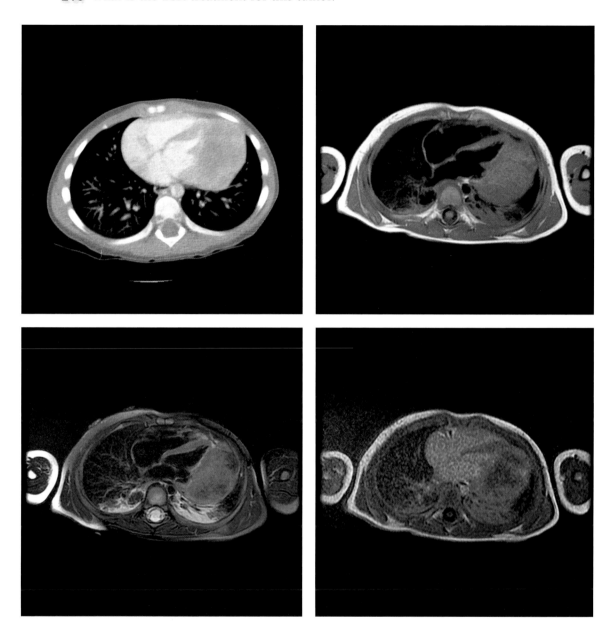

A. Surgical removal
B. Chemotherapy
C. Close follow-up
D. Alcohol ablation

22 If this patient were to undergo PET imaging, what part of the heart would most show abnormal activity?

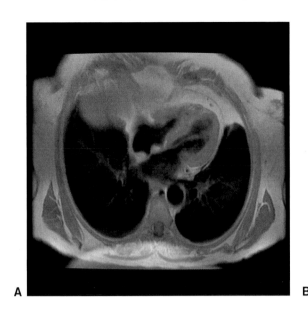

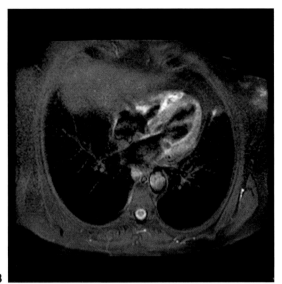

A

B

   A. Right atrial wall
   B. Right ventricular wall
   C. Interatrial septum
   D. Pericardial fat

23 A 55-year-old male presents with shortness of breath. What is the prognosis for this condition?

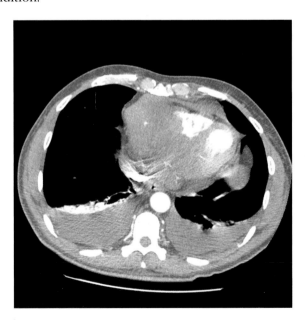

   A. Good, it responds well to chemotherapy.
   B. Fair, it can respond to radiation.
   C. Poor, it typically does not respond to treatment.

24 What is the best next step for this patient?

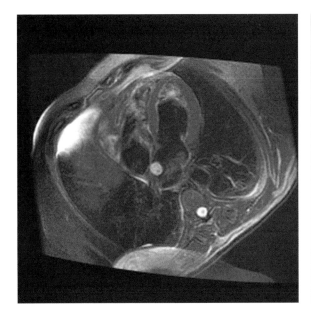
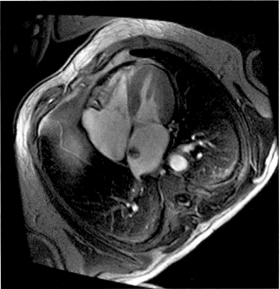

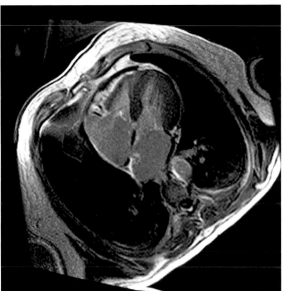

A. Anticoagulation
B. Surgery
C. Chemotherapy
D. Radiation
E. Close observation

25 A 60-year-old female has atrial fibrillation. Which of the following is the most likely diagnosis?

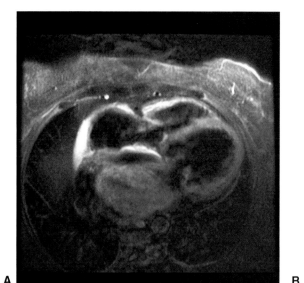

A

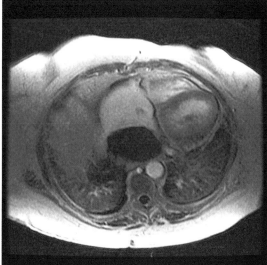

B

A. Myxoma
B. Fibroelastoma
C. Metastatic tumor
D. Thrombus
E. Fibroma

26a Where is the mass located?

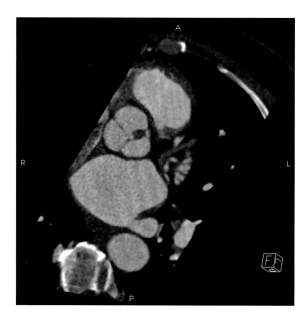

A. Between the noncoronary and right coronary cusp
B. Between the noncoronary and left coronary cusp
C. Between the right and left coronary cusp

26b The patient has no history endocarditis. However, the patient does have a history of transient ischemic attack. What is the best next step?

    A. Anticoagulation
    B. Antibiotics
    C. Surgery
    D. Observation

27 A 49-year-old male presents with a mass seen on echocardiography. What else should you look for in this patient?

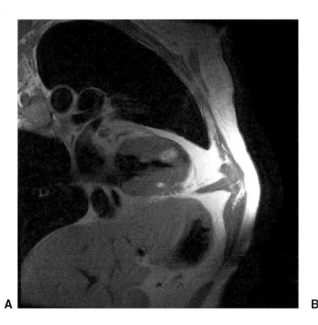

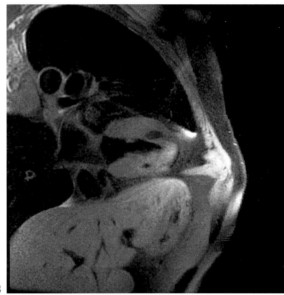

A   B

    A. History of lymphoma
    B. History of infarct
    C. History of renal cysts
    D. History of renal angiomyolipomas
    E. History of echinococcosis infection

28 An 80-year-old male presents with a cardiac mass. What history is most helpful in narrowing the differential?

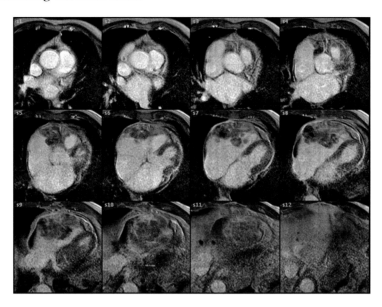

A. Patient has a history of echinococcosis.
B. Patient has a history of lymphoma.
C. Patient has a history of prior PET showing increased uptake in the right heart.
D. Patient has a history of endocarditis.

29a For the images below, select the most likely history.

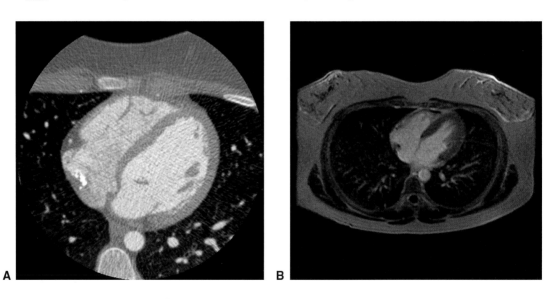

A. A 13-year-old patient with heart failure
B. A 24-year-old patient with a history of central line placement
C. A 40-year-old patient with shortness of breath
D. A 45-year-old patient with unexplained hypertension and tachycardia

29b For the images below, select the most likely history.

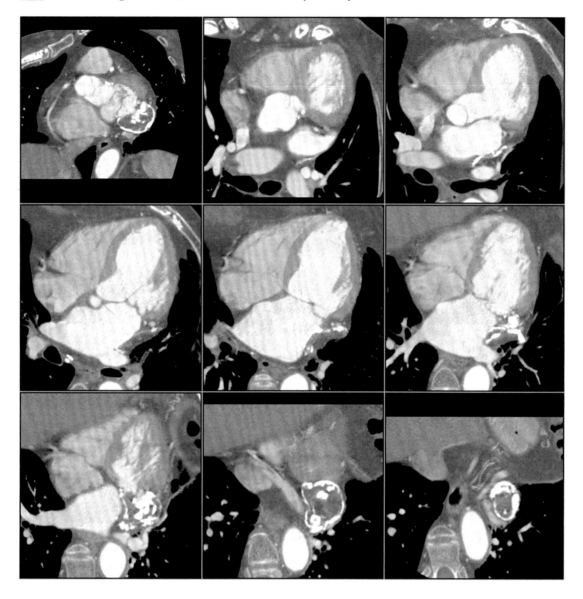

A. A 40-year-old patient with unexplained hypertension and tachycardia
B. A 50-year-old patient with endocarditis
C. A 60-year-old patient, asymptomatic
D. A 77-year-old patient with a history of echinococcus infection

30a A 71-year-old patient is found to have an incidental mass. Based on the PET examination, what should be the next step?

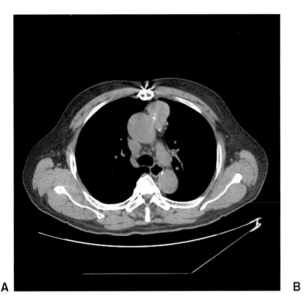

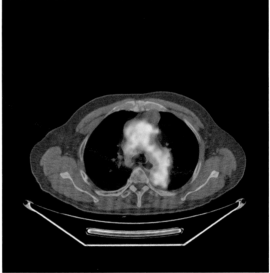

A

B

   A. Biopsy for tissue diagnosis
   B. Contrast-enhanced CTA for further evaluation
   C. Chemotherapy/radiation
   D. No further evaluation necessary, this is benign

30b A 71-year-old patient with abnormality noted on PET-CT now presents for follow-up imaging. This condition most commonly occurs in which vascular territory?

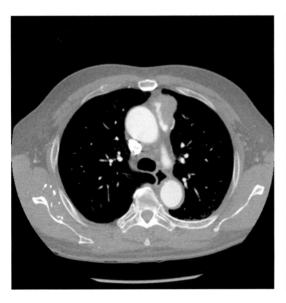

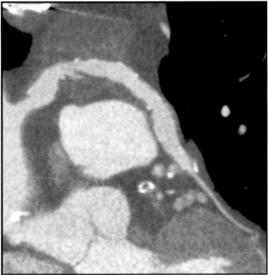

   A. Right coronary artery
   B. Left anterior descending artery
   C. Left circumflex artery

31 An 18-year-old with shortness of breath undergoes a CTA PE protocol with the abnormality shown. Subsequently, a follow-up cardiac MR was obtained after symptoms had resolved. What is the best explanation of the findings?

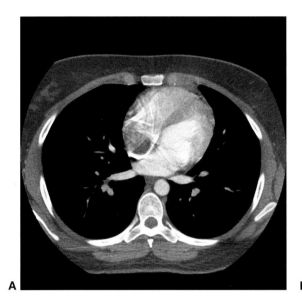
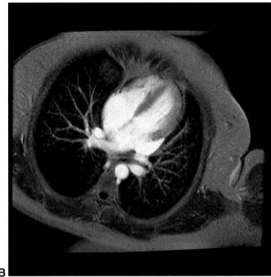

A

B

A. The pathology has embolized in the interval between the CT and MRI study.
B. This was a pseudomass caused by unopacified IVC venous return to the right atrium.
C. The mass shows equal enhancement relative to the blood pool on MRI.

ANSWERS AND EXPLANATIONS

1 **Answer C.** Primary cardiac lymphomas may be identical in histology to extracardiac lymphomas. More than 80% of cases are of the diffuse large B-cell lineage. The prevalence of cardiac lymphoma has increased in recent years due to Epstein-Barr virus–related lymphoproliferative disorders, which are found in patients with acquired immunodeficiency syndrome and transplant recipients. Pericardial effusions can be large and in severe cases may result in tamponade. Aside from the typical pericardial effusion that can arise as a result of cardiac lymphoma involvement, a primary effusion lymphoma (PEL) may also develop. PEL is usually a large cell lymphoma that appears to bridge features of large cell immunoblastic and anaplastic large cell lymphoma.

References: Burke AP, Tavora F. Cardiac lymphoma and metastatic tumors to the heart. In: Burke AP, Tavora F (eds.). *Practical cardiovascular pathology*. Philadelphia, PA: Lippincott Williams & Wilkins, 2010.

Jeudy J, Kirsch J, Tavora F, et al. From the radiologic pathology archives: cardiac lymphoma: radiologic-pathologic correlation. *Radiographics* 2012;32(5):1369–1380.

2 **Answer B.** There has been increasing interest in the role of cardiac MR in breast carcinoma particularly in evaluating cardiotoxicity as a result of chemotherapy. Cardiotoxicity has been described as a decrease in left ventricular ejection fraction by >10% in asymptomatic cancer patients. Left ventricular dysfunction and heart failure due to cancer therapy are associated with a 3.5-fold increase in mortality risk. T1 and T2 mapping measures distinct aspects of myocardial involvement, including edema and fibrosis, which occur in therapy-related cardiotoxicity. Differences in left ventricular end-diastolic volume (LVEDV) and left ventricular end-systolic volume (LVESV) occur before any detectable decline in LVEF and can be shown well by functional sequences. Some studies have reported that aortic pulse wave velocity increases after treatment with an anthracycline and can be readily assessed by phase-contrast sequences, although the full utility is still being explored.

Reference: Jafari F, Safaei AM, Hosseini L, et al. The role of cardiac magnetic resonance imaging in the detection and monitoring of cardiotoxicity in patients with breast cancer after treatment: a comprehensive review. *Heart Fail Rev* 2021;26:679–697.

3 **Answer D.** Delayed enhancement sequences are the most helpful in the evaluation of cardiac thrombus. Thrombus manifests as an absence of gadolinium uptake due to its avascular composition. Cardiac masses demonstrate contrast uptake due to tumor-associated vascularity. At times, poorly vascularized masses may also appear to be similar to thrombus at typical inversion times of myocardial nulling. With prolongation of the inversion time, cardiac masses will increase in signal similar to other tissues, whereas thrombus will continue to have absent signal.

References: Goyal P, Weinsaft JW. Cardiovascular magnetic resonance imaging for assessment of cardiac thrombus. *Methodist Debakey Cardiovasc J* 2013;9(3):132–136.

Whalen H, Dako F, Patel P, et al. Role of imaging for suspected cardiac thrombus. *Curr Treat Options Cardiovasc Med* 2019;21(12):81.

4 **Answer D.** Cardiac metastases are several times more common than primary cardiac tumors. The most common malignancies to spread to the heart are lung and breast cancers, lymphoma, and malignant melanoma. Metastatic spread to the heart can occur by direct invasion (lung, breast, esophagus), hematogenous (melanoma, lymphoma, leukemia), transvenous via the great veins (renal cell carcinoma, hepatoma), or via mediastinal lymphatics.

Reference: Motwani M, Kidambi A, Herzog BA, et al. MR imaging of cardiac tumors and masses: a review of methods and clinical applications. *Radiology* 2013;268(1):26–43.

5 **Answer C.** The above is a true cardiac lipoma. Cardiac lipomas are benign tumors accounting for about 10% of all primary cardiac tumors. Lipomatous hypertrophy (LH) can be confused with lipomas because both have similar imaging characteristics including fatty attenuation on CT, high signal on T1-weighted images, and suppression of signal with fat-saturation techniques. LH classically involves the fossa ovalis, whereas true lipomas can occur throughout the heart, including the visceral and parietal pericardium. True lipomas are histologically composed of mature adipocytes, whereas LH is a mixture of mature and brown fat, which is metabolically active on PET imaging.

References: Burke A, Jeudy J Jr, Virmani R. Cardiac tumours: an update: cardiac tumours. *Heart* 2008;94(1):117–123.

Motwani M, Kidambi A, Herzog BA, et al. MR imaging of cardiac tumors and masses: a review of methods and clinical applications. *Radiology* 2013;268(1):26–43.

6 **Answer C.** This case is a primary left atrial osteosarcoma. Unlike metastatic osteosarcoma, which most often occurs in the right atrium, primary cardiac osteosarcomas arise in the left atrium in the overwhelming majority of cases and are therefore usually accompanied by signs and symptoms of congestive heart failure. The diagnosis of osteosarcoma is more dependent on histopathologic analysis.

Imaging features that may suggest osteogenic sarcoma include a broad base of attachment, an aggressive growth pattern such as extension into the pulmonary veins, invasion of the atrial septum, or infiltrative growth along the epicardium.

The presence of a left atrial mass would most commonly include a cardiac myxoma in the differential. However, calcification is not a feature of lymphomas or myxomas. Cardiac thrombus or myxoma demonstrates the malignant characteristics seen in this mass, including invasion of surrounding structures.

References: Araoz PA, Eklund HE, Welch TJ, et al. CT and MR imaging of primary cardiac malignancies. *Radiographics* 1999;19(6):1421–1434.

Trimble CR, Burke A, Kligerman S. Primary cardiac osteosarcoma: AIRP best cases in radiologic-pathologic correlation. *Radiographics* 2015;35(5):1352–1357.

7 **Answer A.** In this patient, decreased subendocardial attenuation and mild remodeling of the LV is observed at the apex consistent with ischemic injury. Lobulated thrombus is observed at the apex. Thrombus develops as a result of underlying stasis as a consequence of decreased contractility of the heart.

Given the morphology of the heart and location of the abnormality, the other choices would be much more rare. Thrombus is one of the most common intracardiac lesions that is in the differential diagnosis for a cardiac tumor.

Recent thrombus (<2 to 3 weeks) and a chronic (>3 weeks) organized thrombus may have similar appearance on CT demonstrating increased signal intensity on T1-weighted MR sequences. Neither should demonstrate gadolinium contrast enhancement. Chronic thrombi have uniformly low signal on T2-weighted images compared with a tumor.

References: Motwani M, Kidambi A, Herzog BA, et al. MR imaging of cardiac tumors and masses: a review of methods and clinical applications. *Radiology* 2013;268(1):26–43.

Whalen H, Dako F, Patel P, et al. Role of imaging for suspected cardiac thrombus. *Curr Treat Options Cardiovasc Med* 2019;21(12):81.

8 **Answer B.** Cardiac rhabdomyomas are associated with tuberous sclerosis, so one would look for renal angiomyolipomas. Treatment is usually watchful waiting since these lesions tend to regress. However, if the tumor causes significant cardiac chamber obstruction or arrhythmias, the surgery should be considered. Chemotherapy is typically not necessary. Cardiac rhabdomyomas can be diagnosed on prenatal ultrasound.

References: Ghadimi Mahani M, Lu JC, Rigsby CK, et al. MRI of pediatric cardiac masses. *AJR Am J Roentgenol* 2014;202(5):971–981. doi:10.2214/AJR.13.10680. Review.

Tao TY, Yahyavi-Firouz-Abadi N, Singh GK, et al. Pediatric cardiac tumors: clinical and imaging features. *Radiographics* 2014;34(4):1031–1046. doi:10.1148/rg.344135163.

9 **Answer C.** Primary malignant pericardial mesothelioma (PPM) is an exceedingly rare neoplasm arising from the mesothelial surface of the pericardium. Approximately 200 cases have been reported worldwide, most described in case reports or small case series. Unlike peritoneal and pleural mesothelioma, there has been no definite correlation between asbestos exposure and pericardial disease. On microscopy, malignant mesotheliomas of the pericardium resemble pleural mesotheliomas and can be classified into three types: epithelial, sarcomatoid, and biphasic. Malignant mesothelioma carries a poor prognosis with few successful treatment strategies and little benefit from radiation and chemotherapy.

Constrictive pericarditis, pericardial effusion, cardiac tamponade, and heart failure are common clinical presentations of PPM resulting from physical compression or myocardial infiltration. Magnetic resonance imaging and fluorodeoxyglucose positron emission tomography scans are helpful for the diagnosis or staging.

References: Cao S, Jin S, Cao J, et al. Malignant pericardial mesothelioma: a systematic review of current practice. *Herz* 2018;43(1):61–68.

Patel J, Sheppard MN. Primary malignant mesothelioma of the pericardium. *Cardiovasc Pathol* 2011;20(2):107–109.

10 **Answer A.** Although fibromas represent the second most common cardiac neoplasm in children, it is the pediatric cardiac tumor most commonly resected. Approximately 15% of cardiac fibromas occur in adolescents and adults.

Fibromas are round, bulging, well-circumscribed tumors with an intramural location within the ventricular myocardium. Fibromas may often extend into or even completely obliterate the chamber lumen. Singular or multifocal central calcifications are quite common and distinguish them from rhabdomyomas in children. Clinical symptoms of fibroma growth include arrhythmias, vascular obstruction, and heart failure.

References: Grebenc ML, Rosado de Christenson ML, Burke AP, et al. Primary cardiac and pericardial neoplasms: radiologic-pathologic correlation. *Radiographics* 2000;20(4):1073–1103; quiz 1110–1111, 1112.

Maleszewski JJ, Anavekar NS, Moynihan TJ, et al. Pathology, imaging, and treatment of cardiac tumours. *Nat Rev Cardiol* 2017;14(9):536–549.

11 **Answer C.** Cardiac angiosarcomas are the most common primary differentiated cardiac neoplasms. Angiosarcomas consist of irregularly shaped vascular channels lined by anaplastic epithelial cells with sizeable areas of necrosis and hemorrhage.

Given the vascular nature of the lesion, angiosarcomas show a heterogeneous enhancement pattern with intravenous iodinated contrast on CT imaging. Similarly with MRI, gadolinium perfusion imaging in the arterial phase shows immediate enhancement. Late gadolinium enhancement is heterogeneous owing to peripheral fibrosis, which creates an area of increased signal intensity and regions of focal hypointensity associated with central necrosis.

References: Best AK, Dobson RL, Ahmad AR. Best cases from the AFIP: cardiac angiosarcoma. *Radiographics* 2003;23 Spec No:S141–S145.

Tyebally S, Chen D, Bhattacharyya S, et al. Cardiac tumors: JACC cardiooncology state-of-the-art review. *JACC: CardioOncology* 2020;2(2):293–311.

12a Answer B. Coronal postcontrast image shows a mass along the inferior apical left ventricular cavity. Left atrium is not shown in this image. Right atrium appears grossly normal. RVOT is not fully seen but appears normal. Visualized ascending aorta appears normal.

12b Answer D. Left ventricular thrombus is most often associated with postinfarct wall motion abnormalities. Note the enhancement along the infarcted myocardium while there is no enhancement of the mass. Treatment of choice is anticoagulation. This is not a mass that requires surgical resection or chemotherapy. Treatment is necessary to prevent complications of thrombus embolization.

12c Answer C. The most common mass in the heart is thrombus. The most common benign cardiac tumor is myxoma. The most common malignant tumor is angiosarcoma. The most common tumor in children is rhabdomyoma. Melanoma can metastasize to the heart but is not the most common cause of cardiac mass.

References: Grebenc ML, Rosado de Christenson ML, Burke AP, et al. Primary cardiac and pericardial neoplasms: radiologic-pathologic correlation. *Radiographics* 2000;20(4):1073–1103; quiz 1110–1111, 1112. Review.

Sparrow PJ, Kurian JB, Jones TR, et al. MR imaging of cardiac tumors. *Radiographics* 2005;25(5):1255–1276. Review.

13 Answer B. Metastatic involvement of the heart is more common than primary cardiac tumors. The most common site of metastatic involvement is the pericardium. Tumor thrombus will usually show heterogeneous enhancement, while thrombus will show no enhancement. Metastatic tumors (excluding melanoma) tend to show low signal on T1W.

Reference: Sparrow PJ, Kurian JB, Jones TR, et al. MR imaging of cardiac tumors. *Radiographics* 2005;25(5):1255–1276. Review.

14a Answer E. Postcontrast gated coronary CTA shows a low-attenuation filling defect at the tip of the left atrial appendage. The aorta and pulmonary artery appear normal. Left atrium is only partially visualized along with the pulmonary veins, and they appear normal.

14b Answer B. The filling defect seen on the initial CTA at the tip of left atrial appendage is no longer identified on the delayed acquisition image. This is consistent with slow flow in the left atrial appendage, which can be seen in patients with atrial fibrillation and LA enlargement. Thrombus would have shown a persistent low-attenuation filling defect at the tip of the left atrial appendage with a border. It is unlikely that the thrombus could have embolized in the short amount of time between the initial CTA and the second acquisition.

14c Answer C. Left atrial appendage thrombus is most often evaluated by transesophageal echocardiogram (TEE). While CTA can visualize LA appendage thrombus, its specificity is not high given that the false positives can happen with slow flow. A delayed phase may be helpful but adds additional radiation. MRI can also visualize left atrial appendage thrombus but is not used routinely as TEE is more available and performed just prior to pulmonary vein ablation.

Reference: Saremi F, Channual S, Gurudevan SV, et al. Prevalence of left atrial appendage pseudothrombus filling defects in patients with atrial fibrillation undergoing coronary computed tomography angiography. *J Cardiovasc Comput Tomogr* 2008;2(3):164–171. doi:10.1016/j.jcct.2008.02.012.

15 **Answer B.** While the most common type of mass in the heart is thrombus, in this case, there is evidence for metastatic disease (see liver lesions). This patient had hepatocellular carcinoma (HCC) with tumor invasion via the hepatic veins to the right atrium. Other tumors besides HCC with direct invasion to the right atrium include renal cell carcinoma and IVC sarcoma. Myxoma is within the differential and can be in the right atrium, but the liver lesions here make it more likely that this is a metastatic tumor. Endocarditis can cause masses in the valves, but they tend not to be this large. Lymphoma could also cause a mass in the heart but is not the best answer in this case given the liver findings.

References: Grebenc ML, Rosado de Christenson ML, Burke AP, et al. Primary cardiac and pericardial neoplasms: radiologic-pathologic correlation. *Radiographics* 2000;20(4):1073–1103; quiz 1110–1111, 1112. Review.

Sparrow PJ, Kurian JB, Jones TR, et al. MR imaging of cardiac tumors. *Radiographics* 2005;25(5):1255–1276. Review.

16 **Answer A.** This mass is most consistent with a large RCA aneurysm given the history suggesting Kawasaki disease. Catheter angiography is the best next step to better evaluate this aneurysm. One could argue for CABG right away if the diagnosis of giant RCA aneurysm was not in doubt. However, sometimes, the anatomy can be significantly distorted on CT that a catheter angiogram can show the aneurysm better than CT given the ability to directly inject the vessel. Biopsy would not be a wise choice for an aneurysm. Given this is not a tumor, medical treatment would not be helpful. CMR would not provide any more information given the findings are highly suggestive of giant RCA aneurysm already.

Reference: Díaz-Zamudio M, Bacilio-Pérez U, Herrera-Zarza MC, et al. Coronary artery aneurysms and ectasia: role of coronary CT angiography. *Radiographics* 2009;29(7):1939–1954. doi:10.1148/rg.297095048. Review.

17a **Answer D.** The contour abnormality is at the right heart border on the PA view. The lateral view shows it adjacent to the heart and not posterior in the right lower lobe.

17b **Answer A.** This is right pericardial cyst along the right atrial border. It shows T2 prolongation on the T2W image. This mass shows no enhancement, septations, or nodules. Simple pericardial cysts do not require treatment or follow-up.

Reference: Restrepo CS, Vargas D, Ocazionez D, et al. Primary pericardial tumors. *Radiographics* 2013;33(6):1613–1630. doi:10.1148/rg.336135512. Review.

18 **Answer C.** This is a right atrial mass showing T2 prolongation (Image B) and heterogeneous contrast enhancement (Image C). While thrombus is the most common mass in the right atrium, in this case, the contrast enhancement excludes thrombus. The T2 prolongation and enhancement is suggestive of a right atrial myxoma. The best treatment is therefore surgery.

Reference: Grebenc ML, Rosado-de-Christenson ML, Green CE, et al. Cardiac myxoma: imaging features in 83 patients. *Radiographics* 2002;22(3):673–689. Review.

19 **Answer B.** Proton density-weighted (Image A) and post fat-saturated T2W (Image B) images show lipomatous hypertrophy of the interatrial septum (LHIAS). There is a classic barbell shape of the fat in the interatrial septum sparing the fossa ovalis. The right atrial location does not indicate a benign lesion as malignant and metastatic tumors can occur in this chamber. Fat suppression is used here, not fluid suppression. The images are noncontrast images, so nothing can be said about the lack or presence of enhancement.

Reference: Kimura F, Matsuo Y, Nakajima T, et al. Myocardial fat at cardiac imaging: how can we differentiate pathologic from physiologic fatty infiltration? *Radiographics* 2010;30(6):1587–1602. doi:10.1148/rg.306105519.

20a **Answer D.** Proton density-weighted (Image A) and fat-saturated T2W (Image B) images show a right atrial wall mass that loses signal on fat suppression. There is suggestion of a thin capsule. This is most consistent with a right atrial lipoma. No treatment is necessary. This is not a tumor or thrombus that requires anticoagulation or chemotherapy or surgery. Lipomatous hypertrophy of the interatrial septum (LHIAS) can be positive on PET, but the lesion in this case does not involve the interatrial septum and appears to be a simple right atrial lipoma.

Reference: Kimura F, Matsuo Y, Nakajima T, et al. Myocardial fat at cardiac imaging: how can we differentiate pathologic from physiologic fatty infiltration? *Radiographics* 2010;30(6):1587–1602. doi:10.1148/rg.306105519.

20b **Answer C.** Short tau inversion recovery (STIR) is not specific to fat as it will suppress anything with short T1 (including postcontrast T1 shortening). STIR imaging does not require a high field strength magnet. It will have lower signal due to the inversion pulse.

Chemical fat suppression is specific to fat and will not suppress contrast enhancement. However, it is susceptible to field inhomogeneity, which can cause incomplete fat saturation. With a higher-strength magnet, there is greater separation of the fat and water peaks making fat suppression easier.

Reference: Delfaut EM, Beltran J, Johnson G, et al. Fat suppression in MR imaging: techniques and pitfalls. *Radiographics* 1999;19(2):373–382. Review. Erratum in: *Radiographics* 1999;19(4):1092.

21a **Answer B.** The contour abnormality is along the left heart border, which is consistent with a LV abnormality.

21b **Answer A.** The most common type of cardiac tumor in infants and children is a rhabdomyoma. Myxomas are most common in adults. Fibromas are the second most common cardiac tumor in children. Cardiac teratoma is rare in the pediatric population.

21c **Answer C.** This is a large tumor along the LV lateral wall with enhancement most consistent with a cardiac fibroma in this 3-year-old boy. Fibromas are derived from fibroblasts. Treatment is watchful waiting as this cannot be resected due to the large size and involvement of a large portion of the LV. Unlike rhabdomyomas, fibromas do not typically regress, so for this patient, cardiac transplantation may ultimately be required. Alcohol ablation is used for hypertrophic cardiomyopathy patients with left ventricular outflow tract obstruction.

References: Ghadimi Mahani M, Lu JC, Rigsby CK, et al. MRI of pediatric cardiac masses. *AJR Am J Roentgenol* 2014;202(5):971–981. doi:10.2214/AJR.13.10680. Review.

Tao TY, Yahyavi-Firouz-Abadi N, Singh GK, et al. Pediatric cardiac tumors: clinical and imaging features. *Radiographics* 2014;34(4):1031–1046. doi:10.1148/rg.344135163.

22 **Answer C.** Proton density-weighted (Image A) and triple inversion recovery images (Image B) show a dumbbell-shaped lesion in the interatrial septum sparing the fossa ovalis. This is classic for lipomatous hypertrophy of the interatrial septum. This lesion can show PET activity due to the presence of metabolically active brown fat.

Reference: Kimura F, Matsuo Y, Nakajima T, et al. Myocardial fat at cardiac imaging: how can we differentiate pathologic from physiologic fatty infiltration? *Radiographics* 2010;30(6):1587–1602. doi:10.1148/rg.306105519.

23 **Answer C.** CT shows an infiltrative mass in the right atrium and ventricle with a pericardial effusion and a left lung nodule. This is most consistent with a cardiac angiosarcoma, the most common primary malignant tumor of the heart. It is more common in males and carries a poor prognosis with median survival rate of 6 months.

Reference: Araoz PA, Eklund HE, Welch TJ, et al. CT and MR imaging of primary cardiac malignancies. *Radiographics* 1999;19(6):1421–1434. Review.

24 **Answer B.** This is a mass in the left atrium most consistent with a left atrial myxoma. It shows T2 prolongation with gradual postcontrast enhancement. The treatment is surgery.

Reference: Araoz PA, Eklund HE, Welch TJ, et al. CT and MR imaging of primary cardiac malignancies. *Radiographics* 1999;19(6):1421–1434. Review.

25 **Answer D.** This left atrial tumor is most consistent with left atrial thrombus given the lack of enhancement (Image B). Thrombus can have variable signal on T1W, T2W, and PDW images depending on the age of thrombus. The lack of enhancement is essentially diagnostic of thrombus as the other entities should all show enhancement.

Reference: Sparrow PJ, Kurian JB, Jones TR, et al. MR imaging of cardiac tumors. *Radiographics* 2005;25(5):1255–1276. Review.

26a **Answer C.** The mass is located between the left and right coronary cusps. The noncoronary cusp is typically located at the interatrial septum. The right coronary cusp is located anteriorly (look for the sternum/right ventricular outflow tract). The left coronary cusp is adjacent to the left atrial appendage.

Reference: Bennett CJ, Maleszewski JJ, Araoz PA. CT and MR imaging of the aortic valve: radiologic-pathologic correlation. *Radiographics* 2012;32(5):1399–1420. doi:10.1148/rg.325115727.

26b **Answer C.** The image shows an aortic valvular mass most consistent with a papillary fibroelastomas given the lack of history of endocarditis. When it involves the aortic valve, it is more commonly seen on the aortic side, and when it involves the mitral valve, it is more commonly on the left atrial surface. It is much rarely seen in the cardiac chambers. These tumors can cause embolization/coronary occlusion. In symptomatic patients, surgical resection should be considered.

Reference: Mariscalco G, Bruno VD, Borsani P, et al. Papillary fibroelastoma: insight to a primary cardiac valve tumor. *J Card Surg* 2010;25(2):198–205. doi:10.1111/j.1540-8191.2009.00993.x.

27 **Answer D.** Multiple fatty lesions are seen in the LV myocardium. The first image is T1W double inversion recovery (DIR) black blood imaging (Image A) showing myocardial areas of increased signal, which shows fat suppression (Image B). These fatty myocardial lesions can be seen in patients with tuberous sclerosis. These are not fatty changes from prior infarct.

Reference: Kimura F, Matsuo Y, Nakajima T, et al. Myocardial fat at cardiac imaging: how can we differentiate pathologic from physiologic fatty infiltration? *Radiographics* 2010;30(6):1587–1602. doi:10.1148/rg.306105519.

28 **Answer B.** Postcontrast images show a mass along the right atrium and ventricle with heterogeneous enhancement. This is a nonspecific finding and should be correlated with patient's history to narrow the differential. Metastatic involvement of the heart is more common than primary cardiac tumors. Therefore, the most helpful history would be prior lymphoma. Cardiac echinococcosis should show cystic lesions, which are not seen here. Uptake on PET is nonspecific and will not necessarily narrow the differential since this mass already shows enhancement on MRI. However, if PET also shows other areas of abnormal uptake that may be helpful if a primary is suggested. Endocarditis/abscess can show enhancement, but in this case, the appearance is more consistent with mass rather than abscess.

References: Buckley O, Madan R, Kwong R, et al. Cardiac masses, part 1: imaging strategies and technical considerations. *AJR Am J Roentgenol* 2011;197(5):W837–W841. doi:10.2214/AJR.10.7260. Review.

Jeudy J, Kirsch J, Tavora F, et al. From the radiologic pathology archives: cardiac lymphoma: radiologic-pathologic correlation. *Radiographics* 2012;32(5):1369–1380. doi:10.1148/rg.325115126.

O'Donnell DH, Abbara S, Chaithiraphan V, et al. Cardiac tumors: optimal cardiac MR sequences and spectrum of imaging appearances. *AJR Am J Roentgenol* 2009;193(2):377–387. doi:10.2214/AJR.08.1895. Review.

Sparrow PJ, Kurian JB, Jones TR, et al. MR imaging of cardiac tumors. *Radiographics* 2005;25(5):1255–1276. Review.

29a **Answer B.** CT (Image A) shows a calcified lesion along the right atrial wall along the crista terminalis. Postcontrast MRI (Image B) shows a nonenhancing mass in the same location. This is most consistent with an old calcified right atrial thrombus. Most likely history in this case would be a patient with a history of central line placement.

Typical history for a cardiac fibroma could be a 13-year-old patient with heart failure. For angiosarcoma, a 40-year-old patient with shortness of breath may be the best history. For a patient with hypertension and tachycardia, a cardiac paraganglioma may be possible due to the excessive production of catecholamines. If the images showed valvular vegetations, then a history of endocarditis could be likely. For asymptomatic patients, a benign pseudomass such as a prominent crista terminalis could be seen. For patients with a history of echinococcus infection, there could be residuals such as calcified masses.

29b **Answer D.** CT shows a calcified lesion along the inferior lateral heart. The best answer here would be a patient with a history of echinococcus infection as this is most consistent with hydatid cyst residuals. Please see prior discussion for discussion on other answer choices.

Reference: Kantarci M, Bayraktutan U, Karabulut N, et al. Alveolar echinococcosis: spectrum of findings at cross-sectional imaging. *Radiographics* 2012;32(7):2053–2070. doi:10.1148/rg.327125708. Review.

30a **Answer B.** Noncontrast CT (Image A) shows a mass anterior and to the left of the ascending aorta. Note the sternotomy wires. PET (Image B) shows no significant activity in this mass. Given the sternotomy wires, this may be a saphenous graft aneurysm, so the best next step is to evaluate for possible aneurysm with contrast-enhanced CTA. If there is a concern for a vascular pathology, biopsy should not be performed. Lack of PET activity makes this less likely to be a malignancy. This is not a lesion that can be left alone without further evaluation.

30b **Answer A.** Images show a saphenous vein graft aneurysm. These patients typically present with chest pain/angina. However, a significant number of cases are discovered incidentally (up to ⅓ of reported cases). There is no consensus on treatment depending on aneurysm size; however, some have advocated treating the aneurysm >1 cm. Currently, surgery is performed more often than percutaneous treatment (covered stent). SVG aneurysms most often occur in the RCA territory, likely due to larger number of SVGs to the RCA territory and possibly the larger caliber of the RCA grafts.

Reference: Ramirez FD, Hibbert B, Simard T, et al. Natural history and management of aortocoronary saphenous vein graft aneurysms: a systematic review of published cases. *Circulation* 2012;126(18):2248–2256. doi:10.1161/CIRCULATIONAHA.112.101592. Review.

31 **Answer B.** There is a low-attenuation lesion in the right atrium on the CT (Image A). The postcontrast MRI (Image B) shows no mass in the right atrium. This is most consistent with a pseudofilling defect in the right atrium from unopacified blood returning to the right atrium, most likely due to patient doing a Valsalva maneuver as the patient held their breath. This has been described as transient interruption of the contrast in PE studies. It is unlikely for a large mass in the right atrium to embolize without any symptoms. The mass is also unlikely to have equal enhancement to the blood pool and not show up on the any of the images on MRI.

Reference: Wittram C, Yoo AJ. Transient interruption of contrast on CT pulmonary angiography: proof of mechanism. *J Thorac Imaging* 2007;22(2):125–129.

7 Valvular Disease

Jean Jeudy, MD • Sachin Malik, MD

QUESTIONS

1a What type of sequence from a cardiac MR examination was acquired to produce the images shown below?

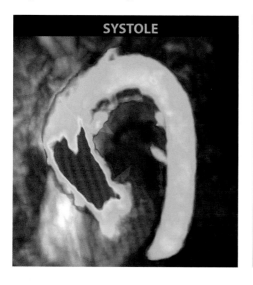
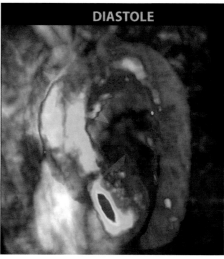

A. Three-dimensional phase contrast
B. Late gadolinium enhancement
C. Two-dimensional phase contrast through plane
D. Two-dimensional phase contrast in plane

1b What abnormality is shown?

A. Aortic stenosis
B. Aortic regurgitation
C. Mitral stenosis
D. Mitral regurgitation

2 Which of the following valvular abnormalities have the worst acute prognosis?

A. Bicuspid aortic valve
B. Drug-induced tricuspid valvulopathy
C. Infarcted papillary muscle with rupture
D. Multivalvular rheumatic fever

3a A 17-year-old female with a history of tetralogy of Fallot postsurgical repair undergoes follow-up cardiac MRI. Coronal (left) and sagittal (right) right ventricular outflow tract views from a four-dimensional flow sequence during diastole are shown. What abnormality is highlighted by the arrows?

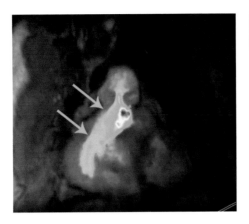 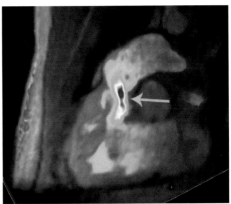

   A. Pulmonic stenosis
   B. Pulmonic regurgitation
   C. Tricuspid stenosis
   D. Tricuspid regurgitation

3b What sequence could be used to directly quantify the abnormality?
   A. Late gadolinium enhancement
   B. Bright blood
   C. Dark blood
   D. Phase contrast

3c In this patient, which of the following is a long-term consequence if this goes untreated?
   A. Right heart failure
   B. Pulmonary artery stenosis
   C. Pulmonary artery aneurysm
   D. Left atrial calcifications

4 Enlargement of which cardiac structure would be the most reliable sign of pulmonary valve stenosis?
   A. Right ventricle
   B. Main pulmonary trunk
   C. Main trunk and left pulmonary artery
   D. Right and left pulmonary arteries

5 Which is the most common cause of mitral stenosis worldwide?
   A. Rheumatic heart disease
   B. Myxomatous degenerative disease
   C. Carcinoid syndrome
   D. Congenital mitral stenosis

6 Which is the most common cause of pulmonic stenosis?
   A. Congenital stenosis
   B. Rheumatic disease
   C. Degenerative thickening
   D. Carcinoid syndrome

7 What would be the primary contributor to this patient's mitral insufficiency?

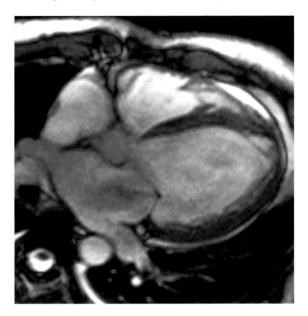

A. Mitral valve prolapse
B. Annular dilation
C. Congenital mitral stenosis
D. Infective endocarditis

8 Rheumatic disease involving the aortic valve is most commonly associated with

A. Aortic insufficiency
B. Isolated involvement
C. Bicuspid aortic valve
D. Aortic stenosis

9 A 67-year-old male with a history of pulmonary hypertension presents with progressively worsening shortness of breath and lower extremity edema. Based on the clinical history and images shown, what abnormality most likely accounts for the patient's symptoms?

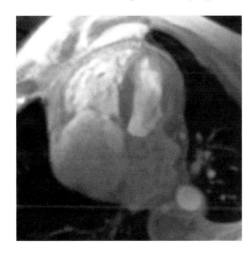
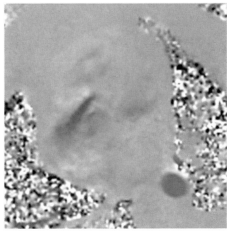

A. Annular enlargement
B. Congenital abnormality
C. Acute traumatic injury
D. Pacemaker-related complication

10a A 77-year-old female with a history of atrial fibrillation and prior heart valve surgery presents after a ground-level fall. A CT angiogram of the chest is performed as part of a trauma scan. Which of the following most likely explains the abnormalities in the image shown?

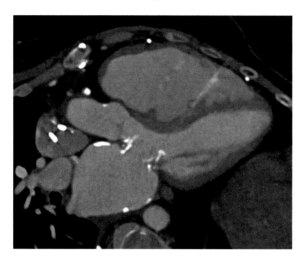

A. Atrial fibrillation
B. Acute trauma
C. Rheumatic heart disease
D. Systemic lupus erythematosus

10b What other abnormality did this patient most likely have?
A. Mitral stenosis
B. Aortic stenosis
C. Pulmonic stenosis
D. Tricuspid stenosis

11 Based on the images below, which of the following best describes the mitral valve?

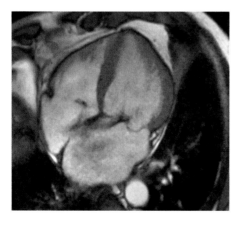 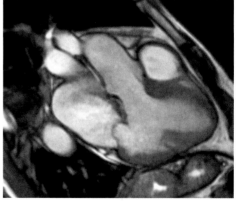

A. Flail
B. Normal
C. Stenosis
D. Prolapse

12a A 47-year-old male presents with syncope and exertional chest pain. Which of the following best describes the abnormality identified by the arrow in the image shown from his cardiac MRI?

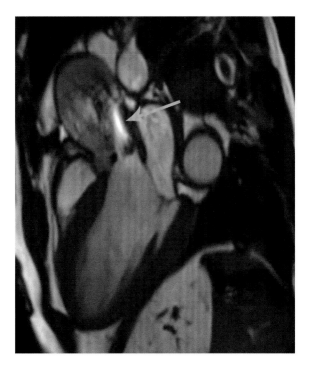

A. Aortic stenosis
B. Aortic regurgitation
C. Aortic aneurysm
D. Aortic pseudoaneurysm

12b Based on the additional images shown below, what is the most likely etiology of the abnormality identified in part 1 of this question?

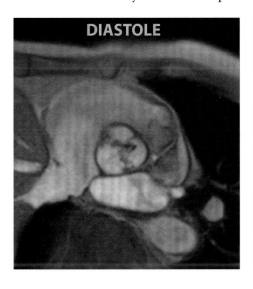 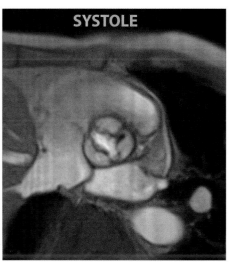

A. Iatrogenic
B. Acute trauma
C. Bicuspid aortic valve
D. Medication side effect

12c Bicuspid aortic valve is most commonly associated with which of the following?

A. Right-sided aortic arch
B. Mitral valve prolapse
C. Aortic coarctation
D. Polysplenia

13 After obtaining a preoperative contrast-enhanced CT, an abnormality was incidentally noted on the aortic valve (below). Patient has no history of fever, leukocytosis, palpitations, or known endocarditis.

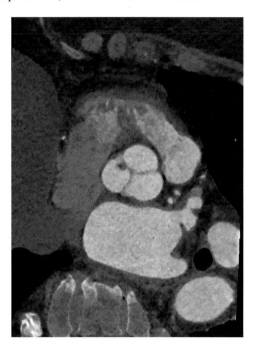

Given the clinical history and imaging findings, the most likely etiology would be

A. Fibroma
B. Metastasis
C. Rhabdomyosarcoma
D. Papillary fibroelastoma

14 Results from the analysis of a phase-contrast sequence are shown below. Which of the following does the patient most likely have?

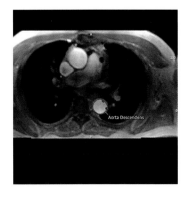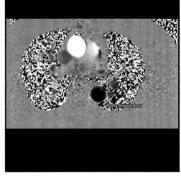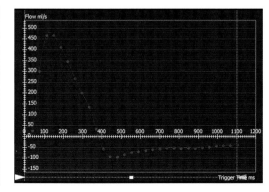

A. Aortic coarctation
B. Aortic regurgitation
C. Aortic aneurysm
D. Aortic stenosis

15 What is the most likely diagnosis?

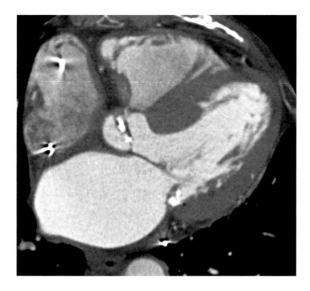

    A. Flail leaflet
    B. Rheumatic mitral valve disease
    C. Mitral valve prolapse
    D. Mitral regurgitation

16a A 59-year-old female presents with fevers, leukocytosis, and palpitations. Based on the history and images shown below, what is the most likely diagnosis?

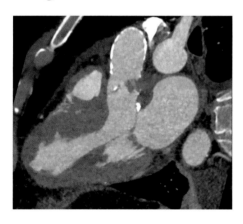 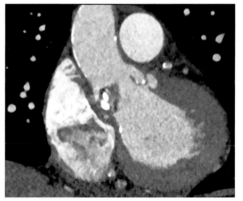

    A. Papillary fibroelastoma
    B. Thrombus
    C. Aortic dissection
    D. Infective endocarditis

16b What complication is seen?
    A. Aneurysm
    B. Dissection
    C. Pseudoaneurysm
    D. Pulmonary emboli

17 An 86-year-old patient with severe aortic stenosis undergoes transcatheter aortic valve implantation. The postoperative course was largely uncomplicated; however, a new left bundle-branch block is observed on telemetry. Which of the following is the most likely etiology?

A. Cardiac sarcoidosis
B. Complication of TAVI surgery
C. Acute myocardial infarction
D. Drug toxicity

18 Basal short-axis (left) and two-chamber (right) views of the heart from a noncontrast chest CT are shown. What is the most likely diagnosis?

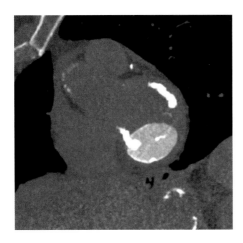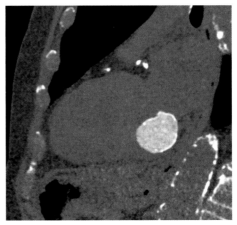

A. Intramyocardial hemorrhage
B. Left circumflex artery aneurysm
C. Left ventricular pseudoaneurysm
D. Caseous necrosis of the mitral annulus

19 A patient with a history of pulmonary valve stenosis undergoes a transcatheter pulmonary valve replacement. Which of the following postprocedural radiographs correctly matches this patient?

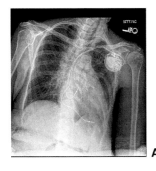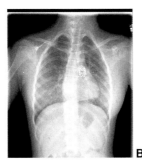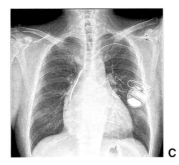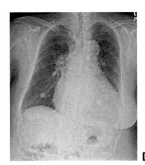

A   B   C   D

20 What is the most optimal cardiac imaging plane for visualizing both atrioventricular valves?

A. Vertical long axis
B. Short axis
C. Horizontal long axis
D. Coronal

21 A 33-year-old patient with a history of murmur undergoes a cardiac MRI. The MR depicts the following:
Which is the most appropriate diagnosis?

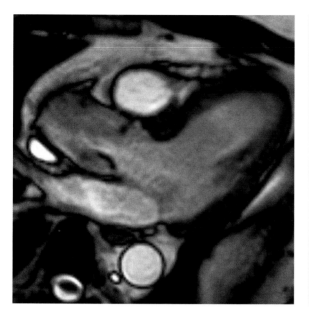 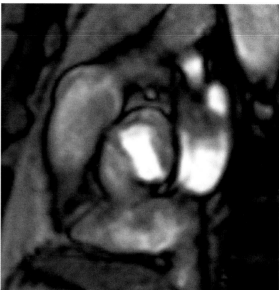

    A. Critical aortic valve stenosis
    B. Bioprosthetic aortic valve
    C. Aortic valve endocarditis
    D. Bicuspid aortic valve

22 A patient with severe tricuspid insufficiency presents for a cardiac CT. Previous echocardiogram reports decreased movement of tricuspid valve leaflets.

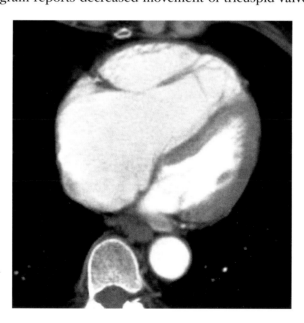

Given the history and imaging, what would be the most likely etiology?

    A. Eisenmenger physiology
    B. Mitral annular calcification
    C. Carcinoid heart disease
    D. Rheumatic heart disease

23 Mitral valve prolapse may occur in association with which condition?

A. Shone syndrome
B. Carcinoid disease
C. Marfan syndrome
D. Rheumatic heart disease

24a A 34-year-old female presents to the emergency department with atypical chest pain. Images from her CT are provided below.

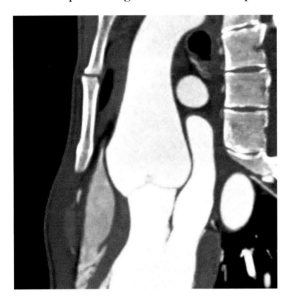 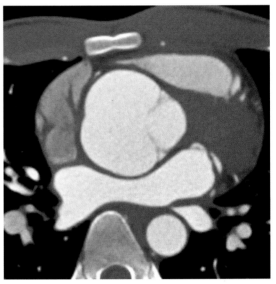

Which best describes the underlying pathology?

A. Acute aortic syndrome
B. Annuloaortic ectasia
C. Subvalvular aortic stenosis
D. Rheumatic heart disease

24b Including Marfan syndrome and Ehlers-Danlos syndrome, which of the following syndromes may also be a cause of annuloaortic ectasia?

A. Loeys-Dietz syndrome
B. Shone syndrome
C. Williams syndrome
D. Heyde syndrome

25 Aortic peak velocity >4 m/sec corresponds to a mean aortic gradient of

A. <20 mm Hg
B. 21 to 40 mm Hg
C. >40 mm Hg

26 Which of the following pathologies most accurately describes the finding?

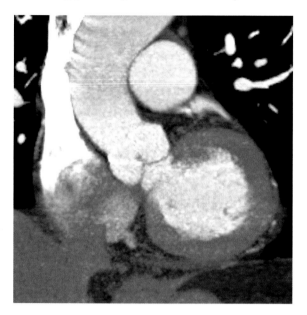

A. Supravalvular aortic stenosis
B. Valvular aortic stenosis
C. Subvalvular aortic stenosis
D. Valvular aortic insufficiency

ANSWERS AND EXPLANATIONS

1a **Answer A.** The images shown are from a three-dimensional phase-contrast image, also referred to as 4D flow. Phase-contrast MRI is a technique used to measure and quantify velocity. This was typically performed in a two-dimensional manner by measuring flow through a slice (through plane) or within a slice (in plane). However, more recently, this technique has been applied in three-dimensions using both electrocardiographic and respiratory gating to image the heart over a long period of time while free breathing. This allows for the creation of three-dimensional images with flow and velocity profiles in all directions as seen here. Some benefits and applications include three-dimensional visualization and flow evaluation of the heart and great vessels and ability to scan the entire heart and then process areas of interest after the scan is complete. Two-dimensional phase-contrast images must be obtained during the scan targeting the area of interest. One of the major limitations of the technique is the relatively long scan time, which can range from 10 to 20 minutes. However, many techniques are being developed that aim to shorten the scan time to 5 minutes or less.

References: Azarine A, et al. Four-dimensional Flow MRI: principles and cardiovascular applications. *Radiographics* 2019;39:632–648.

Markl M, et al. 4D flow MRI. *J Magn Reson Imaging* 2012;36:1015–1036.

1b **Answer B.** Color-coded 4D flow images of the aorta during systole and diastole demonstrate severe aortic regurgitation (arrow in diastole). Aortic stenosis would show a narrow high velocity jet originating from the center of the aortic valve plane. The broad-based flow jet during systole is normal forward flow. Images do not show flow across the mitral valve.

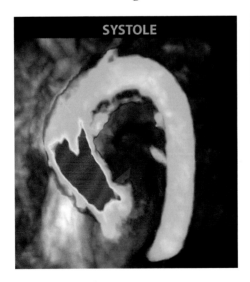
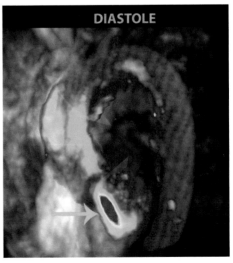

Reference: Azarine A, et al. Four-dimensional flow MRI: principles and cardiovascular applications. *Radiographics* 2019;39:632–648.

2 **Answer C.** All of the other clinical scenarios are related to chronic valvular disease. Patients in this setting will typically have complaints of progressive dyspnea. Infarction of the papillary muscle with rupture, in the setting of myocardial infarction or trauma, is associated with acute mitral insufficiency, shortness of breath, florid pulmonary edema, significant hemodynamic compromise, and death.

Reference: Pawale A, El-Eshmawi A, Torregrossa G, et al. Ruptured papillary muscle causing acute severe mitral regurgitation. *J Card Surg* 2013;28(6):707.

3a **Answer B.** The images show a color-coded representation of flow from a four-dimensional flow sequence during diastole. The arrows highlight a flow jet connecting the pulmonary valve and the right ventricle during diastole compatible with pulmonary regurgitation. Pulmonary stenosis would show an antegrade jet past the pulmonary valve during systole. No tricuspid disease is shown in the images provided.

References: Ahmed S, et al. Role of multidetector CT in assessment of repaired tetralogy of Fallot. *Radiographics* 2013;33:1023–1036.

Ordovas KG, et al. Cardiovascular MR imaging after surgical correction of tetralogy of Fallot: approach based on understanding of surgical procedures. *Radiographics* 2013;33:1037–1052.

3b **Answer D.** Phase-contrast MRI is a technique used to measure and quantify velocity and flow. The technique uses bipolar gradients to measure the phase shift of a moving spin. If the spin is stationary, no net phase shift will be seen, but if the spin is moving, then the net phase shift will be proportional to its velocity. This was typically performed in a two-dimensional manner by measuring flow through a slice (through plane) or within a slice (in plane). However, more recently, this technique has been applied in three-dimensions using both electrocardiographic and respiratory gating to image the heart over a long period of time while free breathing—also referred to as 4D flow.

Late gadolinium enhancement imaging is an inversion recovery technique used after the administration of intravenous contrast material to suppress the signal from normal myocardium and assess for areas of enhancement. Bright blood imaging is a balanced steady-state free precession image in which the blood is bright. This can be used for anatomic imaging and to acquire cine images of the heart. Note that if no other valvular regurgitation or intracardiac shunt exists, bright blood images could *indirectly* quantify the pulmonary regurgitation by quantifying the right and left ventricular stroke volumes. The right ventricular stroke volume could then be subtracted from the left ventricular stroke volume to calculate the pulmonic regurgitant volume. Dark blood imaging is a double-inversion technique designed to suppress signal from the blood. This can be used for anatomic imaging and can be either T1 or T2 weighted for tissue characterization.

Reference: Markl M, et al. 4D flow MRI. *J Magn Reson Imaging* 2012;36:1015–1036.

3c **Answer A.** Pulmonary regurgitation is a common complication in repaired tetralogy of Fallot and is closely monitored on serial imaging. Long-standing pulmonary regurgitation can cause right heart failure and arrhythmias. Pulmonary artery stenosis and aneurysm are not sequelae of long-standing pulmonic regurgitation. Left atrial calcifications are associated with rheumatic heart disease.

References: Ahmed S, et al. Role of multidetector CT in assessment of repaired tetralogy of Fallot. *Radiographics* 2013;33:1023–1036.

Ordovas KG, et al. Cardiovascular MR imaging after surgical correction of tetralogy of Fallot: approach based on understanding of surgical procedures. *Radiographics* 2013;33:1037–1052.

4 **Answer C.** Enlargement of the right ventricle or the main pulmonary artery can occur in volume overload, pulmonary hypertension, or tricuspid valvular disease. Enlargement of the pulmonary trunk can also be seen in the setting of pulmonary stenosis. However, as blood crosses the stenotic pulmonic valve, there is acceleration in flow and asymmetric flow toward the left pulmonary artery with resulting asymmetric enlargement of the left pulmonary artery. Because the right pulmonary artery originates at a 90-degree angle from the main pulmonary artery, it is not exposed to this accelerated flow.

Reference: Chen JJ, Manning MA, Frazier AA, et al. CT Angiography of the cardiac valves: normal, diseased, and postoperative appearances. *Radiographics* 2009;29(5):1393–1412.

5 **Answer A.** Rheumatic heart disease (RHD) is the most common cause of mitral valve stenosis, particularly in the developing world. It usually originates as a streptococcal infection of the upper respiratory tract (rheumatic fever). Acute RHD produces a pancarditis, characterized by endocarditis, myocarditis, and pericarditis. Chronic RHD is characterized by repeated valvular inflammation with subsequent leaflet thickening, commissural fusion, and shortening and thickening of the tendinous cords.

Congenital mitral stenosis is very rare. Carcinoid valvulopathy affects primarily tricuspid and pulmonary valves. Myxomatous degeneration results in mitral valve prolapse and insufficiency.

Reference: Hughes S. Valvular heart disease. In: Suvarna SK (ed.). *Cardiac Pathology.* London, UK: Springer, 2013:147–161.

6 **Answer A.** Pulmonary stenosis is a congenital disorder in 95% of cases and most often an isolated abnormality. Pulmonary stenosis can also be observed as a component of complex congenital heart disease such as tetralogy of Fallot. Acquired pulmonary stenosis whether degenerative or inflammatory is exceedingly rare. Carcinoid syndrome is also rare and typically causes valvular insufficiency.

Reference: Chen JJ, Manning MA, Frazier AA, et al. CT angiography of the cardiac valves: normal, diseased, and postoperative appearances. *Radiographics* 2009;29(5):1393–1412.

7 **Answer B.** Balanced steady-state free precession image demonstrates left ventricular enlargement and mitral insufficiency arising centrally from the valve. The valve leaflets are otherwise unremarkable without evidence of thickening, vegetation, or prolapse. Ventricular dilation commonly leads to subsequent annular dilatation and functional insufficiency.

The mitral valve requires coordinated function of the left atrium, mitral annulus, leaflets, papillary muscles, and left ventricle. Mitral insufficiency often results from dysfunction of one or more of these components. In the setting of ischemic cardiomyopathy, mitral annular dilation is frequently associated with alterations in the subvalvular apparatus and regional or global LV dysfunction. Isolated annular dilatation does not usually result in moderate or severe mitral insufficiency.

Reference: Otsuji Y, Kumanohoso T, Yoshifuku S, et al. Isolated annular dilation does not usually cause important functional mitral regurgitation. *J Am Coll Cardiol* 2002;39(10):1651–1656.

8 **Answer D.** Rheumatic heart disease may result in aortic stenosis or mixed stenosis and insufficiency. Rheumatic involvement of the mitral valve always precedes aortic involvement. Isolated aortic valve disease is very uncommon. Although insufficient valvular disease may result from calcification and fixed positioning of the valve leaflets, most cases of valvular insufficiency are related to damage to the valve leaflets or supporting apparatus.

Bicuspid aortic valves demonstrate early degeneration of the valve leaflets leading to fusion of the commissures, valvular sclerosis, and significant aortic stenosis similar to what one may see in rheumatic heart disease. However, the two entities are not closely associated.

References: Chen JJ, Manning MA, Frazier AA, et al. CT angiography of the cardiac valves: normal, diseased, and postoperative appearances. *Radiographics* 2009;29(5):1393–1412.

Hughes S. Valvular heart disease. In: Suvarna SK (ed.). *Cardiac pathology*. London, UK: Springer, 2013:147–161.

9 **Answer A.** Four-chamber magnitude (left) and phase (right) images from a phase contrast in plane sequence demonstrate tricuspid regurgitation. This is seen on the phase image as the black flow jet extending into the right atrium from the tricuspid valve plane. Tricuspid regurgitation in adults is commonly secondary meaning the underlying valve apparatus is normal and intact. Annular enlargement most likely accounts for the tricuspid regurgitation seen in this patient. This is usually related to right ventricular enlargement with some etiologies including left heart failure, severe mitral disease, pulmonary hypertension, pulmonic stenosis or regurgitation, and hyperthyroidism. Primary tricuspid regurgitation (abnormality of the underlying valve apparatus) causes include injury from trauma, iatrogenic injury, infective endocarditis, marantic endocarditis, Ebstein anomaly, rheumatic valve disease, carcinoid syndrome, myxomatous degeneration resulting in prolapse, connective tissue disease, and drug related.

The images given do not demonstrate any evidence of congenital heart disease, traumatic injury, or a cardiac lead. There is right atrial and right ventricular enlargement suggesting that the etiology of tricuspid regurgitation is annular enlargement from pulmonary hypertension.

Reference: Mulla S, Siddiqui WJ. Tricuspid Regurgitation (Tricuspid Insufficiency) [Updated 2020 Feb 4]. In: *StatPearls [Internet]*. Treasure Island, FL: StatPearls Publishing, 2020. https://www.ncbi.nlm.nih.gov/books/NBK526121/

10a **Answer C.** Three-chamber view of the heart demonstrates left atrial wall calcifications and a mitral valve replacement. Left atrial wall calcifications, sometimes referred to as porcelain left atrium when extensive, are most commonly caused by rheumatic heart disease. Mitral valve stenosis or regurgitation is common chronic valvular sequelae following rheumatic fever. Aortic involvement can also be seen in rheumatic heart disease but is rare in isolation and often preceded by mitral involvement. This patient had developed mitral stenosis, which was surgically repaired. Incidentally, two cardiac leads are seen coursing through the superior vena cava.

Atrial fibrillation may be a consequence of rheumatic mitral valve disease but is not a primary cause of left atrial calcifications and mitral stenosis. Acute trauma does not cause left atrial calcifications. Systemic lupus erythematosus is not typically associated with a calcified left atrium.

References: Carapetis J, Beaton A, Cunningham M, et al. Acute rheumatic fever and rheumatic heart disease. *Nat Rev Dis Primers* 2016;2:15084.

Leacock K, et al. Porcelain Atrium: a case report with literature review. *Case Rep Radiol* 2011;2011:501396.

10b **Answer A.** Rheumatic heart disease is strongly associated with mitral stenosis and is reported in up to 99% of cases. In order to maintain filling of the left ventricle across the narrowed mitral valve, there is an increase in left atrial pressures. If left untreated over the long term, this can result in left atrial enlargement, blunting of the pulmonary venous waveforms, increased pulmonary venous and capillary wedge pressures, pulmonary hypertension, initially right ventricular hypertrophy following by enlargement, and secondary tricuspid regurgitation from annular enlargement.

Rheumatic heart disease has been reported as a cause of aortic, pulmonic, and tricuspid stenosis. However, mitral stenosis is far and away the most commonly associated valvular disease.

References: Carapetis J, Beaton A, Cunningham M, et al. Acute rheumatic fever and rheumatic heart disease. *Nat Rev Dis Primers* 2016;2:15084.

Leacock K, et al. Porcelain atrium: a case report with literature review. *Case Rep Radiol* 2011;2011:501396.

11 **Answer D.** Four-chamber (left) and three-chamber (right) bright blood images of the heart from a cardiac MRI demonstrate prolapse of the posterior mitral valve leaflet (arrowhead) with associated regurgitation (arrows).

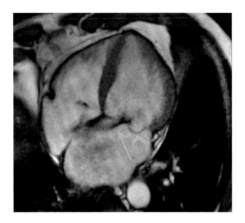 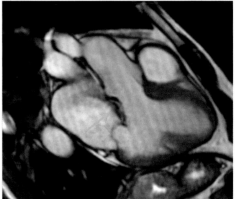

Mitral valve prolapse is defined as extension of one or both leaflets at least 2 mm beyond the mitral annular plane. Prolapse is most commonly caused by myxomatous degeneration of the valve leaflets. Clinically, the importance of prolapse lies in its association with mitral regurgitation. In this case, the patient has an eccentric jet directed anteriorly and toward the interatrial septum. The direction of the regurgitant jet can be used to predict which leaflet is abnormal. An anteriorly directed jet implies posterior leaflet pathology and vice versa. Note that although the prolapse can be seen on the four-chamber view in this case, prolapse should always be assessed on the three-chamber view since the other views can overcall this abnormality.

A flail leaflet is when the tip of the leaflet is pointed toward the left atrium during systole and is usually caused by a ruptured chordae tendineae or papillary muscle. The mitral valve is clearly not normal in this case. Mitral stenosis would show a high velocity jet going into the left ventricle during diastole.

Reference: Hayek E, Gring CN, Griffin BP. Mitral valve prolapse. *Lancet* 2005;365(9458):507–518.

12a **Answer A.** The three-chamber bright blood image of the heart demonstrates a turbulent flow jet extending from the aortic valve into the ascending aorta compatible with aortic stenosis. A regurgitant jet would extend from the aortic valve into the left ventricle. This patient does have an ascending aortic aneurysm, but the arrow does not point at this abnormality, and it is hard to assess without measurements. No pseudoaneurysm is shown.

Reference: Singh A, McCann GP. Cardiac magnetic resonance imaging for the assessment of aortic stenosis. *Heart* 2019;105:489–497.

12b **Answer C.** Short-axis gradient recall echo images of the aortic valve in systole and diastole demonstrate a bicuspid aortic valve (Sievers 1 LR) with fusion (arrow) of the left (LCC) and right (RCC) coronary cusps.

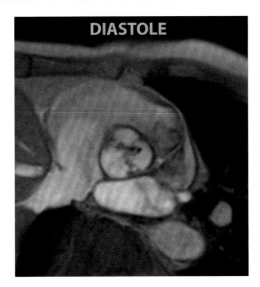

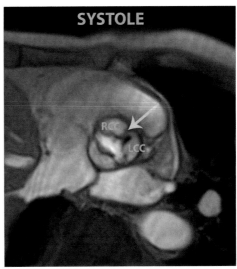

Studies suggest around 75% of patients with a bicuspid aortic valve will go on to develop fibrocalcific stenosis requiring surgery. The Sievers classification system describes three major categories of bicuspid aortic valve. Type 0 has no raphe. This is the classic "fish-mouth" appearance of the aortic valve often taught in medical school. Type 1 has one raphe. Type 2 has two raphes. The images show a Sievers 1 LR bicuspid aortic valve, which is the most common type of bicuspid. The L and R refer to which raphes are fused—in this case, the left (L) and right (R) raphes.

There is no evidence shown to suggest that this bicuspid aortic valve is iatrogenic or as a result of acute trauma. Some medications have been associated with the development of aortic stenosis but that would not explain the congenital bicuspid aortic valve.

References: Sievers HH, Schmidtke C. A classification system for the bicuspid aortic valve from 304 surgical specimens. *J Thorac Cardiovasc Surg* 2007;133(5):1226–1233.

Singh A, McCann GP. Cardiac magnetic resonance imaging for the assessment of aortic stenosis. *Heart* 2019;105:489–497.

12c **Answer C.** Bicuspid aortic valve is most commonly associated with aortic coarctation.

Reference: Mordi I, Tzemos N. Bicuspid aortic valve disease: a comprehensive review. *Cardiol Res Pract* 2012;2012:196037.

13 **Answer D.** Short-axis view of the aortic valve from a gated CT of the chest demonstrates a small well-circumscribed soft tissue mass on the noncoronary cusp of the aortic valve abutting the raphe of the noncoronary and right cusps.

Papillary fibroelastomas are the third most common primary cardiac tumor in adults and the most common tumor of the cardiac valves. Papillary fibroelastomas can become quite large and occur on any valve surface or area of the endocardium. Histologically, they are composed of a core of myxoid connective tissue containing abundant mucopolysaccharide matrix and elastic fibers that is covered by a surface endothelium. Recurrences are rare, and valve-sparing surgery should be considered whenever possible, as regrowth of partially resected lesions does not always occur.

The remaining pathologies rarely involve the valves primarily. Cardiac rhabdomyomas are the most frequently encountered primary cardiac tumor in infants and children. Cardiac rhabdomyoma arises more commonly in the ventricles, although up to 30% of cases can involve either atrium.

Patients with tuberous sclerosis have a 40% to 86% incidence of cardiac rhabdomyomas so it is an important association to screen for.

Fibromas of the heart are connective tissue tumors derived from fibroblasts and are very similar to soft tissue fibromas. About 90% of the reported cases occur in children before the age of 1 year, although fibromas can occur in any age group. Fibromas are associated with Gorlin syndrome in which patients develop odontogenic cysts, epidermal cysts, multiple nevi, and basal cell carcinomas of the skin.

Reference: Burke A, Jeudy J, Virmani R. Cardiac tumours: an update. *Heart* 2008;94(1): 117–123.

14 **Answer B.** Images show holodiastolic flow reversal in the descending thoracic aorta, which is strongly suggestive of aortic regurgitation in patients without congenital heart disease. The magnitude (left) and phase (middle) images were obtained at the level of the mid chest. The circular contours show that flow in the descending thoracic aorta was being evaluated. Holodiastolic flow reversal is seen on the flow diagram (right) as negative flow (i.e., below the X-axis) beginning at approximately 400 ms in this patient. The positive flow (i.e., above the X-axis) from approximately 0 to 400 ms on the flow diagram is the forward flow during systole.

Severe aortic coarctation may show increased flow in the distal descending thoracic aorta compared to the arch or proximal descending thoracic aorta due to reversal of flow in the intercostal arteries, which drain into the thoracic aorta. There are no findings shown to suggest an aortic aneurysm or aortic stenosis.

Reference: Bolen MA, et al. Cardiac MR assessment of aortic regurgitation: holodiastolic flow reversal in the descending aorta helps stratify severity. *Radiology* 2011;260(1):98–104.

15 **Answer B.** CT of the chest demonstrates thickening and calcification of both mitral and aortic valve leaflets, most consistent with rheumatic heart disease.

Rheumatic fever is an immunologically mediated, multisystem inflammatory disorder that occurs after an episode of group A streptococcal pharyngitis. A rheumatic carditis occurs during the active phase of rheumatic fever and may progress over time to chronic rheumatic heart disease. Significant valve thickening and commissural fusion and thickening of the chordae tendineae are characteristic by histology.

The mitral valve is most commonly affected in 65% to 70% of cases and along with the aortic valve in another 25% of cases. Tricuspid valve involvement is infrequent, and the pulmonary valve is very rarely affected.

Reference: Schoen FJ, Mitchell RN. The heart. In: Kumar V, Abbas AK, Fausto N, et al. (eds.). *Robbins and Cotran pathologic basis of disease*. Philadelphia, PA: Saunders, 2009:529–588.

16a **Answer D.** Three-chamber (left) and coronal left ventricular outflow tract (right) views of the heart from a coronary CT angiogram demonstrate a large vegetation on the noncoronary cusp of the aortic valve (arrows) and a paravalvular pseudoaneurysm with the neck just below the left aortic cusp (arrowhead). The imaging findings in conjunction with the clinical history of fevers, leukocytosis, and palpitations are consistent with infective endocarditis.

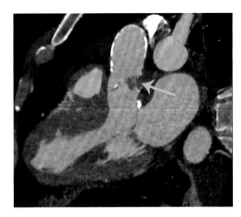 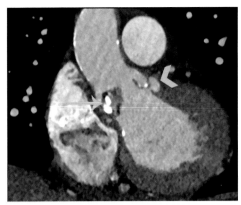

Papillary fibroelastomas are the most common primary tumor of the cardiac valves and typically involve the aortic or mitral valve. Due to the risk of embolization, they are usually surgically resected. This is not a good choice in this case due to the fevers, leukocytosis, and presence of a paravalvular pseudoaneurysm. Thrombus is the most common cardiac mass and can occur on the valves. However, they do not cause paravalvular pseudoaneurysms. In addition, with the given clinical history, an infected vegetation should always be considered first. No aortic dissection is seen.

References: Burke A, Jeudy J, Virmani R. Cardiac tumours: an update. *Heart* 2008;94(1): 117–123.

Murillo H, Restrepo CS, Marmol-Velez JA, et al. Infectious diseases of the heart: pathophysiology, clinical and imaging overview. *Radiographics* 2016;36(4):963–983.

16b **Answer C.** Best seen on the coronal left ventricular outflow tract view is a paravalvular pseudoaneurysm with the neck just below the left aortic cusp (arrowhead). Infective endocarditis can involve a native valve, prosthetic valve, or implanted cardiac device. There are many associated complications with some of the more common ones being valvular stenosis or regurgitation, paravalvular abscess, paravalvular pseudoaneurysm, arrhythmia, and distal embolic phenomenon. While echocardiography is typically the initial imaging examination, gated CT of the heart has been shown to be an excellent second-line modality particularly in the evaluation of both native and prosthetic valve complications from infective endocarditis. The images do not show an aneurysm, dissection, or pulmonary emboli.

Reference: Murillo H, Restrepo CS, Marmol-Velez JA, et al. Infectious diseases of the heart: pathophysiology, clinical and imaging overview. *Radiographics* 2016;36(4):963–983.

17 **Answer B.** Transcatheter aortic valve implantation (TAVI) has become an established treatment option for patients with aortic stenosis at prohibitive risk to undergo conventional surgical aortic valve replacement. Among potential complications that may arise with TAVI surgery, new conduction abnormalities and arrhythmias frequently occur.

New left bundle-branch block has been reported in 29% to 65% of patients after Medtronic CoreValve system and in 4% to 18% of patients receiving the balloon-expandable Edwards SAPIEN valve. In the PARTNER study, new-onset atrial fibrillation was present in 41% of patients acutely after TAVI and 9% within 30 days from the procedure.

Reference: van der Boon RMA, Houthuizen P, Nuis R-J, et al. Clinical implications of conduction abnormalities and arrhythmias after transcatheter aortic valve implantation. *Curr Cardiol Rep* 2013;16(1):1–7.

18 **Answer D.** Images show mitral annular calcifications with a large area of caseous necrosis (arrows).

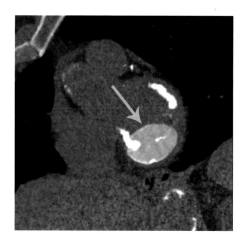 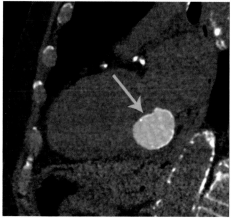

Mitral annular calcifications almost always affect the posterior annulus but can grow to involve the anterior annulus as well. This is a benign condition and not typically resected, but there are rare case reports of systemic embolization and conduction abnormalities. Caseous necrosis is a rare type of mitral annular calcification. In this case, this is seen as the large rounded high-density mass, though note that it is not as dense as the pure calcifications along the rest of the mitral annulus. This is a common pitfall encountered on cardiac MRI because the areas of caseous necrosis can have mixed T1 or T2 signal intensity rather than the absence of signal expected from a purely calcified lesion on MR.

The mixed calcifications and C-shaped distribution along the posterior mitral annulus make this most consistent with mitral annular calcifications rather than intramyocardial hemorrhage. Neither a coronary artery aneurysm nor pseudoaneurysm would be expected to be this uniformly hyperdense on a noncontrast image, and they would not be in the mitral annulus.

Reference: Shriki J, et al. Caseous mitral annular calcifications: multimodality imaging characteristics. *World J Radiol* 2010;2(4):143–147.

19 **Answer B.** The chest x-ray in Image B shows a transcatheter pulmonary valve replacement. Pulmonary valve stenosis is almost always congenital in etiology with some etiologies including tetralogy of Fallot, Williams syndrome, and Noonan syndrome. Noncongenital etiologies are rare and include rheumatic heart disease, inflammatory and infectious endocarditis, and carcinoid heart disease.

Image A shows a transcatheter aortic valve replacement. Image C shows a transcatheter tricuspid valve replacement. This patient also has a surgically repaired mitral valve. Image D shows two MitraClips, which are for repair of mitral regurgitation.

References: Arora S, Misenheimer JA, Ramaraj R. Transcatheter aortic valve replacement: comprehensive review and present status. *Tex Heart Inst J* 2017;44(1):29–38.

Asmarats L, et al. Transcatheter tricuspid valve interventions: landscape, challenges, and future directions. *J Am Coll Cardiol* 2018;71(25).

Idrizi S, Milev I, Zafirovska P, et al. Interventional treatment of pulmonary valve stenosis: a single center experience. *Open Access Maced J Med Sci* 2015;3(3):408–412.

Maggiore P, et al. Transcatheter mitral valve repair and replacement: current evidence for intervention and the role of CT in preprocedural planning—a review for radiologists and cardiologists alike. *Radiol Cardiothoracic Imaging* 2020;2(1).

Yadav, S. The diagnosis and treatment of pulmonary valve stenosis in children. *Asian J Med Sci* 2015;6(6):1–5.

20 Answer C. The horizontal long axis (four-chamber view) provides a view of both atria, atrioventricular valves, and both ventricles. The short axis may provide a supplemental view of the valves but remains limited since the leaflets move in and out of plane. Vertical long axis may provide depiction of one of the valves, depending upon which ventricle the plane passes through. Coronal projections are also suboptimal in visualizing of the valves.

Reference: Miller SW. *Cardiac imaging: the requisites.* Maryland Heights, MO: Elsevier Health Sciences, 2009.

21 Answer D. Balanced steady-state free precession images in three-chamber view (left) and en face view through the valve (right) demonstrate thickening of the aortic valve with "fish-mouth" morphology consistent with a bicuspid aortic valve.

Bicuspid aortic valve (BAV) is the most frequent congenital cardiovascular malformation in humans with a prevalence of approximately 1%. Structural abnormalities of the aortic wall commonly accompany bicuspid valves even when the valve is hemodynamically normal, potentiating aortic dilation or aortic dissection. The other available choices typically present with additional clinical history and complaints.

Reference: Schoen FJ, Mitchell RN. The heart. In: Kumar V, Abbas AK, Fausto N, et al. (eds.). *Robbins and Cotran pathologic basis of disease.* Philadelphia, PA: Saunders, 2009:529–588.

22 Answer C. Cardiac CT demonstrates marked enlargement of right-sided cardiac chambers with thickening and tethering of the anterior tricuspid leaflet, consistent with the diagnosis of carcinoid valvular disease. Notably, there is also deviation of the interventricular septum toward the left compatible with elevated right-sided pressures.

Cardiac involvement from carcinoid disease is a rare and unique manifestation typically inducing abnormalities of the right side of the heart. Valvular dysfunction in carcinoid heart disease is caused by proliferation of endocardial fibroblasts in response to chronic inflammation or induced by a number of circulating vasoactive mediators. Plaque deposition leads to thickening, retraction, and impaired leaflet motion. Compared to the right side of the heart, the left-sided valves are rarely affected because of the pulmonary metabolism and deactivation of the hormonal substances.

Eisenmenger syndrome is a complication of uncorrected large intracardiac left-to-right shunts. Long-standing shunts lead to increased pulmonary resistance leading to bidirectional shunting and then to right-to-left shunting. Rheumatic heart disease causes significant thickening of valve leaflets and valvular stenosis; however, superimposed insufficiency may result when leaflets remain fixed in an open position. Calcified deposits on the mitral valve annulus do not typically affect valvular function or otherwise become clinically important.

References: Grozinsky-Glasberg S, Grossman AB, Gross DJ. Carcinoid heart disease: from pathophysiology to treatment "something in the way it moves." *Neuroendocrinology* 2015;101(4):263–273.

Miles LF, Leong T, McCall P, Weinberg L. Carcinoid heart disease: correlation of echocardiographic and histopathological findings. *BMJ Case Reports* 2014;2014:bcr2014207732.

23 Answer C. Mitral valve prolapse (MVP) is a variable clinical syndrome that results from diverse pathogenic mechanisms. MVP occurs as a primary condition that is not associated with other diseases and can be familial or nonfamilial. It can also be associated with heritable disorders of connective tissue including Marfan syndrome, which is usually caused by mutations in fibrillin-1 (FBN-1).

Carcinoid heart disease generally involves the endocardium and valves of the right heart and is the cardiac manifestation associated with carcinoid tumors. These changes are restricted to the right side of the heart due to inactivation of both serotonin and bradykinin during passage through the lungs.

Shone syndrome classically presents with four cardiovascular defects: a supravalvular mitral membrane, valvular mitral stenosis due to a parachute mitral valve, subaortic stenosis (membranous or muscular), and aortic coarctation. Most presenting cases are incomplete with only two or three of these components present.

References: Otto CM, Bonow RO. Valvular heart disease. In: Bonow RO, Braunwald E (eds.). *Braunwald's heart disease: a textbook of cardiovascular medicine.* Philadelphia, PA: Saunders, 2012:1468–1539.

Schoen FJ, Mitchell RN. The heart. In: Kumar V, Abbas AK, Fausto N, et al. (eds.). *Robbins and Cotran pathologic basis of disease.* Philadelphia, PA: Saunders, 2009:529–588.

24a **Answer B.** The image demonstrates dilatation of the aortic root with effacement of the sinotubular junction, consistent with annuloaortic ectasia. Annuloaortic ectasia (AE) is symmetric dilation of the aortic root and ascending aorta with effacement of the sinotubular junction. AE may cause aortic regurgitation, aortic dissection, and rupture. It is most often associated with Marfan syndrome, but it can also be seen in other conditions, such as Ehlers-Danlos syndrome, osteogenesis imperfecta, or homocystinuria, or be idiopathic. Ascending aortic aneurysm is also seen in syphilis, bicuspid aortic valve, aortitis, and postoperative patients.

Rheumatic heart disease causes thickening of the aortic valve and aortic stenosis. Subvalvular aortic stenosis is the second most common form of AS and refers to narrowing at the outlet of the left ventricle just below the aortic valve.

Reference: Litmanovich D, Bankier AA, Cantin L, et al. CT and MRI in diseases of the aorta. *AJR Am J Roentgenol* 2009;193(4):928–940.

24b **Answer A.** Loeys-Dietz syndrome (LDS) is an autosomal dominant connective tissue disorder defined as those with mutations in transforming growth factor–β (TGF-β) receptor TGFBR1 (predominantly presenting with craniofacial features) and TGFBR2 (predominantly presenting with cutaneous features). LDS is characterized by the triad of arterial tortuosity and aneurysms, hypertelorism, and bifid uvula or cleft palate. Aortic root aneurysms are present in up to 98% of patients with LDS, with thoracic aortic dissection being the leading cause of death (67%), followed by abdominal aortic dissection (22%) and cerebral hemorrhage (7%).

Shone syndrome is a rare congenital heart disease comprising a series of four obstructive or potentially obstructive left-sided cardiac lesions: supravalvular mitral membrane, parachute mitral valve, subaortic stenosis (membranous or muscular), and coarctation of the aorta.

Heyde syndrome is a syndrome of aortic valve stenosis associated with gastrointestinal bleeding from colonic angiodysplasia.

Williams syndrome is a rare genetic disorder that affects a child's growth, physical appearance, and cognitive development. Cardiovascular defects include supravalvular aortic stenosis, pulmonary arterial stenosis, aortic coarctation, cardiomyopathy, tetralogy of Fallot, aortic valve defect (aortic stenosis or insufficiency), and mitral valve defect (mitral stenosis or mitral insufficiency).

References: Chu LC, Johnson PT, Dietz HC, et al. CT angiographic evaluation of genetic vascular disease: role in detection, staging, and management of complex vascular pathologic conditions. *AJR Am J Roentgenol* 2014;202(5):1120–1129.

Eronen M, Peippo M, Hiippala A, et al. Cardiovascular manifestations in 75 patients with Williams syndrome. *J Med Genet* 2002;39(8):554–558.

Islam S, Cevik C, Islam E, Attaya H, et al. Heyde's syndrome: a critical review of the literature. *J Heart Valve Dis* 2011;20(4):366–375.

Roche KJ, Genieser NB, Ambrosino MM, et al. MR findings in Shone's complex of left heart obstructive lesions. *Pediatr Radiol* 1998;28(11):841–845.

25 **Answer C.** The gradient across a valve can be estimated using the peak velocity and the Bernoulli equation ($4 \times v^2$). With a peak velocity of >4.0 m/s, the mean aortic gradient corresponds to a mean aortic valve gradient of >40 mm Hg. The peak gradient would be estimated at 64 mm Hg.

Reference: Nishimura RA, Otto CM, Bonow RO, et al.; ACC/AHA Task Force Members. 2014 AHA/ACC guideline for the management of patients with valvular heart disease: a report of the American College of Cardiology/American Heart Association Task Force on practice guidelines. *Circulation* 2014;129(23):e521–e643. doi: 10.1161/CIR.0000000000000031. Epub 2014 Mar 3. Erratum in: *Circulation* 2014;129(23):e651.

26 **Answer C.** Coronal MPR of a cardiac CT demonstrates a linear but incomplete web arising in the left ventricular outflow tract, below the level of the aortic valve.

Left ventricular outflow tract obstruction includes a spectrum of stenotic lesions that are generally categorized as subvalvular, valvular, or supravalvular. These obstructions to forward flow may present alone or in concert, as in the frequent association of a bicuspid aortic valve with coarctation of the aorta. All of these lesions impose increased afterload on the left ventricle and, if severe and untreated, result in hypertrophy and eventual dilatation and failure of the left ventricle.

Subaortic stenosis (SAS) may be focal, as in a discrete membrane, or more diffuse, resulting in a tunnel leading out of the left ventricle. Fibromuscular SAS is most frequently encountered (90%), but the tunnel-type lesions are associated with a greater degree of stenosis. Congenital valvular stenosis due to bicuspid aortic valve (BAV) occurs with an estimated incidence of 1% to 2%. BAV usually occurs in isolation but is associated with other abnormalities, the most common being coarctation of the aorta, patent ductus arteriosus, or ascending aortopathy. Supravalvular aortic stenosis (SVAS) is obstruction constriction occurring above the level of the aortic valve. SVAS is frequently associated with Williams syndrome. Aortic insufficiency results from malcoaptation of the aortic leaflets due to abnormalities of the aortic leaflets, their supporting structures (aortic root and annulus), or both.

Reference: Aboulhosn J, Child JS. Left ventricular outflow obstruction subaortic stenosis, bicuspid aortic valve, supravalvular aortic stenosis, and coarctation of the aorta. *Circulation* 2006;114(22):2412–2422.

Pericardial Disease

Alan Ropp, MD, MS • Amar B. Shah, MD, MPA • Jean Jeudy, MD

QUESTIONS

1 A patient presents with a history of dyspnea and cardiomegaly. The patient underwent a cardiac MRI. Which of the following cardiac findings is shown on the four-chamber balanced steady-state free precession image below?

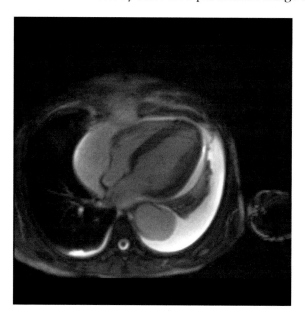

A. Atrial septal defect
B. Enlarged left ventricle
C. Mitral regurgitation
D. Pericardial effusion
E. Pericarditis

2 Assessment of pericardial thickness using cardiac MRI can be challenging due to which of the following?

A. Chemical shift artifact at the fat fluid interface
B. Higher spatial resolution compared to CT
C. Lack of motion of the pericardial layers
D. Low temporal resolution
E. Paramagnetic susceptibility

3 The pericardial abnormality shown below most likely represents which of the following?

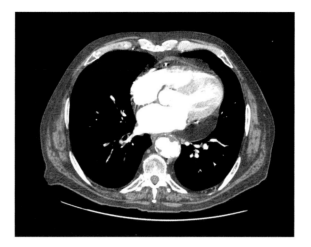

A. Constrictive pericarditis
B. Pericardial lipoma
C. Pericardial lymphoma
D. Pericarditis
E. Pneumopericardium

4 The pericardial mass can be associated with which of the following findings?

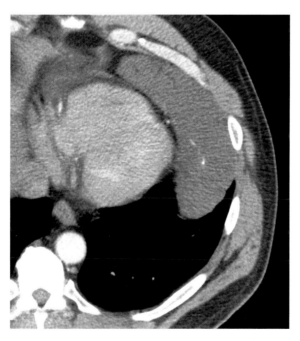

A. Fluid–fluid levels on MRI
B. Serous pericardial effusion
C. Restrictive physiology
D. Systemic malignancy
E. Prior pleurodesis

5a The image below shows which finding?

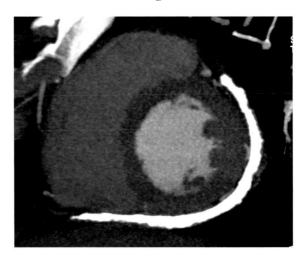

    A. Absent pericardium
    B. Calcific pericarditis
    C. Pericardial effusion
    D. Pericardial metastasis
    E. Acute pericardial hematoma

5b Physiologic and morphologic changes of constrictive pericarditis are most likely to include which of the following?

    A. Decreased right ventricular volume
    B. Decreased IVC caliber
    C. Normal-sized liver
    D. Rightward displacement of the interventricular septum
    E. Thin, distended pericardium

6 Which of the following radiographic findings is most suggestive of the underlying diagnosis?

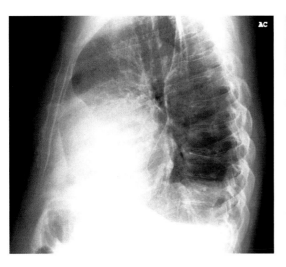
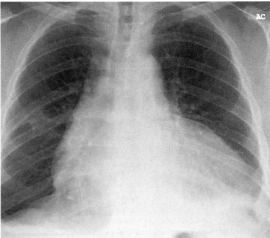

    A. Elevation of the right mainstem bronchus
    B. Pericardial calcification
    C. Separation of the epicardial and pericardial fat
    D. Widening of the mediastinum
    E. Left pleural effusion

7 The mass in the image below is best characterized by which of the following?

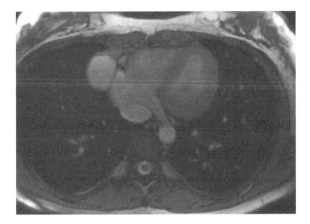

A. Compression of the cardiac chambers
B. Enhancement on postcontrast MRI
C. Intermediate signal on T1 MRI, if it is simple
D. Most commonly located at the right cardiophrenic angle
E. Septations on T2 MRI

8 Which of the following is the most likely diagnosis?

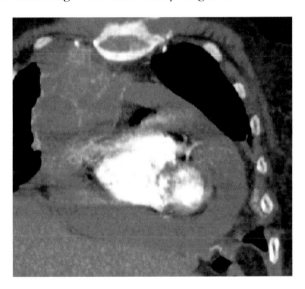

A. Calcific pericarditis
B. Constrictive pericarditis
C. Malignant pericardial effusion
D. Pericardial effusion
E. Pericardial lymphangioma

9 Based on the imaging findings, which of the following procedures would be most appropriate for treatment?

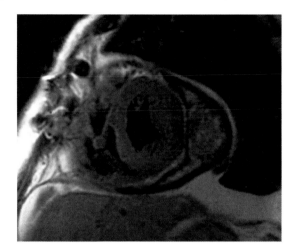

A. Aneurysmectomy
B. CABG
C. Pericardiectomy
D. Radiation therapy
E. Left atrial ablation

10 Which of the following is best associated with the image finding?

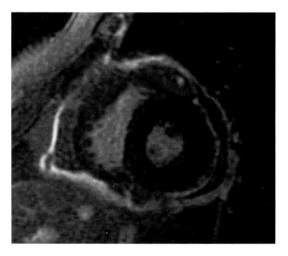

A. Absent inflammation
B. Mild disease
C. Macrophage proliferation
D. Increased neovascularization
E. Ischemia

11 What best describes the principle of ventricular interdependence as it relates to the septal bounce?

A. Increase in volume of one ventricle results in a reduced volume in the opposite ventricle.
B. The finding is decreased during inspiration.
C. Abnormal septal contractility causes a rapid shift toward the left ventricle.
D. The finding is decreased when venous return to the right heart increases.
E. Asymmetry in the His-Purkinje system plays an important role.

12a Which is the most likely diagnosis?

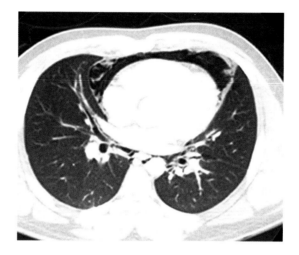

   A. Atrioesophageal fistula
   B. Bronchopleural fistula
   C. Pneumothorax
   D. Pneumopericardium
   E. Pneumoperitoneum

12b Which of the following best characterizes the physiologic findings of cardiac tamponade?

   A. Bradycardia
   B. Hypertension
   C. Normal central venous pressure
   D. Decrease in systolic blood pressure
   E. Increased heart sounds

13 A pericardial window can be performed to drain a pericardial effusion. Which of the following is true regarding a pericardial window procedure?

   A. Removal of a small segment of the pericardium
   B. Chylopericardium is a contraindication.
   C. It is performed when the pericardium is compliant.
   D. A tube should remain in place when drainage is <200 cc/24 h.
   E. Requires sternotomy

14 Restrictive and constrictive cardiac physiology can be difficult to differentiate because they share similar clinical findings. Which of the following are common in both pathologies?

   A. Systolic dysfunction
   B. Diastolic dysfunction
   C. Thickened pericardium
   D. Abnormal myocardium
   E. Ventricular discordance

15 Acute pericarditis can be a challenging diagnosis with several clinical criteria, including chest pain, pericardial friction rub, pericardial effusion, and EKG changes. Which EKG changes are most suggestive of acute pericarditis?

   A. Upward concave ST elevation and PR segment depression
   B. ST depression
   C. Delta wave
   D. Q waves

16 The image below shows pericardial fluid measuring 50 Hounsfield units in a patient with a recent left ventricular pseudoaneurysm repair presenting with chest pain and decreasing hematocrit. This most likely represents which of the following?

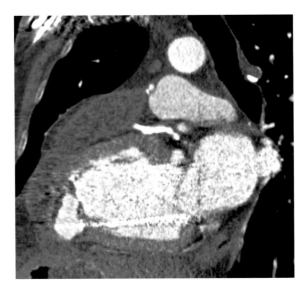

    A. Simple pericardial effusion
    B. Hemopericardium
    C. Pericardial metastasis
    D. Pneumopericardium
    E. Uremic pericarditis

17 The abnormality of the pericardium shown in the image below is most likely secondary to which of the following?

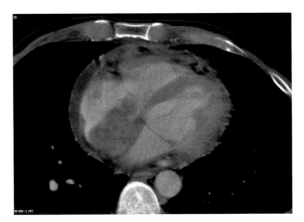

    A. Hematogenous extension
    B. Lymphangitic extension
    C. Primary pericardial origin
    D. Direct seeding of a biopsy tract
    E. Synchronous primary malignancy

18a The image below shows that the pericardial effusion is most likely secondary to which of the following?

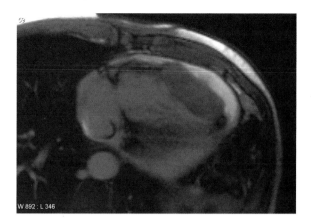

    A. Trauma
    B. Metastatic disease
    C. Infection
    D. Medication
    E. Idiopathic

18b What percentage of patients with malignant cytology will be positive?
    A. 10% to 20%
    B. 20% to 30%
    C. 50% to 60%
    D. 80% to 90%
    E. 90% to 100%

19 The rate of change of pericardial fluid volume can impact the degree of change in pericardial pressure. A sudden increase in volume will be more likely to cause acute cardiac tamponade due to pericardial pressure exceeding 30 mm Hg. This occurs because of the principle of
    A. Pericardial compliance
    B. Ventricular interdependence
    C. Ventricular dyssynchrony
    D. Ventricular compliance
    E. Systolic dysfunction

20 Increased epicardial fat deposition is associated with
    A. Acute myocarditis
    B. Cardiovascular disease
    C. Metastatic disease
    D. Prior inflammation
    E. Prior trauma

21 Which best describes the role of CT compared with MRI in the diagnosis of pericarditis?
    A. CT more accurately measures pericardial thickness.
    B. CT more accurately measures pericardial enhancement.
    C. CT more accurately measures changes in SVC flow.
    D. CT more accurately evaluates restriction of pericardial movement.
    E. CT more accurately depicts fluid from pericardial thickening.

22 Pericardial thickness measuring greater than what value is associated with pericarditis?

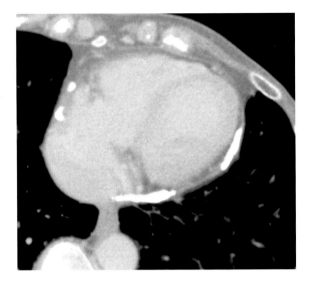

A. 2 mm
B. 3 mm
C. 4 mm
D. 5 mm
E. Pericardial thickening is not associated with pericarditis.

23 The patient in the image below presents with a history of acute chest pain. What is the cause of the abnormality?

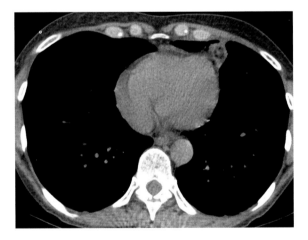

A. Calcific pericarditis
B. Epicardial fat necrosis
C. Hemorrhagic pericardial effusion
D. Pericardial metastasis
E. Lymphoma

24 The pericardial mass imaged below demonstrates what feature that is atypical of a simple pericardial cyst?

A. Fat signal
B. Fluid signal
C. Invasion of the pulmonary artery
D. Septations
E. Internal hemorrhage

25 What is the underlying abnormality shown in the images below?

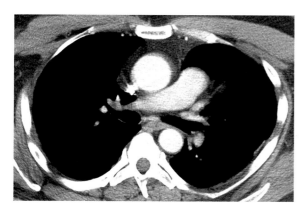 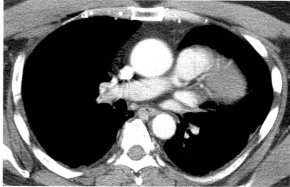

    A. Lung torsion
    B. The luftsichel sign
    C. Pneumomediastinum
    D. Congenital absence of the pericardium
    E. Pneumopericardium

26 The patient is a 63-year-old male with a history of primary lung adenocarcinoma. What is the most likely explanation for the finding designated by the arrow in the image below?

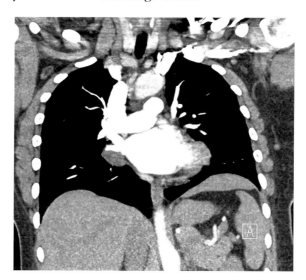

    A. Hamartoma
    B. Azygos vein
    C. Prominent thoracic duct
    D. Metastatic lymph node
    E. Fluid in a pericardial recess

27 Which of the following complications would this patient be most at risk for?

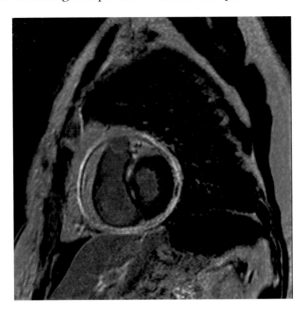

A. Pericardial tamponade
B. Cardiac torsion
C. Increased ventricular interdependence
D. Acute valvular insufficiency
E. Ventricular aneurysm

28 What is the most likely cause of the pericardial abnormality shown in the image below of a patient with surfactant deficiency and pulmonary interstitial emphysema?

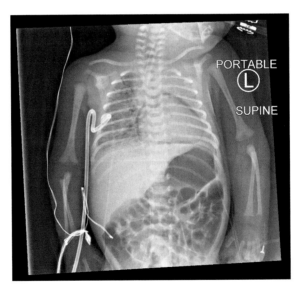

A. Positive pressure ventilation
B. Pericardial hemorrhage
C. Infection with gas-forming organism
D. Artifact
E. Mediastinal lipomatosis

29 The dynamic finding in the cine MRI below occurs due to what underlying change in physiology?

   A. Reduced left ventricular contractility
   B. Ventricular interdependence
   C. Left to right shunting
   D. Severe tricuspid stenosis
   E. Right to left shunting

30 Which of the following images with stars designates the superior aortic pericardial recess?

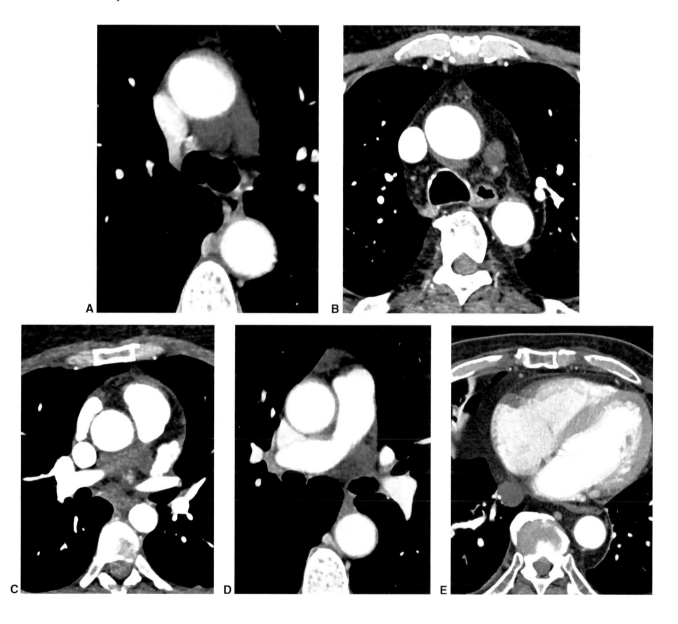

31 What is the arrow pointing to in the image below?

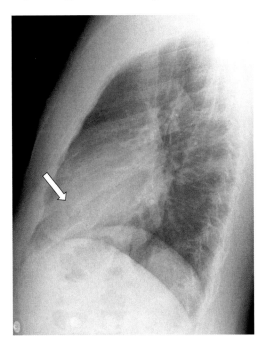

A. Epicardial fat
B. Pneumopericardium
C. Mediastinal fat
D. Pneumomediastinum
E. Artifact

ANSWERS AND EXPLANATIONS

1 **Answer D.** Note the moderate volume T2 hyperintense fluid surrounding the heart, within the pericardium. The normal pericardium is a thin sac composed of two layers enveloping the heart (an inner serous membrane and an outer fibrocollagenous layer). Normally, the pericardium contains only 10 to 50 mL of an ultrafiltrate of plasma. Pericardial fluid exceeding this volume is considered an effusion. This effusion is large enough to exert mass effect on the right heart.

References: Bogaert J, Francone M. Cardiovascular magnetic resonance in pericardial diseases. *J Cardiovasc Magn Reson* 2009;11:14.

Roberts WC, Spray TL. Pericardial heart disease: a study of its causes, consequences, and morphologic features. *Cardiovasc Clin* 1976;7:11–65.

2 **Answer A.** The pericardium normally measures up to 2 mm in systole and 1 mm at diastole. However, accurate measurement of the pericardium on MRI can be challenging. MRI has been shown to overestimate the pericardial thickness, which may be secondary to chemical shift artifact, spatial resolution limits, and motion of the pericardial layers.

References: Bogaert J, Francone M. Cardiovascular magnetic resonance in pericardial diseases. *J Cardiovasc Magn Reson* 2009;11:14.

Sechtem U, Tscholakoff D, Higgins CB. MRI of the abnormal pericardium. *AJR Am J Roentgenol* 1986;147:245–252.

3 **Answer B.** Primary pericardial tumors are uncommon. Pericardial lipomas have been reported to account for 10% of all primary pericardial neoplasms. The mass will be of fat attenuation and well encapsulated. These tumors are usually incidental and asymptomatic. Tumors may become symptomatic if there is significant compression of the cardiac chambers.

References: Steger CM. Intrapericardial giant lipoma displacing the heart. *ISRN Cardiol* 2011;2011:4. http://dx.doi.org/10.5402/2011/243637

Stoian I, et al. Rare tumors of the heart-angiosarcoma, pericardial lipoma, leiomyosarcoma, three case reports. *J Med Life* 2010;3(2):178–182. Published online 2010 May 25.

4 **Answer A.** The above mass is low density, septated, and contains calcifications, most characteristic of pericardial lymphangioma. The mass contains no areas of nodularity or enhancement, indicating it is not due to a primary cardiac malignancy or metastatic disease. Pericardial lymphangiomas are uncommon primary tumors usually diagnosed as an incidental finding. Pericardial lymphangiomas can display fluid–fluid levels of high signal intensity on T2-weighted images due to cystic spaces. They may extend into the mediastinum, potentially causing compression of cardiac or adjacent mediastinal structures. If severe enough, this can cause respiratory distress or altered cardiac function.

References: Shaheen F, Lone N. A rare case of pericardial lymphangioma causing tamponade: routine and dynamic MR findings. *Eur J Radiol Extra* 2009;69(1):e9–e10.

Zakaria RH, et al. Imaging of pericardial lymphangioma. *Ann Pediatr Cardiol* 2011;4(1):65–67. doi:10.4103/0974-2069.79628.

5a **Answer B.** The image shows the pericardium is thickened (measuring >4 mm) and densely calcified along the lateral and inferior wall of the heart. These findings are compatible with calcific pericarditis. Calcific pericarditis can be secondary to prior inflammation, infection (tuberculosis), connective tissue disease, radiation therapy, or uremia. The finding of calcifications can be associated with constrictive physiology.

References: Macgregor JH, Chen JT, Chiles C, et al. The radiographic distinction between pericardial and myocardial calcifications. *AJR Am J Roentgenol* 1987;148(4):675–677.

Wang ZJ, Reddy GP, Gotway MB, et al. CT and MR imaging of pericardial disease. *Radiographics* 2003;23:S167–S180.

5b **Answer A.** Constrictive pericarditis can be associated with decreased right ventricular volume, dilation of the IVC and SVC, hepatomegaly, and ascites. The interventricular septum can be displaced toward the left ventricle or develop a sigmoid shape.

References: Higgins CB. Acquired heart disease. In: Higgins CB, Hricak H, Helms CA (eds.). *Magnetic resonance imaging of the body*. Philadelphia, PA: Lippincott-Raven, 1997:409–460.

Wang ZJ, Reddy GP, Gotway MB, et al. CT and MR imaging of pericardial disease. *Radiographics* 2003;23:S167–S180.

6 **Answer C.** The patient has a large pericardial effusion. While radiography is not sensitive for the diagnosis of a pericardial effusion, large effusions can be identified using several radiographic findings. In the above example, the effusion is best visualized on the lateral view and is outlined by the epicardial and pericardial fat ("oreo cookie sign"). Other findings suggestive of a pericardial effusion include a dilated cardiac silhouette and widening of the subcarinal angle (splaying of the carina).

References: Chen JT, Putman CE, Hedlund LW, et al. Widening of the subcarinal angle by pericardial effusion. *AJR Am J Roentgenol* 1982;139(5):883–887.

Wang ZJ, Reddy GP, Gotway MB, et al. CT and MR imaging of pericardial disease. *Radiographics* 2003;23:S167–S180.

7 **Answer D.** The image shows a mass at the right cardiophrenic angle that is most compatible with a pericardial cyst. Pericardial cysts are most commonly located at the right cardiophrenic angle, have increased T2 signal, are not typically septated, and have no enhancement. Pericardial cysts are formed during development of the pericardial sac and while most common at the right cardiophrenic angle, can be located in the anterior and posterior mediastinum. Less commonly, pericardial cysts can cause compression or become infected.

References: Patel J, Park C, Michaels J, et al. Pericardial cyst: case reports and a literature review. *Echocardiography* 2004;21:269–272.

White CS. MR evaluation of the pericardium. *Top Magn Reson Imaging* 1995;7:258–266.

8 **Answer C.** The image shows a large pericardial effusion with septations and nodular enhancement of the pericardium, compatible with a malignant pericardial effusion. Nodular pericardial thickening in addition to enlarged mediastinal lymph nodes indicates a malignant pericardial effusion. While the above imaging findings are suggestive of malignant effusions, fluid-based sampling is helpful to confirm the diagnosis of a malignant effusion.

References: Rienmüller R, Gröll R, Lipton MJ. CT and MR imaging of pericardial disease. *Radiol Clin North Am* 2004;42:587–601.

Sun JS, Park KJ, Kang DK. CT findings in patients with pericardial effusion: differentiation of malignant and benign disease. *Am J Roentgenol* 2010;194(6):W489–W494.

9 **Answer C.** The above patient has a thickened pericardium with a pericardial hematoma and compression of the right heart, indicating constrictive pericarditis. The patient underwent a pericardiectomy. Pericardiectomy can be performed via either a median sternotomy or anterolateral thoracotomy and is the definitive treatment for constrictive pericarditis. During the procedure, the pericardium is removed to the greatest extent possible. However, despite technical success, hemodynamics may not return to normal.

References: Maisch B, Seferovic PM, Ristic AD, et al. Guidelines on the diagnosis and management of pericardial diseases. *Eur Soc Cardiol* 2004;25(7):587–610.

Tiruvoipati R, Naid RD, Loubani M, et al. Surgical approach for pericardiectomy: a comparative study between median sternotomy and left anterolateral thoracotomy. *Cardiovasc Thorac Surg* 2003;2(3):322–326. doi:10.1016/S1569-9293(03)00074-4.

10 **Answer D.** The patient has pericarditis with a thickened pericardium and late gadolinium enhancement of the underlying epicardium. The presence of late gadolinium enhancement in pericarditis is associated with increased inflammation, neovascularization, proliferation of fibroblasts, and granulation tissue, indicating ongoing inflammation. Patients without late gadolinium enhancement but a thickened pericardium are more likely to be associated with mild or absent inflammation.

References: Srichai MB. CMR imaging in constrictive pericarditis: is seeing believing? *J Am Coll Cardiol Imaging* 2011;4(11):1192–1194. doi:10.1016/j.jcmg.2011.09.009.

Young PM, Glockner JF, Williamson EE. MR imaging findings in 76 consecutive surgically proven cases of pericardial disease with CT and pathologic correlation. *Int J Cardiovasc Imaging* 2012;28(5):1099–1109.

11 **Answer A.** The principle of ventricular interdependence defines how the increase in volume of one ventricle causes a decreased volume in the opposite ventricle. The septal bounce is characterized by the movement of the interventricular septum, initially toward the left ventricle and subsequently away from the left ventricle during early diastole. Since right ventricular filling occurs before left ventricular filling, the increased right ventricular volume will shift the septum toward the left. This will reverse as the left ventricle subsequently fills. In the setting of increased venous return, such as during inspiration, the septal bounce will be exaggerated.

References: Giorgi B, Mollet NR, Dymarkowski S, et al. Clinically suspected constrictive pericarditis: MR imaging assessment of ventricular septal motion and configuration in patients and healthy subjects. *Radiology* 2003;228:417–424.

Walker CM, Chung JH, Reddy GP. Septal bounce. *J Thorac Imaging* 2012;27(1):w1. doi:10.1097/RTI.0b013e31823fdfbd.

12a **Answer D.** The patient has extensive pneumopericardium with air between the pericardium and right atrium and ventricle. Pneumopericardium can be secondary to trauma (blunt or penetrating), postoperative, infectious, or a fistula. Pneumomediastinum is also present.

References: Bejvan SM, Bejvan SM, Godwin JD. Pneumomediastinum: old signs and new signs. *AJR Am J Roentgenol* 1996;166(5):1041–1048.

Karoui M, Bucur PO. Images in clinical medicine. Pneumopericardium. *N Engl J Med* 2008;359(14):e16. doi:10.1056/NEJMicm074422.

12b **Answer D.** Patients with cardiac tamponade physiology will have dyspnea, tachycardia, and elevated jugular venous pressure. Several other clinical finding complexes have also been reported, including the following:

Beck triad—hypotension, elevated jugular venous pressure, and muffled heart sounds

Pulsus paradoxus—>10 mm Hg decrease in systolic blood pressure during inspiration

Kussmaul sign—paradoxical increase in jugular venous pressure during inspiration

References: Roy CL, Minor MA, Brookhart MA, et al. Does this patient with a pericardial effusion have cardiac tamponade? *JAMA* 2007;297(16):9.

Yarlagadda C. Cardiac tamponade clinical presentation. *Medscape*. November 28, 2018. http://emedicine.medscape.com/article/152083-clinical#a0256

13 **Answer A.** A pericardial window is performed either for diagnosis or therapy to drain the accumulated pericardial fluid. The procedure is performed by placing a drain after a small amount of the pericardium has been removed, usually via a subxiphoid approach. Indications include symptomatic or asymptomatic effusion, chylous effusion, purulent effusion, delayed hemopericardium, or reaccumulating effusion. Concomitant surgery requiring a sternotomy and full pericardiectomy is a contraindication to a pericardial window.

References: Komanapalli C, Sukumar M. *Thoracoscopic pericardial window*. August 30, 2010. http://www.ctsnet.org/sections/clinicalresources/thoracic/expert_tech-32.html

Muller DK. Pericardial window. *Medscape*. December 02, 2016. http://emedicine.medscape.com/article/1829679-overview

14 **Answer B.** Constrictive pericarditis and restrictive cardiomyopathy may have overlapping clinical findings, which include diastolic dysfunction and normal to near-normal systolic function. Imaging plays a key role in diagnosis by distinguishing between a thickened and enhancing pericardium in pericarditis and abnormal myocardium with late gadolinium enhancement in restrictive cardiomyopathy. Constrictive physiology will typically demonstrate LV-RV discordance, while restrictive cardiomyopathy will not.

References: Chinnaiyan KM, Leff CB, Marsalese DL. Constrictive pericarditis versus restrictive cardiomyopathy: challenges in diagnosis and management. *Cardiol Rev* 2004;12(6):314–320.

Mookadam F, Jiamsripong P, Raslan SF, et al. Constrictive pericarditis and restrictive cardiomyopathy in the modern era. *Future Cardiol* 2011;7(4):471–483. doi:10.2217/fca.11.18.

15 **Answer A.** EKG changes in pericarditis include upward, concave ST elevation and PR segment depression. The ST elevation reflects underlying epicardial inflammation and along with the PR depression occurs early in the disease process. Over time, the ST and PR segments will return to normal and may lead to T-wave inversion, which can normalize. Delta waves are associated with Wolff-Parkinson white syndrome, while Q waves are associated with prior myocardial infarction.

References: Ginzton LE, Laks MM. The differential diagnosis of acute pericarditis from the normal variant: new electrocardiographic criteria. *Circulation* 1982;65(5):1004–1009.

Khandaker MH, Espinosa RE, Nishimura RA, et al. Pericardial disease: diagnosis and management. *Mayo Clin Proc* 2010;85(6):572–593. doi:10.4065/mcp.2010.0046.

16 **Answer B.** Hemopericardium is the accumulation of blood in the pericardial sac. Hemopericardium can be secondary to aneurysm rupture, trauma (blunt or penetrating), dissection, anticoagulation, or iatrogenic. If the volume of blood accumulates rapidly, cardiac tamponade can occur.

References: Krejci CS, Blackmore CC, Nathens A. Hemopericardium an emergent finding in a case of blunt cardiac injury. *Am J Roentgenol* 2000;175:250–250. http://www.ajronline.org/doi/full/10.2214/ajr.175.1.1750250

Levis JT, Delgado MC. Hemopericardium and cardiac tamponade in a patient with an elevated international normalized ratio. *West J Emerg Med* 2009;10(2):115–119.

17 **Answer B.** Cardiac metastases can involve the heart via hematogenous or lymphatic pathways and usually occur late in the disease process. Lymphatic pathways lead to pericardial involvement, while hematogenous pathways lead to cardiac involvement. Lung cancer, breast cancer, lymphoma, and melanoma are the most common cause of cardiac metastasis and often also involve the pericardium.

References: Chiles C, Woddard PK, Gutierrez FR, et al. Metastatic involvement of the heart and pericardium: CT and MR imaging. *Radiographics* 2001;21(2):439–449.

Reynen K, Kockeritz U, Strasser RH. Metastases to the heart. *Ann Oncol* 2004;15(3):375–381. doi:10.1093/annonc/mdh086.

18a **Answer B.** The image shows a mass in the free wall of the right ventricle representing cardiac metastasis. A malignant pericardial effusion is also present. The diagnosis of a malignant pericardial effusion can be confirmed via pericardiocentesis. Treatment options include pericardial window, radiation therapy, or infusion of a sclerosing agent.

References: Chiles C, Woddard PK, Gutierrez FR, et al. Metastatic involvement of the heart and pericardium: CT and MR imaging. *Radiographics* 2001;21(2):439–449.

Millaire A, Wurtz A, De Groote P, et al. Malignant pericardial effusions: usefulness of pericardioscopy. *Am Heart J* 1992;124:1030–1034.

18b **Answer D.** Malignant pericardial effusions can be diagnosed via pericardiocentesis. Cytology studies are positive in 80% to 90% of patients with malignant pericardial effusions. The finding of a malignant effusion has been associated with decreased survival.

References: Maher EA, Shepherd FA, Todd TJ. Pericardial sclerosis as the primary management of malignant pericardial effusion and cardiac tamponade. *J Thorac Cardiovasc Surg* 1996;112:637–643.

Meyers DG, Bouska DJ. Diagnostic usefulness of pericardial fluid cytology. *Chest* 1989;95:1142–1143.

19 **Answer A.** If pericardial fluid accumulates rapidly, a volume of 100 can lead to pericardial pressure increasing by >30 mm Hg. The sudden rise in pressure is secondary to limits of pericardial compliance, as the rapid change does not allow for the pericardium to stretch to accommodate the increasing volume.

References: Holt JP, Rhode EA, Kines H. Pericardial and ventricular pressure. *Circ Res* 1960;8:1171–1181.

Shabetai R. Pericardial effusion: haemodynamic spectrum. *Heart*. 2004;90(3):255–256. doi:10.1136/hrt.2003.024810.

20 **Answer B.** Increased epicardial fat deposition (fat between the heart and visceral pericardium) has been suggested to contribute to coronary artery disease, increased coronary plaque burden, adverse cardiac events, and atrial fibrillation.

Reference: Dey D, Nakazato R, Li D, et al. Epicardial and thoracic fat-noninvasive measurement and clinical implications. *Cardiovasc Diagn Ther* 2012;2(2):85–93. doi:10.3798/j.issn.2223-3652.2012.04.03.

21 **Answer A.** CT is more accurate than MR to identify pericardial thickening and pericardial enhancement in patients with suspected pericarditis. MRI can better identify delayed pericardial enhancement, restricted movement of the pericardium, and changes in blood flow. Distinguishing between small effusion and mild pericardial thickening can be a limitation of CT.

References: Feng D, Glockner J, Kim K, et al. Cardiac magnetic resonance imaging pericardial late gadolinium enhancement and elevated inflammatory markers can predict the reversibility of constrictive pericarditis after anti-inflammatory medical therapy: a pilot study. *Circulation* 2011;124(17):1830–1837. doi:10.1161/circulationaha.111.026070.

Wang ZJ, Reddy GP, Gotway MB, et al. CT and MR imaging of pericardial disease. *Radiographics* 2003;23:S167–S180. doi:10.1148/rg.23si035504.

22 **Answer B.** The normal pericardium will measure <4 mm on CT and will usually measure between 1 and 2 mm. A thickened pericardium can be suggestive of acute pericarditis. However, this should be interpreted in the context of clinical findings. Evaluation for the presence of late gadolinium enhancement on MRI will also help to confirm the diagnosis.

References: Ling LH, Oh JK, Breen JF, et al. Calcific constrictive pericarditis: is it still with us? *Ann Intern Med* 2000;132(6):444–450.

Maisch B, Seferovic PM, Ristic AD, et al. Guidelines on the diagnosis and management of pericardial diseases executive summary: the task force on the diagnosis and management of pericardial diseases of the European Society of Cardiology. *Eur Heart J* 2004;25(7):587–610.

23 Answer B. Epicardial fat necrosis is a self-limited cause of acute chest pain. It is an uncommon cause of pain and can be associated with mass adjacent to the pericardium on CT. The image will show infiltrated/necrotic fat. The mass may be mistaken for a diaphragmatic hernia, fat-containing thymic tumor, sarcoma, or lipoma.

References: Fred HL. Pericardial fat necrosis: a review and update. *Texas Heart Inst J* 2010;37(1):82–84.

Van den Heuvel DAF, Van Es HW, Cirkel GA, et al. Images in thorax: acute chest pain caused by pericardial fat necrosis. *Thorax* 2010;65(2):188. doi:10.1136/thx.2009.114637.

24 Answer D. The balanced steady state free precession image shows a septated pericardial mass. The septations indicate that the mass is not a simple pericardial cyst. Balanced steady state free precessions' sequences have both fat and fluid weighing.

Reference: Bogaert J, Francone M. Pericardial disease: value of CT and MR imaging. *Radiology* 2013;267(2):340–356.

25 Answer D. The image demonstrates leftward rotation of the cardiac apex with interposition of lung between the aorta and pulmonary artery. This is a characteristic appearance of congenital absence of the pericardium. With pneumomediastinum or pneumopericardium curvilinear lucency can be observed outlining the pericardium, cardiac, or mediastinal structures, which remain intact.

Lung torsion occurs when there is free rotation of the lung parenchyma around its bronchovascular pedicle, with the appearance of atelectatic lung and most notably occurring in the setting of previous lobectomy or pneumonectomy. The Luftsichel sign occurs in the setting of left upper lobe collapse and subsequent hyperinflation of the left lower lobe. On plain radiographs, this has the appearance of curvilinear lucency between the lung and aortic arch.

Reference: Cipriani A, Brunetti G, Bernardinello G, et al. Expert Analysis: Congenital Pericardial Agenesis. American College of Cardiology. Latest in Cardiology > Congenital Pericardial Agenesis. July 27, 2020. https://www.acc.org/latest-in-cardiology/articles/2020/07/27/09/25/congenital-pericardial-agenesis

26 Answer E. The right inferior pulmonary vein pericardial sleeve recess is a common location for the accumulation of a small amount of physiologic pericardial fluid. It may be mistaken for lymphadenopathy but will typically measure as simple fluid with a Hounsfield unit range of 0 to 10.

Reference: Truong MT, Erasmus JJ, Sabloff BS, et al. Pericardial "sleeve" recess of right inferior pulmonary vein mimicking adenopathy: computed tomography findings. *J Comput Assist Tomogr* 2004;28 (3):361–365.

27 Answer C. The image shows diffuse pericardial thickening and gadolinium enhancement of the pericardium. This could lead to constrictive pericarditis, a possible cause of increased ventricular interdependence.

Reference: Wang ZJ, Reddy GP, Gotway MB, et al. CT and MR imaging of pericardial disease. *Radiographics* 2003;23:S167–S180.

28 Answer A. The image depicts pneumopericardium. Of the options listed, positive pressure ventilation is the most likely cause.

Reference: O'Neill D, Symon D. Pneumopericardium and pneumomediastinum complicating endotracheal intubation. *Postgrad Med J* 1979;55:273–275.

29 **Answer B.** In the setting of constrictive pericarditis or pericardial tamponade, a global increase in the external pressure exerted on the heart results in an increase in ventricular interdependence. This occurs when an increase in volume of one ventricle results in a decrease in volume of the opposite ventricle. During inspiration, negative intrathoracic pressure results in increased venous return to the heart. In the setting of constrictive pericarditis or tamponade, this increased blood volume results in the "septal bounce" appreciated when the septum briefly, and seemingly paradoxically, deviates toward the left ventricle as the right ventricular volume exceeds the left. This effect is reversed during exhalation.

Reference: Walker C, Chung J, Reddy G. Septal bounce. *J Thorac Imaging* 2012;27(1):1.

30 **Answer A.** This is the superior aortic pericardial recess containing a small amount of fluid. These may be mistaken for lymph nodes but are normal anatomic structures that may contain a small amount of physiologic fluid.

Reference: Truong MT, Erasmus EJ, Gladish GW, et al. Anatomy of pericardial recesses on multidetector CT: implications for oncologic imaging. *AJR Am J Roentgenol* 2003;181: 1109–1113.

31 **Answer A.** This lateral radiograph shows a large pericardial effusion. The inner or deep lucent stripe along the heart border represents the epicardial fat. The fluid density surrounding the heart represents the pericardial effusion, and the outer or superficial lucent stripe represents the surrounding mediastinal fat and lung. This is known as the "oreo cookie" sign.

Reference: Li I, Greenstein J, Hahn B. Pericardial effusion with oreo cookie sign. *J Emerg Med* 2017;52(5):756–757.

Joe Y. Hsu, MD • Jean Jeudy, MD

QUESTIONS

1 What cardiac abnormality is suggested by the following image?

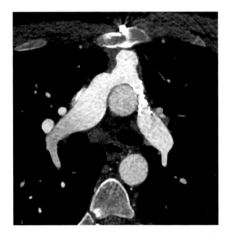 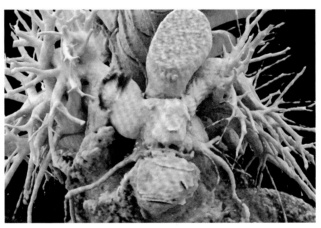

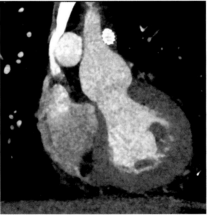

A. Ebstein anomaly
B. Tetralogy of Fallot
C. Transposition of great arteries
D. Shone syndrome

2 In this patient with hypoplastic left heart syndrome, the creation of this shunt reflects which stage of surgical palliation?

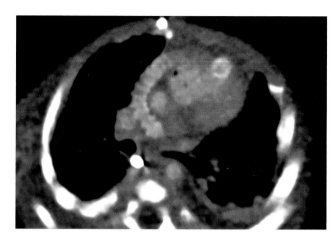 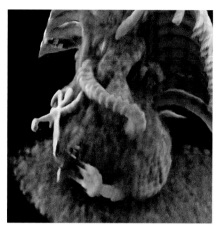

    A. Norwood procedure
    B. Modified Glenn procedure
    C. Fontan procedure
    D. Blalock-Taussig procedure

3 Patient with a history of surgically corrected congenital heart disease presents as an adult with portal hypertension and liver failure? Which congenital disorder could be implicated as an etiology for the current pathology?

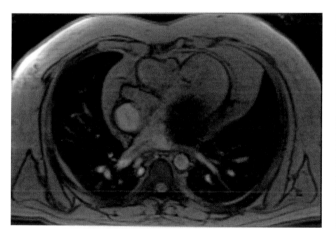 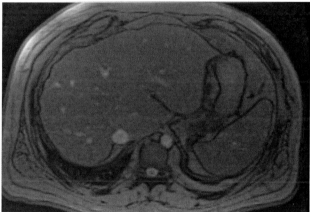

    A. Tetralogy of Fallot
    B. Tricuspid atresia
    C. Truncus arteriosus
    D. Transposition of the great arteries

4 A patient presenting with the following anatomy (images below). Which of the following associations may be seen with this abnormality?

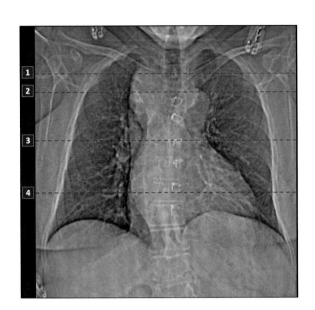

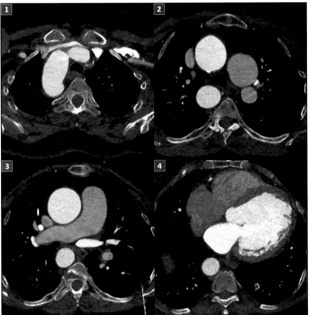

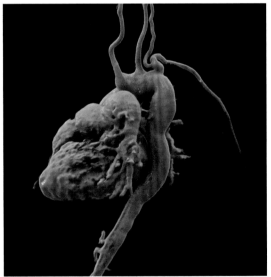

A. Dysphagia and tracheal compression
B. Conotruncal anomalies
C. Circumflex variant with contralateral left-sided descending thoracic aorta
D. Aortic outpouching called diverticulum of Kommerell

5 A 25-year-old patient presents with increasing shortness of breath and signs of early heart failure. Echocardiography demonstrates no evidence of intracardiac shunt. Cardiac MRI confirms and reveals normal pulmonary veins and normal vena cava. Phase-contrast imaging demonstrates $Q_p/Q_s < 0.4$.
Which of the following would be the most likely diagnosis?

A. Ventricular septal defect
B. Unroofed coronary sinus
C. Anomalous pulmonary vein
D. Patent ductus arteriosus

6 A patient has a history of tetralogy of Fallot status post surgical correction as a child. The patient was lost to follow up and now presents for new baseline imaging. Which of the following would be an unexpected finding?

A. Aortic root dilatation
B. Atrial and ventricular arrhythmias
C. Supravalvular aortic stenosis
D. Pulmonic insufficiency

7a A patient without any significant past medical history presents to the emergency department with mild chest pressure. Which of the following best characterizes the image findings?

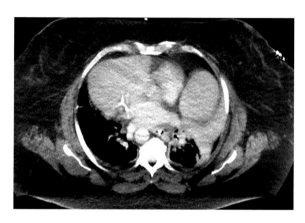 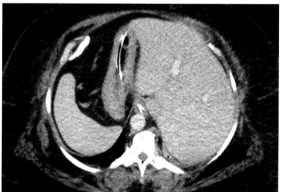

A. Levocardia, situs inversus
B. Levocardia, situs solitus
C. Dextrocardia, situs inversus
D. Dextrocardia, situs solitus

7b A rotating medical student reviews the anatomy of the case with you after you report the findings to the emergency physician. How would you characterize the bronchial anatomy to pulmonary artery?

A. Right eparterial; left eparterial
B. Right hyparterial; left eparterial
C. Right eparterial; left hyparterial
D. Right hyparterial; left hyparterial

8a A 48-year-old presents with heart murmur. What is the most likely underlying condition based on the chest radiographs?

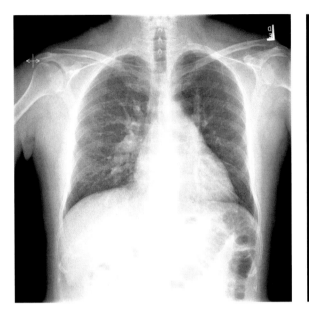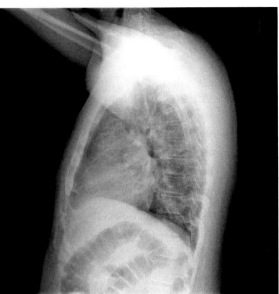

A. Aortic stenosis
B. Mitral stenosis
C. Atrial septal defect (ASD)
D. Normal
E. Ebstein anomaly

8b Patient has a follow-up chest radiograph months later. Which of the following is a contraindication to the procedure that was done?

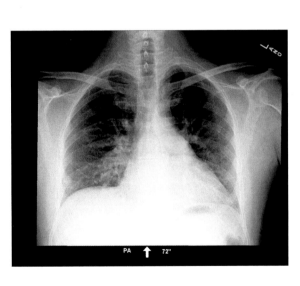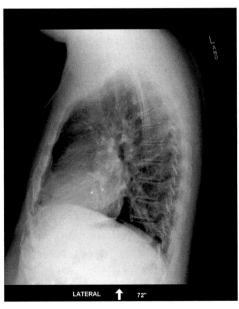

A. $Q_p/Q_s > 2$
B. Atrial fibrillation
C. Lack of adequate rims
D. Bilateral iliac artery thrombosis

8c Which of the following is a potential long-term complication of septal occluder device placement?

A. Atrial fibrillation
B. Heart block
C. Embolization/malpositioning
D. Erosion of the device

9 What is the treatment for this condition?

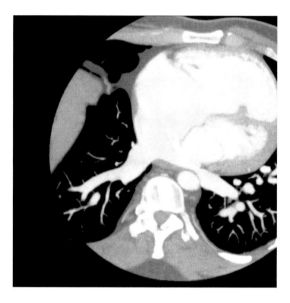

A. Medical
B. Surgical
C. Endovascular
D. None

10a This was an incidental finding on a gated CTA of an asymptomatic patient. What is the best next step?

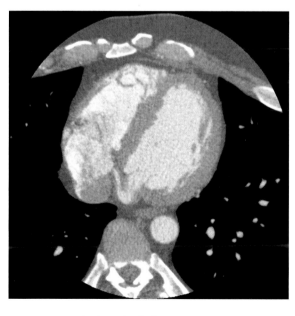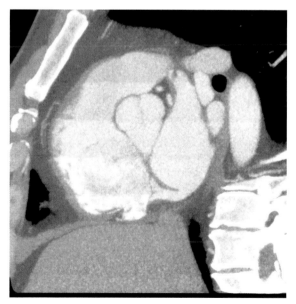

A. Surgical closure
B. Catheter-based closure
C. Leave it alone.

10b Unroofed coronary sinus is associated with which of the following vascular abnormalities?

    A. Azygos continuation of the IVC

    B. Coarctation of the aorta

    C. Anomalous right pulmonary venous return

    D. Left-sided SVC

11 How many types of atrial septal defects (ASD) are there?

    A. There are two types of ASD.

    B. There are three types of ASD.

    C. There are four types of ASD.

    D. There are five types of ASD.

12 What is a major difference between membranous versus muscular ventricular septal defects (VSD)?

    A. Muscular VSD can undergo spontaneous closure.

    B. Membranous VSD can undergo spontaneous closure.

    C. Endocarditis prophylaxis is not required for muscular VSD.

    D. Endocarditis prophylaxis is not required for membranous VSD.

13a A 61-year-old female presents with shortness of breath. What is the best next step?

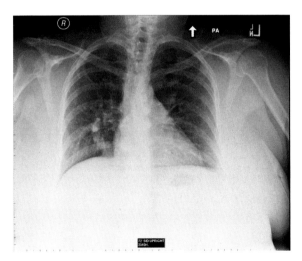 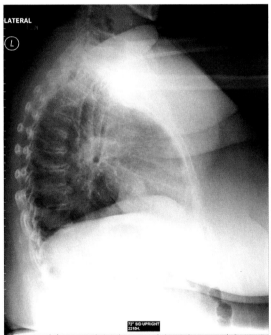

    A. Biopsy

    B. CT of the chest without contrast

    C. CTA of the chest

    D. VQ scan

    E. No further imaging necessary

13b No atrial septal defect was seen in this patient. What type of shunt does the patient have?

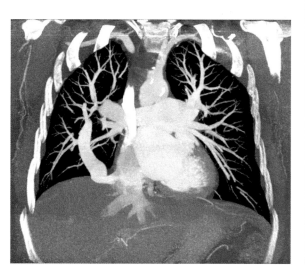 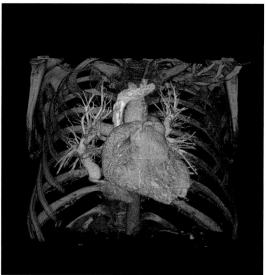

    A. Left to right
    B. Right to left
    C. No shunt

14 A patient with subaortic stenosis presents for a CTA of the chest demonstrating the following additional finding. What other abnormality should you also look for to exclude Shone complex/syndrome?

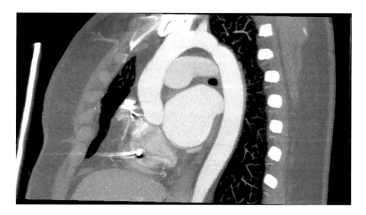

    A. Parachute mitral valve
    B. Bicuspid aortic valve
    C. Sex chromosomal abnormality (XO)
    D. Cor triatriatum

15 What valves are switched in Ross procedure?

    A. Mitral to tricuspid
    B. Aortic to pulmonic
    C. Pulmonic to aortic
    D. Mitral to pulmonic

16   A 51-year-old presents with shortness of breath and significant pulmonary hypertension. What is the diagnosis?

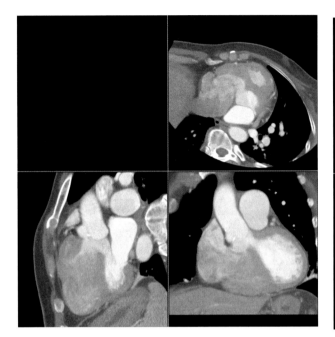

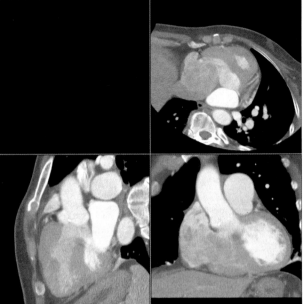

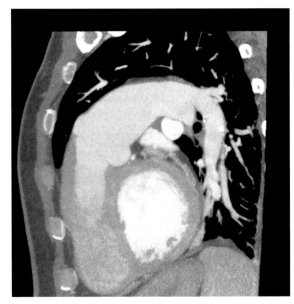

A. Muscular ventricular septal defect without Eisenmenger syndrome
B. Muscular ventricular septal defect with Eisenmenger syndrome
C. Membranous ventricular septal defect without Eisenmenger syndrome
D. Membranous ventricular septal defect with Eisenmenger syndrome

17a A 19-year-old female presents with chest pain. Where is the abnormality?

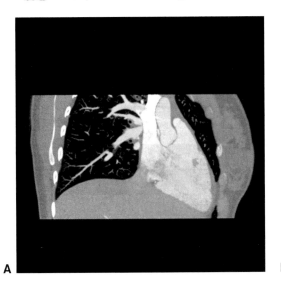 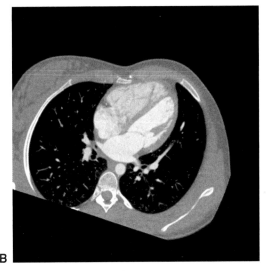

A   B

    A. Left atrium
    B. Aorta
    C. Pulmonary vein
    D. Left ventricle

17b A cardiac catheterization was subsequently performed. The Q_p/Q_s was determined to be 2.1. The patient became symptomatic and developed atrial fibrillation. What is the best treatment?

    A. Stent
    B. Surgical repair
    C. Medical treatment
    D. Device closure

18a An 86-year-old female presents with shortness of breath. Where is the abnormality?

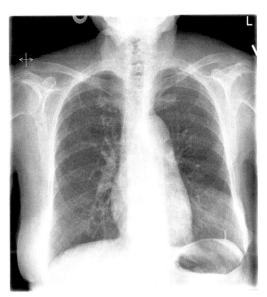

    A. Aorta
    B. Main pulmonary trunk
    C. Left atrium
    D. No abnormality

18b What type of shunt is this?

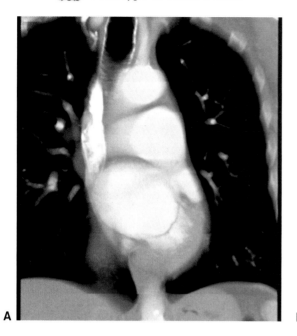

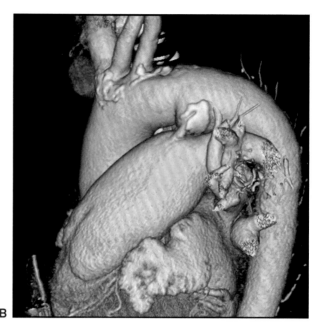

A

B

A. Left-to-left shunt
B. Right-to-left shunt
C. Left-to-right shunt
D. Right-to-right shunt
E. Mixed shunt

19a A 56-year-old female presents with shortness of breath. What is commonly associated with this condition?

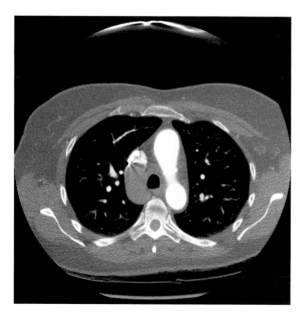

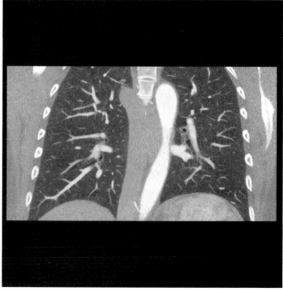

A. Polysplenia
B. Asplenia
C. Bicuspid aortic valve
D. Unicuspid aortic valve

19b This is the identical patient from 19a. What underlying condition does she have?

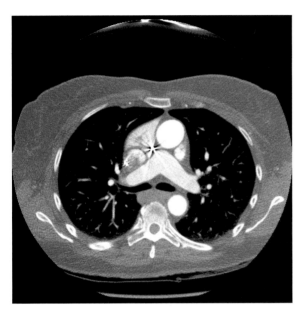
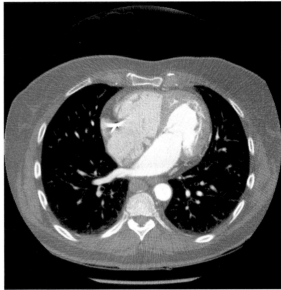

    A. Dextrotransposition of the great arteries (D-TGA)
    B. Levotransposition of the great arteries (L-TGA)
    C. Truncus arteriosus
    D. Normal anatomy

19c This patient also has this abnormality. What should be done?

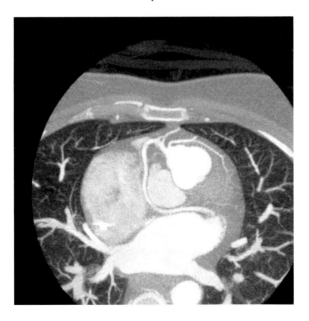

    A. Surgical correction
    B. No treatment
    C. No contact sports
    D. ICD placement

20 A 36-year-old female presents with congenital heart disease. What procedure did she have?

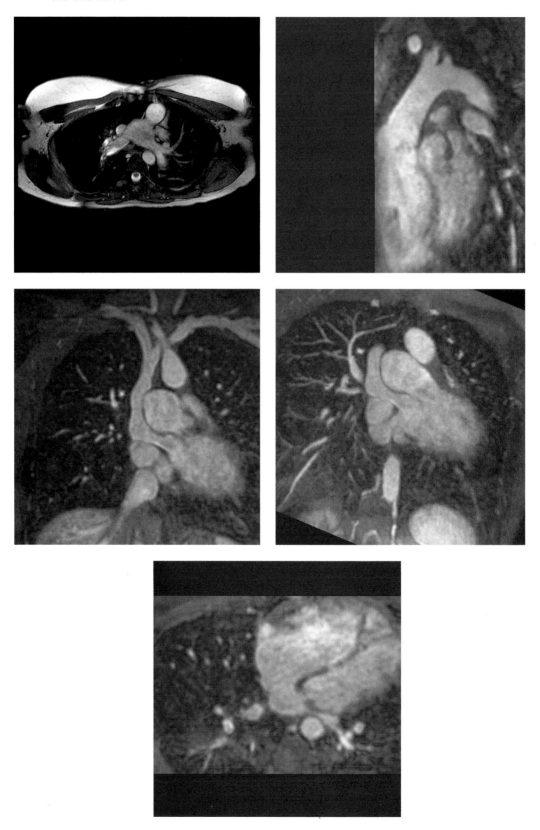

    A. Tetralogy of Fallot repair
    B. Mustard/Senning procedure
    C. Jatene arterial switch
    D. Rastelli procedure

21 In truncus arteriosus, what is the most common morphology of the truncal valve?

    A. Unicuspid
    B. Bicuspid
    C. Tricuspid
    D. Quadricuspid

22a What type of aortic abnormality is most associated with this condition?

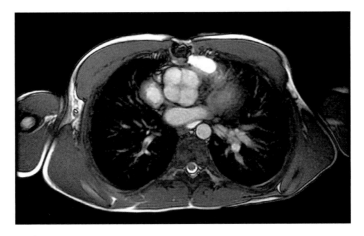

    A. Aortic insufficiency
    B. Aortic stenosis
    C. Aortic coarctation
    D. Aortic aneurysm

22b Which congenital heart disease is most associated with this abnormality?

    A. Tetralogy of Fallot
    B. Truncus arteriosus
    C. Dextrotransposition of the great vessels
    D. Levotransposition of the great vessels

23 What type of shunt is this?

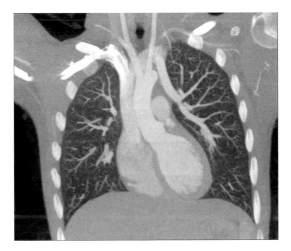

    A. Left to right
    B. Right to left
    C. Mixed

24 The depicted venous anatomy drains into which structure?

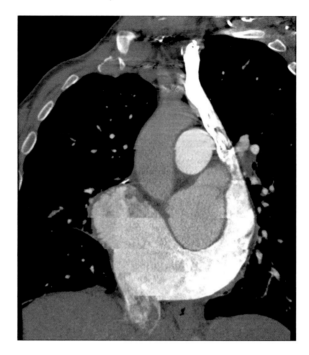

A. Left atrium
B. Left ventricle
C. Coronary sinus
D. IVC

25 Which commissures are fused?

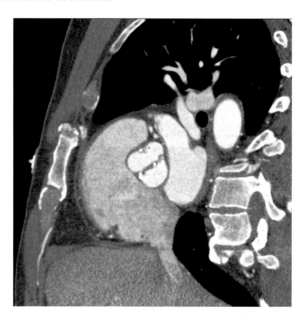

A. Left and noncoronary sinus
B. Noncoronary and right coronary sinus
C. Right and left coronary sinus

26 Mitral valve clefts are associated with

    A. Primum atrial septal defect
    B. Secundum atrial septal defect
    C. Sinus venosus atrial septal defect
    D. Unroofed coronary sinus atrial septal defect

27 What tricuspid valvular abnormality is seen?

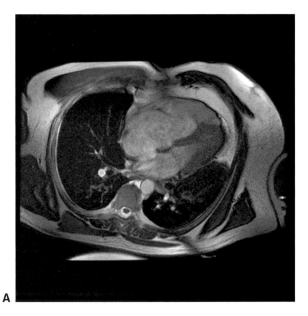

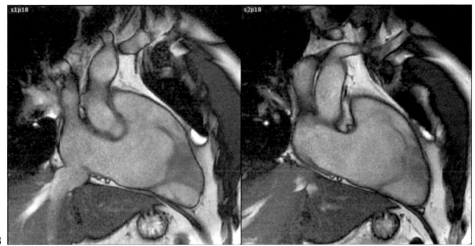

    A. Posteriorly displaced septal leaflets
    B. Sail-like anterior leaflet
    C. Fusion of the anterior and septal leaflets
    D. Hockey stick of the anterior leaflet

28 Common complications after this procedure include baffle obstruction, baffle leak, arrhythmias, and which of the following?

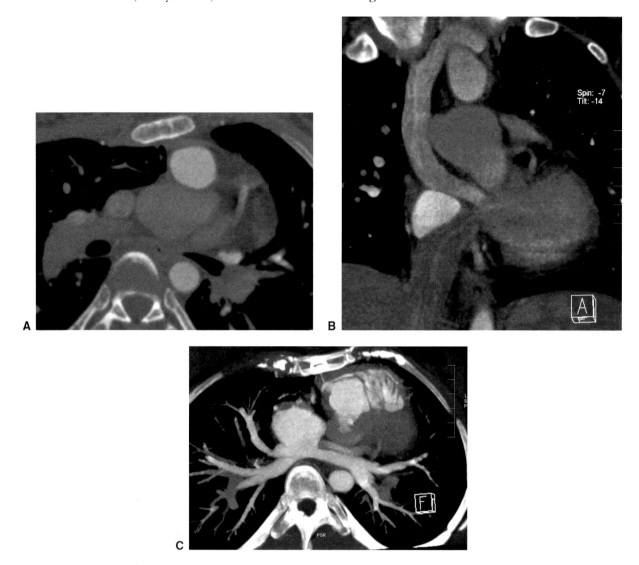

A. Left ventricular dysfunction
B. Right ventricular dysfunction
C. Mitral regurgitation
D. Mitral stenosis

29 A 75-year-old male undergoes a cardiac CTA. What is the best next step?

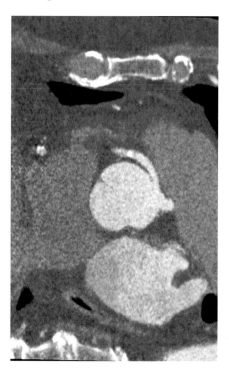

A. Surgical correction
B. ICD placement
C. No treatment
D. Stress test

30 What is the diagnosis?

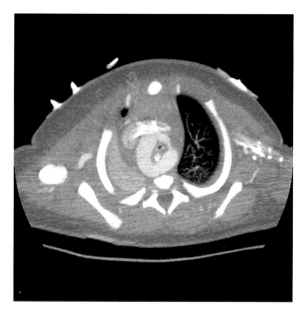

A. Right arch with aberrant left subclavian artery
B. Right arch with mirror image branching
C. Double aortic arch with dominant right arch
D. Double aortic arch with dominant left arch

31 What is the best overall diagnosis?

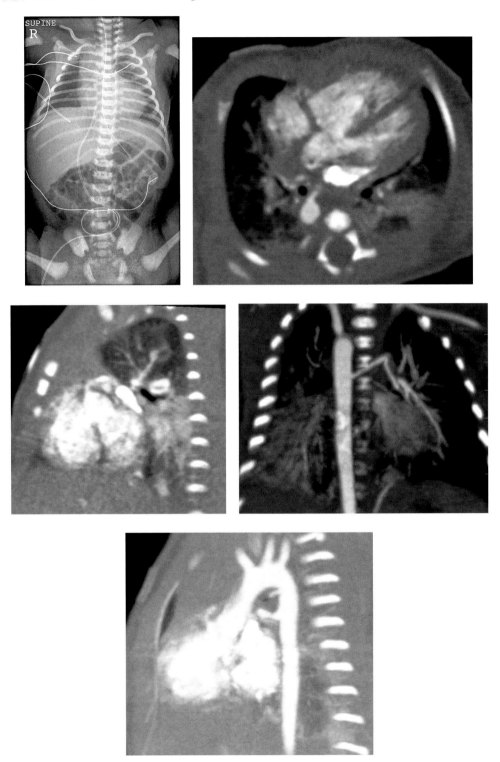

A. Tetralogy of Fallot (overriding aorta, ventricular septal defect, right ventricular hypertrophy, right ventricular outflow obstruction)

B. Pulmonary atresia with ventricular septal defect (PA-VSD), multiple aortopulmonary collateral arteries (MAPCAs)

C. Right arch with aberrant left subclavian artery, bronchial artery hypertrophy, ventricular septal defect

D. Right arch with mirror image branching, bronchial artery hypertrophy, ventricular septal defect

32 An 18-year-old male presents with chest pain. Which of the following is the best diagnosis?

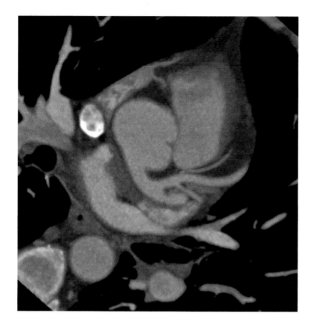

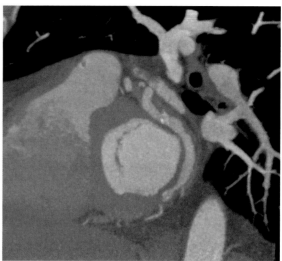

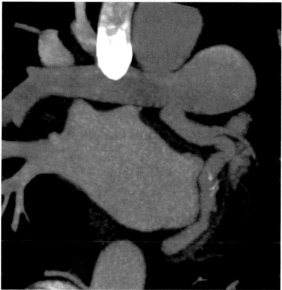

A. Normal coronary arteries post nitroglycerin
B. Premature atherosclerosis
C. Kawasaki disease
D. Coronary fistula

33 Where is the most common location of rupture for this condition?

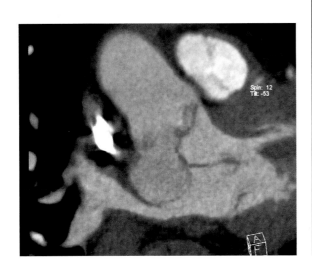
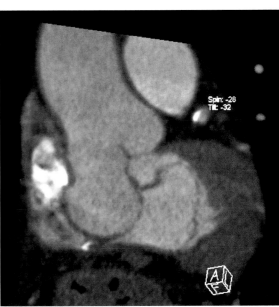

A. Right atrium
B. Right ventricle
C. Left atrium
D. Left ventricle

ANSWERS AND EXPLANATIONS

1 **Answer C.** This patient is status post surgical repair of D-transposition of the great arteries. D-TGA is a form of cyanotic congenital heart disease (CHD) representing approximately 3% of all CHD and almost 20% of all cyanotic CHD. The congenital abnormality is characterized by the aorta arising from the right ventricle and the pulmonary artery from the left ventricle (ventriculoarterial discordance). This results in two parallel circulations, the first of which sends deoxygenated blood to the right atrium and then back to the systemic circulation via the right ventricle and aorta. The second circuit sends oxygenated pulmonary venous blood to the left atrium and back to the lungs via the left ventricle and pulmonary artery.

The dextro term of D-TGA refers to the anatomic relationship of the aortic origin, which is anterior and rightward of the pulmonary artery. The ventriculoarterial discordance of D-TGA is incompatible with life without communication between the two parallel circuits, typically through intracardiac or extracardiac communication.

Classic surgical management is the atrial switch procedure (Mustard or Senning operation), which redirects the parallel circuits into a circulation in series. The atrial switch procedure has largely been replaced since the 1980s by the arterial switch operation. The procedure first successfully performed by Jatene and colleagues includes switching of the aorta and coronary arteries from the systemic RV and of the PA from the LV and reattaching both great arteries to the appropriate ventricles. The Lecompte maneuver (depicted in this case) modifies the Jatene procedure by placing the bifurcation of pulmonary arteries anterior to the aorta allowing for improved orientation of the branch pulmonary arteries and a reduction in tension created from the anterior translocation of the pulmonary arterial root. This provides the characteristic imaging appearance as noted in this case.

Ebstein anomaly and tetralogy of Fallot are congenital abnormalities that preferentially involve right-sided cardiac structures. Shone syndrome is a constellation of cardiac abnormalities involving left-sided cardiac structures: coarctation of the aorta, subaortic stenosis, supravalvular mitral ring, and a parachute mitral valve.

Reference: Hornung T, O'Donnell C. 51-Transposition of the great arteries. In: Gatzoulis MA, Webb GD, Daubeney PEF (eds.). *Diagnosis and management of adult congenital heart disease*, 3rd ed. Elsevier, 2018:513–527.

2 **Answer A.** Hypoplastic left heart syndrome (HLHS) is the abnormal development of the left-sided cardiac structures, typically associated with underdevelopment of the left ventricle, aorta, and aortic arch, as well as mitral atresia or stenosis. The subsequent decrease in systemic perfusion results in hypoxemia, acidosis, and shock.

Surgical palliation of the abnormality takes staged series of reconstructive open heart procedures:

- Stage 1—Norwood procedure: The procedure is performed within 2 weeks of birth. A neo-aorta is surgically constructed from the aortic arch, descending aorta, and main pulmonary artery, which is then connected to the right ventricle. Blood is directed to the lungs through either a modified Blalock-Taussig or right ventricle to PA conduit (Sano modification).

- Stage 2—hemi-Fontan or bidirectional Glenn operation: The second stage is usually performed between 4 and 12 months. This procedure creates a direct connection between the pulmonary artery and the superior vena cava returning oxygen-poor blood from the upper part of the body to the heart.

- Stage 3—Fontan procedure: The third stage is usually performed between 18 months and 3 years. The Fontan procedure allows oxygen-poor blood from the IVC.

Although there have been significant refinements in surgical technique and marked improvement in survival rates, staged surgical procedures are only palliative and not curative. Cardiac transplantation or initial hybrid procedure with pulmonary artery banding and stenting of the atrial septum and ductus arteriosus are other potential choices for therapy.

References: Bardo DM, Frankel DG, Applegate KE, et al. Hypoplastic left heart syndrome. *Radiographics* 2001;21:705–717.

Feinstein JA, Benson DW, Dubin AM, et al. Hypoplastic left heart syndrome: current considerations and expectations. *J Am Coll Cardiol* 2012;59:S1–S42.

3 **Answer B.** The Fontan procedure refers to any surgical procedure that leads to systemic flow of venous blood to the lungs without passing through a ventricle. The most common congenital heart defects palliated with the creation of Fontan circulation include tricuspid atresia, pulmonary atresia with an intact ventricular septum, hypoplastic left heart syndrome, and a double-inlet ventricle.

Fontan-associated liver disease (FALD) is a common complication of the Fontan circulation, which has been recognized with increasing frequency in adolescents and adults. The spectrum of subsequent pathology ranges from mild histologic changes to fulminant liver failure. Systemic venous pressure elevation caused by passive pulmonary blood flow results in elevated systemic venous pressure, likely causing liver congestion.

Patients after Fontan with cirrhosis have reduced life expectancy, even after cardiac transplant. It remains to be seen what effect on long-term survival milder forms of hepatic fibrosis have in Fontan patients. Magnetic resonance imaging is the best modality for postoperative evaluation of patients with Fontan circulation, and cardiac transplantation remains the only definitive treatment for those with failing Fontan circulation.

Surgical correction of truncus arteriosus requires separation of the pulmonary arteries from the conotruncus, closure of VSD, and creation of a surgical conduit from the RV to the pulmonary arteries. Neither tetralogy of Fallot nor dextroposed transposition of the great arteries is ever palliated with Fontan circulation.

References: Emamaullee J, Zaidi AN, Schiano T, et al. Fontan-associated liver disease: screening, management, and transplant considerations. *Circulation* 2020;142:591–604.

Fredenburg TB, Johnson TR, Cohen MD. The Fontan procedure: anatomy, complications, and manifestations of failure. *Radiographics* 2011;31:453–463.

Kay WA, Moe T, Suter B, et al. Long term consequences of the fontan procedure and how to manage them. *Prog Cardiovasc Dis* 2018;61:365–376.

4 **Answer B.** Congenital aortic arch malformations form a large spectrum of variations and anomalies as a consequence of disordered embryogenesis of branchial arches. Right-sided aorta with mirror image branching is the second most common form of a right-sided arch, after right arch with aberrant left subclavian artery. This anomaly rarely produces symptoms and is usually an incidental radiologic finding. However, it is strongly associated with CHD in the majority of cases, including tetralogy of Fallot, truncus arteriosus, tricuspid atresia, and transposition of the great arteries with pulmonary valve stenosis.

The other answers reflect other arch anomalies that are morphologically distinct.

References: Hanneman K, Newman B, Chan F. Congenital variants and anomalies of the aortic arch. *Radiographics* 2017;37:32–51.

Priya S, Thomas R, Nagpal P, et al. Congenital anomalies of the aortic arch. *Cardiovasc Diagn Ther* 2018;8:S26–S44.

5 **Answer D.** A patent ductus arteriosus (PDA) connects the proximal descending aorta to the main pulmonary artery near the origin of the left branch pulmonary artery. This PDA classically closes spontaneously after birth. After the first few weeks of life, persistence of ductal patency is abnormal.

The clinical presentation of a persistent PDA largely depends on the size and magnitude of the shunt and the status of the pulmonary vasculature. Patients with small ductus arteriosus never have signs of significant hemodynamic impairment and, other than the risk of endarteritis, have a normal prognosis. Left-to-right shunting through a larger ductus arteriosus results in pulmonary overcirculation and left heart volume overload.

All of the other pathologies will demonstrate an intracardiac communication.

Reference: Schneider DJ, Moore JW. Patent ductus arteriosus. *Circulation* 2006;114:1873–1882.

6 **Answer C.** Tetralogy of Fallot (TOF) is one of the most common cyanotic congenital heart malformations. Complete corrective TOF surgery is usually performed before 6 months of age. Although long-term result of repaired TOF has historically improved, postoperative sequelae are not rare and persist with aging.

Pulmonary regurgitation is common and results in a variety of findings, including right ventricular dilation, right ventricular dysfunction, tricuspid regurgitation, and exercise intolerance. Right ventricular dilatation and RV outflow patch aneurysms may also occur. A significant subset of adults exhibit progressive aortic root dilatation late after repair of TOF, which may lead to aortic valve regurgitation, aortic dissection, and aortic rupture.

Supravalvular aortic stenosis is typically an abnormality that occurs before birth and is often associated with other congenital malformations or syndromes, such as Williams syndrome, or present in a nonsyndromic condition including previous surgery (e.g., the suture site in the ascending aortic wall after arterial switch for TGA).

References: Masuda M. Postoperative residua and sequelae in adults with repaired tetralogy of Fallot. *Gen Thorac Cardiovasc Surg* 2016;64:373–379.

Smith CA, McCracken C, Thomas AS, et al. Long-term outcomes of tetralogy of Fallot: a study from the pediatric cardiac care consortium. *JAMA Cardiol* 2019;4:34–41.

Zeppenfeld K, Jongbloed M, Schalij MJ. 102—Ventricular arrhythmias in congenital heart disease. In: Zipes DP, Jalife J, Stevenson WG (eds.) *Cardiac electrophysiology: from cell to bedside*, 7th ed. Elsevier, 2018:970–982.

7a **Answer C.** Levocardia refers to the heart being located at the left hemithorax. Mesocardia (from the Greek word mesi, middle) refers to a middle position of the heart inside the chest cavity, and dextrocardia suggest that the heart is located in the right hemithorax. Situs solitus suggests a normal location of the abdominal viscera, whereas situs inversus is the term used to describe the mirror image of the abdominal contents.

Reference: Jacobs JP, Anderson RH, Weinberg PM, et al. The nomenclature, definition and classification of cardiac structures in the setting of heterotaxy. *Cardiol Young* 2007;17(Suppl 2): 1–28.

7b **Answer D.** The eparterial bronchus is a synonymous term for the right superior lobar bronchus, which arises above the point where the right pulmonary artery crosses the right main bronchus. A hyparterial bronchus is morphologically a left lung in which the left main bronchus passes beneath the left pulmonary artery before it gives rise to the left upper lobe bronchus.

Situs solitus corresponds to the usual arrangement of these organs, whereas in situs inversus (as we see in this case), mirror image anatomic arrangement is apparent.

Reference: Chassagnon G, Morel B, Carpentier E, et al. Tracheobronchial branching abnormalities: lobe-based classification scheme. *Radiographics* 2016;36:358–373.

8a **Answer C.** Frontal and lateral chest radiographs demonstrate an enlarged pulmonary artery trunk and increased vascular flow. This is suggestive of underlying left to right shunting, which can be caused by an atrial septal defect. Both aortic and mitral stenosis should not give an enlarged pulmonary artery trunk nor increased vascular flow. The findings are not normal given the enlarged pulmonary trunk and increased pulmonary flow. Ebstein anomaly would give a markedly enlarged right heart (e.g., boxed-shaped heart).

References: Baron MG, Book WM. Congenital heart disease in the adult: 2004. *Radiol Clin North Am* 2004;42(3):675–690, vii. Review.

Steiner RM, Gross GW, Flicker S, et al. Congenital heart disease in the adult patient: the value of plain film chest radiology. *J Thorac Imaging* 1995;10(1):1–25. Review.

8b **Answer C.** An Amplatzer septal occluder is now seen on the chest radiograph. Indications for percutaneous atrial septal defect (ASD) closure include hemodynamically significant ASD (such as $Q_p/Q_s > 2$) and paradoxical emboli. It is not indicated in patients with small secundum ASD of no hemodynamic significance. It is also not indicated in septum primum, sinus venosus, and unroofed coronary sinus type of ASDs. Atrial fibrillation is not a contraindication to ASD closure. Adequate rims are required for the placement of the Amplatzer device. Only venous access is needed to deploy the device.

References: Kazmouz S, Kenny D, Cao QL, et al. Transcatheter closure of secundum atrial septal defects. *J Invasive Cardiol* 2013;25(5):257–264. Review.

Lee EY, Siegel MJ, Chu CM, et al. Amplatzer atrial septal defect occluder for pediatric patients: radiographic appearance. *Radiology* 2004;233(2):471–476.

8c **Answer D.** Complications of ASD occlusion include atrial fibrillation, SVT, heart block, device malposition, embolization, and erosion. The most common immediate complication is device embolization and malpositioning. Atrial fibrillation and heart block also typically occur early. Cardiac erosion is a long-term complication that can be difficult to detect.

References: Crawford GB, Brindis RG, Krucoff MW, et al. Percutaneous atrial septal occluder devices and cardiac erosion: a review of the literature. *Catheter Cardiovasc Interv* 2012;80(2):157–167. doi: 10.1002/ccd.24347. Review.

Lee T, Tsai IC, Fu YC, et al. MDCT evaluation after closure of atrial septal defect with an Amplatzer septal occluder. *AJR Am J Roentgenol* 2007;188(5):W431–W439.

9 **Answer B.** This is an inferior type of sinus venosus atrial septal defect (ASD) associated with anomalous pulmonary venous return of the right inferior pulmonary vein. The treatment is surgical. While secundum ASD can potentially be treated endovascularly with closure devices, sinus venosus ASD cannot be treated endovascularly due to the lack of rims for the device to attach to.

Reference: Vyas HV, Greenberg SB, Krishnamurthy R. MR imaging and CT evaluation of congenital pulmonary vein abnormalities in neonates and infants. *Radiographics* 2012;32(1):87–98. doi: 10.1148/rg.321105764.

10a **Answer C.** Images demonstrate unroofed coronary sinus (note the connection between the left and right atrium and the coronary sinus). In this case, the shunt appears small without evidence of left heart enlargement. Given the small shunt, no treatment is required. Surgical treatment would be considered if there is a significant shunt ($Q_p/Q_s > 2$). There is no role for catheter-based closure in unroofed coronary sinus.

10b **Answer D.** Unroofed coronary sinus is associated with left-sided SVC. Azygos continuation of the IVC is associated with polysplenia and many other congenital heart diseases. Coarctation is classically associated with bicuspid aortic valve. Anomalous right pulmonary venous return can be associated with sinus venosus atrial septal defects.

Reference: Shah SS, Teague SD, Lu JC, et al. Imaging of the coronary sinus: normal anatomy and congenital abnormalities. *Radiographics* 2012;32(4):991–1008. doi: 10.1148/rg.324105220.

11 **Answer C.** There are four types of ASD: sinus venosus, ostium secundum, ostium primum, and unroofed coronary sinus.

Reference: Rojas CA, El-Sherief A, Medina HM, et al. Embryology and developmental defects of the interatrial septum. *AJR Am J Roentgenol* 2010;195(5):1100–1104. doi: 10.2214/AJR.10.4277. Review.

12 **Answer A.** Muscular VSD can undergo spontaneous closure, while membranous VSD will not close spontaneously. Endocarditis prophylaxis is necessary for both muscular and membranous VSDs.

Reference: Minette MS, Sahn DJ. Ventricular septal defects. *Circulation* 2006;114(20):2190–2197. Review. Erratum in: Circulation 2007;115(7):e205.

13a **Answer C.** PA and lateral chest radiographs show an abnormal vertical linear opacity along the right lower lung. On the lateral view, it appears to course inferiorly toward the IVC region. This is consistent with the "scimitar sign," which is suggestive of anomalous pulmonary venous return (scimitar vein). The differential also includes anomalous single pulmonary vein, which would drain normally into the left atrium. These conditions have different treatments (surgical for scimitar, no treatment for anomalous single pulmonary vein). The best next step would be to define the anatomy with a CTA chest. Biopsy would not be helpful and may even be dangerous. CT without IV contrast would not define the vascular anatomy well. VQ scan would not clarify what the tubular structure is. No further imaging would also not be helpful given we need to further define the abnormality.

References: Ferguson EC, Krishnamurthy R, Oldham SA. Classic imaging signs of congenital cardiovascular abnormalities. *Radiographics* 2007;27(5):1323–1334. Review.

Nazarian J, Kanne JP, Rajiah P. Scimitar sign. *J Thorac Imaging* 2013;28(4):W61.

13b **Answer A.** A scimitar vein is draining into the IVC. This is a type of anomalous pulmonary venous return and a left to right shunt (remember that the pulmonary veins carry oxygenated blood, so it is part of the left circulation).

In classic scimitar syndrome, there is anomalous right pulmonary vein, hypoplasia of the right lung along with pulmonary artery hypoplasia, dextrocardia, and systemic arterial supply to the lungs. These features are not always present on all patients. Atrial septal defect (ASD) is not part of the syndrome but can sometimes occur concurrently. If patient is symptomatic due to significant shunting, surgical correction to redirect the vein into the left atrium can be performed.

References: Ferguson EC, Krishnamurthy R, Oldham SA. Classic imaging signs of congenital cardiovascular abnormalities. *Radiographics* 2007;27(5):1323–1334. Review.

Nazarian J, Kanne JP, Rajiah P. Scimitar sign. *J Thorac Imaging* 2013;28(4):W61.

14 Answer A. Shone syndrome/complex has four components—supravalvular mitral membrane (SVMM), parachute mitral valve, subaortic stenosis (membranous or muscular), and coarctation of the aorta. Bicuspid aortic valve, coarctation, and sex chromosomal abnormality are associated with Turner syndrome.

Reference: Bittencourt MS, Hulten E, Givertz MM, et al. Multimodality imaging of an adult with Shone complex. *J Cardiovasc Comput Tomogr* 2013;7(1):62–65. doi: 10.1016/j.jcct.2012.10.009.

15 Answer C. In a Ross procedure, the pulmonic valve is switched to the aortic position and a prosthetic valve is placed in the pulmonic position.

Reference: Lakoma A, Tuite D, Sheehan J, et al. Measurement of pulmonary circulation parameters using time-resolved MR angiography in patients after Ross procedure. *AJR Am J Roentgenol* 2010;194(4):912–919. doi: 10.2214/AJR.09.2897.

16 Answer D. Images show a membranous VSD with evidence of both left to right and right to left shunting (note the mixing of the contrast material at the site of ventricular septal defect). This is consistent with Eisenmenger syndrome with suprasystemic right heart pressures causing right to left shunting. Note the marked right ventricular hypertrophy from the pulmonary hypertension due to long-standing shunt. Muscular ventricular septal defects are located along the muscular septum, which is not shown here.

Reference: Peña E, Dennie C, Veinot J, et al. Pulmonary hypertension: how the radiologist can help. *Radiographics* 2012;32(1):9–32. doi: 10.1148/rg.321105232.

17a Answer C. Image A shows anomalous pulmonary venous return with right superior pulmonary vein (RSPV) returning to SVC. Note the right heart appears enlarged (Image B). Left atrium and ventricle appear normal. Visualized ascending aorta also appears normal.

Reference: Kafka H, Mohiaddin RH. Cardiac MRI and pulmonary MR angiography of sinus venosus defect and partial anomalous pulmonary venous connection in cause of right undiagnosed ventricular enlargement. *AJR Am J Roentgenol* 2009;192(1):259–266. doi: 10.2214/AJR.07.3430.

17b Answer B. The images show anomalous pulmonary venous return with the right superior pulmonary vein (RSPV) entering to the SVC. There is significant shunting as evidenced by Q_p/Q_s of 2.1 and right heart enlargement. In addition, the presence of atrial fibrillation suggests significant volume overloading and chamber remodeling. The best treatment therefore is surgery. Note there is an association between right partial anomalous pulmonary venous return and sinus venosus atrial septal defects. Device closure is not feasible since the anomalous vein needs to be redirected to the left atrium. Medical treatment is not advisable given the significant shunting ($Q_p/Q_s > 1.5$) and development of atrial fibrillation. Stenting would not fix this problem.

References: Dillman JR, Yarram SG, Hernandez RJ. Imaging of pulmonary venous developmental anomalies. *AJR Am J Roentgenol* 2009;192(5):1272–1285. doi: 10.2214/AJR.08.1526. Review.

Kafka H, Mohiaddin RH. Cardiac MRI and pulmonary MR angiography of sinus venosus defect and partial anomalous pulmonary venous connection in cause of right undiagnosed ventricular enlargement. *AJR Am J Roentgenol* 2009;192(1):259–266. doi: 10.2214/AJR.07.3430.

18a **Answer B.** Frontal CXR shows an enlarged pulmonary trunk. The left mediastinal contour is composed of, starting superiorly, the left subclavian artery, left arch, main pulmonary trunk, left atrial appendage (if enlarged), and left ventricle. In this case, the contour below the arch is enlarged suggesting enlarged pulmonary trunk. Aortic enlargement can occur throughout its course so can involve the ascending aorta, arch, or descending aorta. Left atrial enlargement can be seen with enlarged left atrial appendage contour, or in extreme left atrial enlargement, a double contour is seen along the right heart border (double density sign). There can also be splaying of the carina.

Reference: Ferguson EC, Krishnamurthy R, Oldham SA. Classic imaging signs of congenital cardiovascular abnormalities. *Radiographics* 2007;27(5):1323–1334. Review.

18b **Answer C.** Coronal reformat shows enlarged PA contour (Image A). 3D volume-rendered images show a PDA (Image B). Patent ductus arteriosus is a type of left-to-right shunt. However, it does not involve the right heart since the connection is between the aorta and pulmonary artery (so the right heart will not be enlarged). It is associated with rubella infection during pregnancy. It can lead to Eisenmenger syndrome in long-standing shunts.

References: Goitein O, Fuhrman CR, Lacomis JM. Incidental finding on MDCT of patent ductus arteriosus: use of CT and MRI to assess clinical importance. *AJR Am J Roentgenol* 2005;184(6):1924–1931.

Morgan-Hughes GJ, Marshall AJ, Roobottom C. Morphologic assessment of patent ductus arteriosus in adults using retrospectively ECG-gated multidetector CT. *AJR Am J Roentgenol* 2003;181(3): 749–754.

Schneider DJ, Moore JW. Patent ductus arteriosus. *Circulation* 2006;114(17):1873–1882.

19a **Answer A.** The images show enlarged azygos vein seen in interrupted IVC with azygos continuation. This condition is associated with polysplenia. Bicuspid aortic valve is associated with coarctation but also aortic aneurysm from bicuspid aortopathy. Unicuspid aortic valve is associated with aortic stenosis.

Reference: Applegate KE, Goske MJ, Pierce G, et al. Situs revisited: imaging of the heterotaxy syndrome. *Radiographics* 1999;19(4):837–852; discussion 853–854. Review.

19b **Answer B.** The images show transposition of the vessels with the aorta arising anterior to the pulmonary artery. This is a levo-type of transposition of the great arteries (L-TGA) with ventricular inversion (morphologic RV on the left side, morphologic LV on the right side). With the ventricles switched in position, there is a transposition of the great arteries. However, the flow circuit is normal with the systemic blood going into the pulmonary artery and oxygenated pulmonary venous blood to the aorta. The systemic ventricle on the left is a morphologic right ventricle containing the tricuspid valve. This can cause problems later as the morphologic RV can fail and the tricuspid valve can be leaky. There is also a higher rate of arrhythmia from the systemic RV. As a result, these patients can sometimes present at a young age with already an ICD and valvular replacement.

Reference: Cohen MD, Johnson T, Ramrakhiani S. MRI of surgical repair of transposition of the great vessels. *AJR Am J Roentgenol* 2010;194(1):250–260. doi: 10.2214/AJR.09.3045. Review.

19c **Answer B.** A retroaortic left circumflex artery is seen. This is a benign coronary anomaly and no surgery is necessary. There is no need for activity restriction or ICD placement.

References: Kim SY, Seo JB, Do KH, et al. Coronary artery anomalies: classification and ECG-gated multi-detector row CT findings with angiographic correlation. *Radiographics* 2006;26(2):317–333; discussion 333–334. Review.

Shriki JE, Shinbane JS, Rashid MA, et al. Identifying, characterizing, and classifying congenital anomalies of the coronary arteries. *Radiographics*. 2012;32(2):453–468. doi: 10.1148/rg.322115097. Review.

20 **Answer B.** There is D-TGA with Mustard/Senning baffle. The great vessels are switched, so the procedure switches the inflow to redirect systemic blood to the left ventricle and the pulmonary venous return to the right atrium. Tetralogy repair involves closing the VSD and alleviating the right ventricular outflow tract obstruction. Arterial switch typically show a characteristic draping of the pulmonary artery over the aorta. Rastelli procedure would involve a right ventricular outflow conduit.

References: Cohen MD, Johnson T, Ramrakhiani S. MRI of surgical repair of transposition of the great vessels. *AJR Am J Roentgenol* 2010;194(1):250–260. doi: 10.2214/AJR.09.3045. Review.

Lu JC, Dorfman AL, Attili AK, et al. Evaluation with cardiovascular MR imaging of baffles and conduits used in palliation or repair of congenital heart disease. *Radiographics* 2012;32(3):E107–E127. doi: 10.1148/rg.323115096.

21 **Answer C.** A truncal valve is most often tricuspid, followed by quadricuspid and bicuspid. There is often a ventricular septal defect. Collette and Edwards described four types of truncus arteriosus.

Reference: Kimura-Hayama ET, Meléndez G, Mendizábal AL, et al. Uncommon congenital and acquired aortic diseases: role of multidetector CT angiography. *Radiographics* 2010;30(1): 79–98. doi: 10.1148/rg.301095061.

22a **Answer A.** A quadricuspid aortic valve is most associated with aortic insufficiency. It can also be seen with truncus arteriosus. There is no reported association with aortic stenosis, aortic coarctation, or aortic aneurysm.

22b **Answer B.** A quadricuspid aortic valve is most often seen with truncus arteriosus.

Reference: Bennett CJ, Maleszewski JJ, Araoz PA. CT and MR imaging of the aortic valve: radiologic–pathologic correlation. *Radiographics* 2012;32(5):1399–1420. doi: 10.1148/rg. 325115727.

23 **Answer A.** Partial anomalous venous return is seen with the left superior pulmonary vein returning to the left brachiocephalic vein. This is a left-to-right shunt (pulmonary veins carry oxygenated blood). This can be incidental with treatment not considered unless there is evidence for a significant shunt ($Q_p/Q_s > 1.5$).

Reference: Wang ZJ, Reddy GP, Gotway MB, et al. Cardiovascular shunts: MR imaging evaluation. *Radiographics* 2003;23:S181–S194. Review.

24 **Answer C.** Reformatted oblique image shows a left-sided SVC returning to the coronary sinus. This is a benign anatomical variant that requires no treatment. In rare cases, the left-sided SVC can drain into the left atrium and be associated with unroofed coronary sinus, a type of atrial septal defect.

Reference: Martinez-Jimenez S, Heyneman LE, McAdams HP, et al. Nonsurgical extracardiac vascular shunts in the thorax: clinical and imaging characteristics. *Radiographics* 2010;30(5):e41. doi: 10.1148/rg.e41.

25 Answer C. Bicuspid aortic valve is seen with fusion of the right and left coronary cusps. One can identify the sinuses by the following. The noncoronary sinus typically straddles the interatrial septum. The right sinus is anterior, so look for the sternum while left sinus is adjacent to the left atrial appendage.

Reference: Bennett CJ, Maleszewski JJ, Araoz PA. CT and MR imaging of the aortic valve: radiologic-pathologic correlation. *Radiographics* 2012;32(5):1399–1420. doi: 10.1148/rg.325115727.

26 Answer A. Mitral valve clefts are seen with primum atrial septal defects (ASD). The ASD is a result of endocardial cushion defects, which result in an atrioventricular canal defect including a septum primum defect. Endocardial cushion defects and mitral valve clefts are associated with Down syndrome (trisomy 21). The other types of ASDs are not associated with mitral valvular abnormalities. A secundum ASD can often be seen in patients with Ebstein anomaly. Sinus venosus ASDs are often seen with right-sided partial anomalous venous return. An unroofed coronary sinus is associated with left-sided SVC.

Reference: Morris MF, Maleszewski JJ, Suri RM, et al. CT and MR imaging of the mitral valve: radiologic-pathologic correlation. *Radiographics* 2010;30(6):1603–1620. doi: 10.1148/rg.306105518. Review.

27 Answer B. Cardiac MRI in horizontal (Image A) and vertical long-axis (Image B) views show abnormal location of the septal tricuspid leaflet, which is apically displaced (not posteriorly). There is also "atrialization" of the right ventricle due to the abnormal morphology of the tricuspid leaflet. The anterior leaflet is redundant and sail-like. The septal leaflet is anteriorly displaced. This is consistent with an Ebstein anomaly. Note that Ebstein anomaly has a high association with secundum ASD. There is also an association with maternal lithium and benzodiazepine use.

There is no fusion of the anterior and septal leaflets. The hockey stick appearance of the anterior leaflet is seen in mitral stenosis.

Reference: Attenhofer Jost CH, Connolly HM, Dearani JA, et al. Ebstein's anomaly. *Circulation* 2007;115(2):277–285. Review.

28 Answer B. Axial image shows the aorta to be directly anterior to the pulmonary artery (Image A). This is typically seen with dextrotransposition of the great arteries (ᴅ-TGA). The coronal image (Image B) shows the intra-atrial baffle with the SVC baffle directing the upper venous return to the left atrium. Lower extremity venous return from IVC is also redirected to the left atrium. The axial MIP image (Image C) shows the pulmonary veins baffled to the right atrium, which is connected to the systemic right ventricle. Complications of the baffle repair include baffle obstruction, baffle leak, arrhythmias, and right ventricular dysfunction. The morphologic right ventricle is not made for systemic pressures and will tend to fail. There is no reported increased pathology of the mitral valve. There is increased tricuspid insufficiency due to the systemic pressures.

Reference: Lu JC, Dorfman AL, Attili AK, et al. Evaluation with cardiovascular MR imaging of baffles and conduits used in palliation or repair of congenital heart disease. *Radiographics* 2012;32(3):E107–E127. doi: 10.1148/rg.323115096.

29 **Answer D.** An anomalous RCA from the left sinus of Valsalva is seen. The RCA takes an interarterial course between the pulmonary artery and aortic root. Unlike an interarterial anomalous LAD, which is classically associated with sudden death and thus surgically treated, current treatment of this coronary anomaly is more nuanced. In this case, a stress test to see if there is any inducible ischemia from this anomaly is the best choice. ICD would not be indicated for primary prevention.

References: Angelini P. Coronary artery anomalies: an entity in search of an identity. *Circulation* 2007;115(10):1296–1305. Review.

Shriki JE, Shinbane JS, Rashid MA, et al. Identifying, characterizing, and classifying congenital anomalies of the coronary arteries. *Radiographics* 2012;32(2):453–468. doi: 10.1148/rg.322115097. Review.

30 **Answer C.** Axial maximal intensity projection (MIP) image shows a double arch with a dominant right arch. A right arch with aberrant left subclavian artery can have a similar appearance but would not have the connecting vessel on the left. A right arch with mirror image branching would not have the posterior vessel to the trachea and esophagus. In a double aortic arch with a dominant left arch, the caliber of the left arch would be larger.

References: Kimura-Hayama ET, Meléndez G, Mendizábal AL, et al. Uncommon congenital and acquired aortic diseases: role of multidetector CT angiography. *Radiographics* 2010;30(1):79–98. doi: 10.1148/rg.301095061.

Ramos-Duran L, Nance JW Jr, Schoepf UJ, et al. Developmental aortic arch anomalies in infants and children assessed with CT angiography. *AJR Am J Roentgenol* 2012;198(5):W466–W474. doi: 10.2214/AJR.11.6982. Review.

31 **Answer B.** Multiple images demonstrate a baby with complex congenital heart disease. There is a right arch with mirror image branching, VSD, overriding aorta, and multiple aortopulmonary collateral arteries (MAPCAs). This is most consistent with pulmonary atresia with ventricular septal defect (PA-VSD). This condition has been previously called as pseudotruncus and classified as type IV of truncus arteriosus. However, this condition is now considered its own entity and can have similar abnormalities as tetralogy of Fallot (TOF) except with pulmonary atresia and MAPCAS. TOF has the following four features: overriding aorta, ventricular septal defect, right ventricular hypertrophy, and right ventricular outflow obstruction.

References: Boechat MI, Ratib O, Williams PL, et al. Cardiac MR imaging and MR angiography for assessment of complex tetralogy of Fallot and pulmonary atresia. *Radiographics* 2005;25(6): 1535–1546. Review.

Rajeshkannan R, Moorthy S, Sreekumar KP, et al. Role of 64-MDCT in evaluation of pulmonary atresia with ventricular septal defect. *AJR Am J Roentgenol* 2010;194(1):110–118. doi: 10.2214/AJR.09.2802. Review.

32 **Answer C.** Multiple oblique reformatted MIP images show dilated coronary arteries with calcification. In a young patient, this is most consistent with history of Kawasaki disease. While the coronary arteries can dilate post nitroglycerin administration, this degree of diffuse ectasia should not be seen along the evidence for atherosclerosis. Premature atherosclerosis would typically not involve 18-year-old patients. Coronary fistula is within the differential for dilated coronary arteries, but there is no evidence for abnormal connections on the images provided.

Reference: Díaz-Zamudio M, Bacilio-Pérez U, Herrera-Zarza MC, et al. Coronary artery aneurysms and ectasia: role of coronary CT angiography. *Radiographics* 2009;29(7): 1939–1954. doi: 10.1148/rg.297095048. Review.

33 **Answer B.** Images show a sinus of Valsalva (SOV) aneurysm involving the noncoronary cusp. SOV aneurysms most often occur in the right and noncoronary cusps. They are associated with aortic regurgitation and supracristal ventricular septal defects. They tend to rupture into the right ventricular outflow tract (RVOT), followed by the right atrium and rarely in the left atrium or ventricle.

Reference: Bricker AO, Avutu B, Mohammed TL, et al. Valsalva sinus aneurysms: findings at CT and MR imaging. *Radiographics* 2010;30(1):99–110. doi: 10.1148/rg.301095719.

10 Acquired Disease of the Thoracic Aorta and Great Vessels

Joe Y. Hsu, MD • Amar B. Shah, MD, MPA • Jean Jeudy, MD

QUESTIONS

1 Which of the following indications would be the LEAST appropriate indication for TEVAR?

A. Acute type B aortic dissection with malperfusion
B. Descending aortic caliber of 4.5 cm
C. Contained aortic transection
D. Aortoesophageal fistula

2 What is the following abnormality?

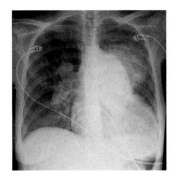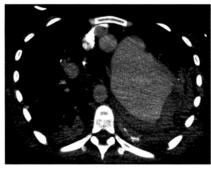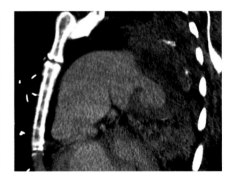

A. Pulmonary artery dissection
B. Pulmonary sarcoma
C. Pulmonary embolism
D. Loculated pericardial fluid

3 What is the most common cause of an ascending thoracic aortic aneurysm?

A. Aortitis
B. Marfan syndrome
C. Aortic stenosis
D. Atherosclerosis

4 What is the most common risk factor for aortic dissection?

A. Marfan syndrome
B. Cystic medial degeneration
C. Hypertension
D. Aortic aneurysm

5 What type of endoleak is demonstrated?

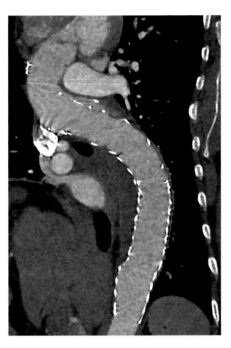

A. Type 1
B. Type 2
C. Type 3
D. Type 4

6 Patient presents with abrupt onset of left facial weakness. Previous reports from outside hospital reveals recurrent GI bleeding, frequent epistaxis, and occasional hemoptysis. CT was performed. Which of the following syndromes should be considered?

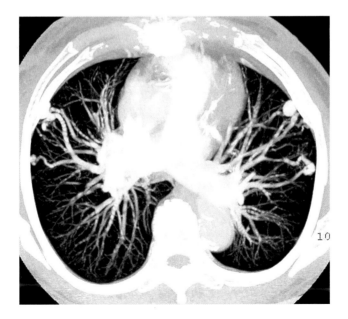

A. Pulmonary AVM
B. Essential hypertension
C. Aortic dissection
D. Pulmonary hypertension

7 Which is the best diagnosis?

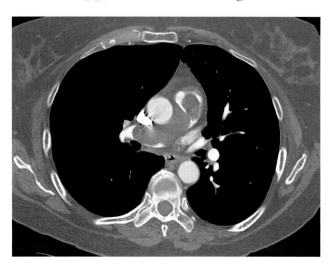

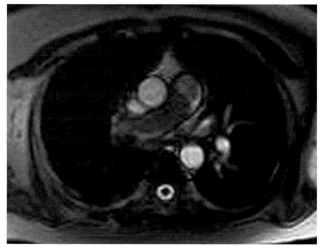

A. Acute pulmonary embolism
B. Pulmonary artery sarcoma
C. Lung cancer extension
D. Pulmonary artery intramural hematoma (IMH)

8 Annuloaortic ectasia is most commonly associated with Marfan syndrome. What other condition can also produce similar findings?

A. Syphilis
B. Bicuspid aortic valve
C. Takayasu arteritis
D. Ehlers-Danlos syndrome

9a A patient presents with nonradiating, harsh crescendo–decrescendo ejection murmur by auscultation. Subsequent cardiac MR with phase-contrast imaging was obtained. Which of the following is the most likely diagnosis?

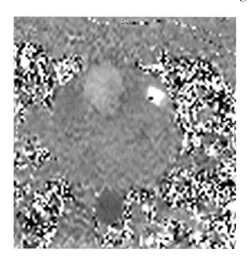

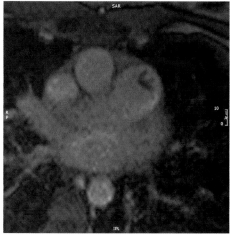

A. Pulmonic stenosis
B. Aortic stenosis
C. Pulmonary dissection
D. Aortic dissection

9b In the MR evaluation of the previous patient, which parameter would be most significantly altered by this acquisition.

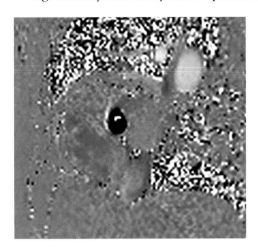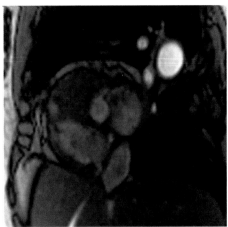

    A. Diastolic flow volume
    B. Aortic valve area
    C. Peak gradient
    D. Aortic distensibility

10 Patients presents for a repeat CTA study after the initial study was reported suboptimal. The CT technician calls you for protocolling. How would you instruct the technician in acquiring the repeat study?

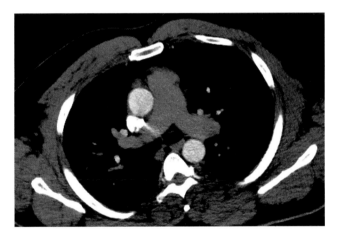

    A. Increase total volume of contrast
    B. Small breath hold without deep inspiration
    C. Decrease delay between start of injection and start of scan
    D. Increase rate of contrast injection

11 Dissection at the aortic arch is considered what type of dissection using the Stanford classification?

    A. Type A
    B. Type B
    C. Type C
    D. Type D

12   Patient with back pain presents with the following imaging. The best diagnosis is

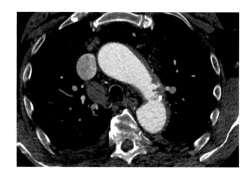 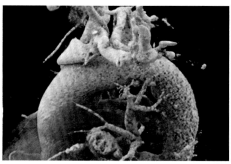

A. Aortic dissection
B. Aortic aneurysm
C. Aortic ulceration
D. Aortic coarctation

13a   What is the most likely diagnosis?

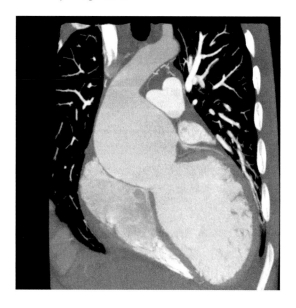

A. Atherosclerosis
B. Marfan syndrome
C. Bicuspid aortopathy
D. Hypertension

13b   In patients with Marfan syndrome, what associated valvular abnormality can be seen?

A. Tricuspid stenosis
B. Tricuspid valve prolapse
C. Mitral stenosis
D. Mitral valve prolapse

14 Which of the following characteristics favor traumatic pseudoaneurysm versus ductus diverticulum?

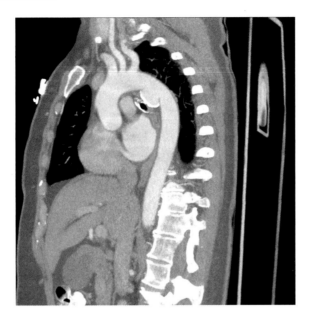

A. Aortic wall outer continuity
B. Smooth margins
C. Location at aortic isthmus
D. Intimal flap
E. Calcification

15 A 57-year-old presents with chest pain. These images were obtained 4 months apart. What is the most likely cause of this aneurysm?

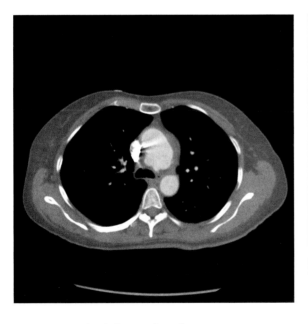 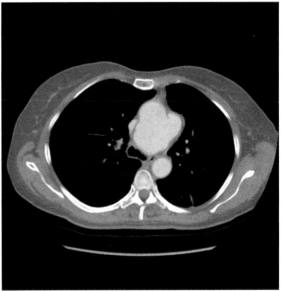

A. Atherosclerotic
B. Takayasu aortitis
C. Posttraumatic
D. Mycotic

16 This is the patient reimaged a few hours later. What is the best next step in the management of this patient?

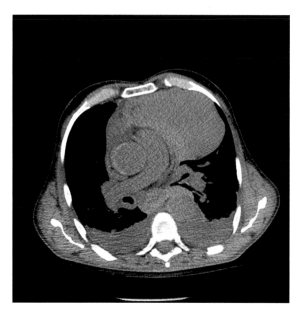 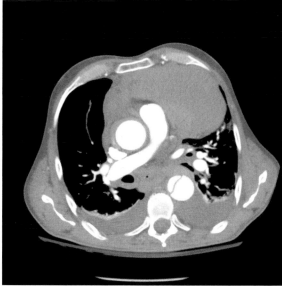

A. Medical management
B. Immediate surgery
C. Endovascular
D. Additional imaging

17 What is the most likely underlying condition that the 56-year-old patient has?

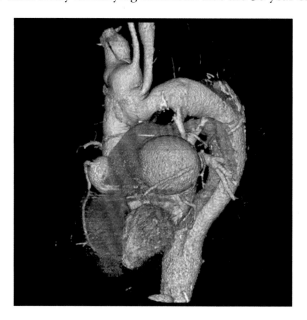

A. Premature atherosclerosis
B. Marfan syndrome
C. Takayasu arteritis
D. Prior syphilis infection

18 What complication is depicted in the following set of images?

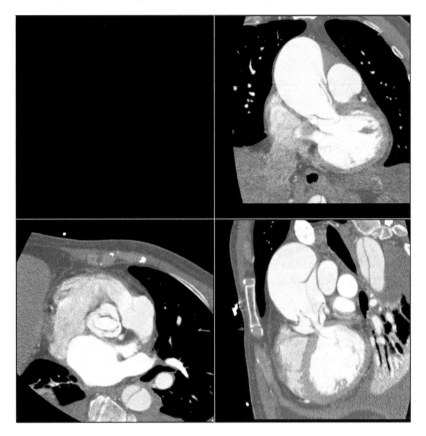

A. Aortic regurgitation
B. Aortic stenosis
C. Aortic valve endocarditis
D. Aortic rupture

19a In this condition, which layer of the aortic wall is intact?

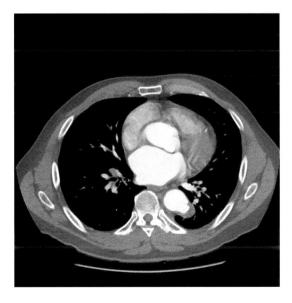

A. Intima
B. Media
C. Adventitia
D. Muscularis propria

19b The patient remains asymptomatic, what is the next step?

    A. Medical therapy

    B. Surgical graft replacement

    C. Endovascular stenting

    D. Axillary–distal femoral bypass

20 A 62-year-old presents with leg pain. What is the best next step?

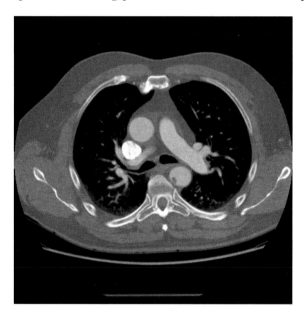

    A. Endovascular thrombectomy

    B. Surgical thrombectomy

    C. Medical treatment

    D. Extracorporeal membrane oxygenation

21 What measurements can be obtained on these images to best assess for severity of pulmonary embolism?

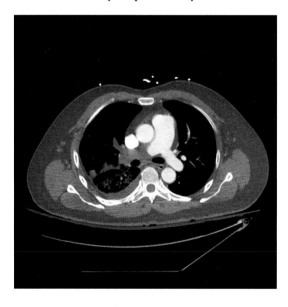 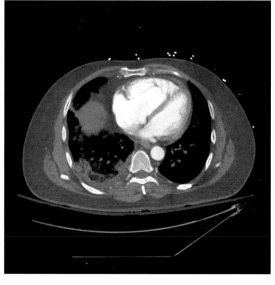

    A. Right ventricle to left ventricle short-axis ratio

    B. Left ventricle to right ventricle short-axis ratio

    C. Interventricular septal wall thickness

    D. Right ventricular wall thickness

22a A 28-year-old male presents with shortness of breath. What is the most likely cause of these findings?

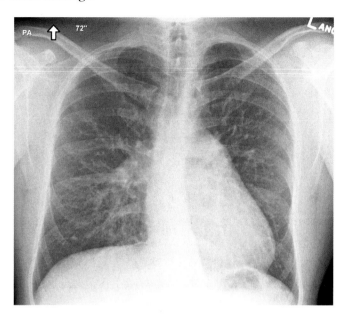

A. Pulmonary edema due to right heart failure
B. Pulmonary edema due to mitral regurgitation
C. Pulmonary hypertension due to left to right shunting
D. Pulmonary hypertension due to idiopathic cause

22b How is this complication best treated?

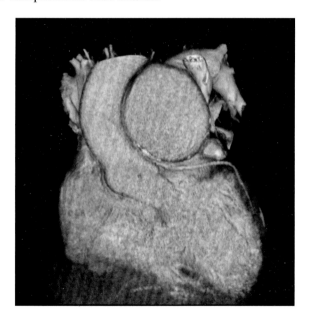

A. Observation
B. Stent
C. Medical

23   What type of arteriovenous malformation is this?

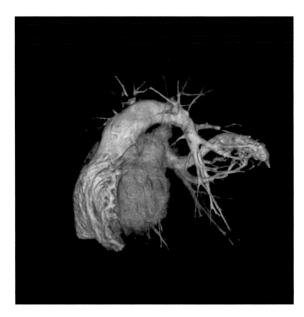

    A. Simple malformation
    B. Intermediate malformation
    C. Complex malformation

24   What type of shunt is pulmonary AVM?
    A. Right to left
    B. Left to right
    C. Right to right
    D. Left to left

25   Multiple pulmonary AVMs are associated with which of the following condition?
    A. Hereditary hemorrhagic telangiectasia (HHT)
    B. Von Hippel-Lindau
    C. Tuberous sclerosis
    D. Marfan syndrome

26   Traditionally, what has been the feeding vessel size cutoff for treatment of pulmonary AVMs?
    A. 1 mm
    B. 2 mm
    C. 3 mm
    D. 4 mm

27   What is the most common pulmonary vein anatomical variant?
    A. Common right pulmonary trunk
    B. Common left pulmonary trunk
    C. Separate trunk of right middle pulmonary vein
    D. Separate trunk of lingular pulmonary vein

28 A 33-year-old male is status post pulmonary vein ablation. What complication has occurred?

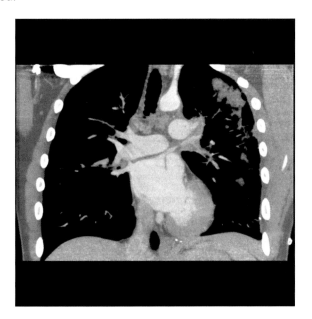

   A. Esophagoatrial fistula
   B. Pulmonary artery thrombosis
   C. Pulmonary vein stenosis
   D. Traumatic atrial septal defect

29 What is the most likely cause of the arch abnormality?

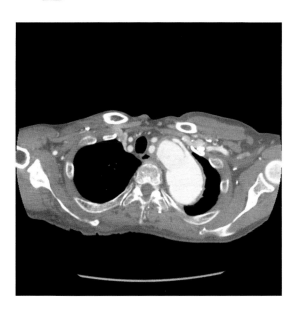
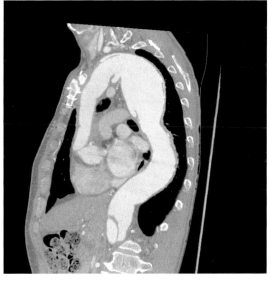

   A. Residual dissection flap
   B. Elephant trunk type repair
   C. Limited intimal tear
   D. Graft infection

30 The differentials for this imaging finding include Takayasu arteritis and which of the following?

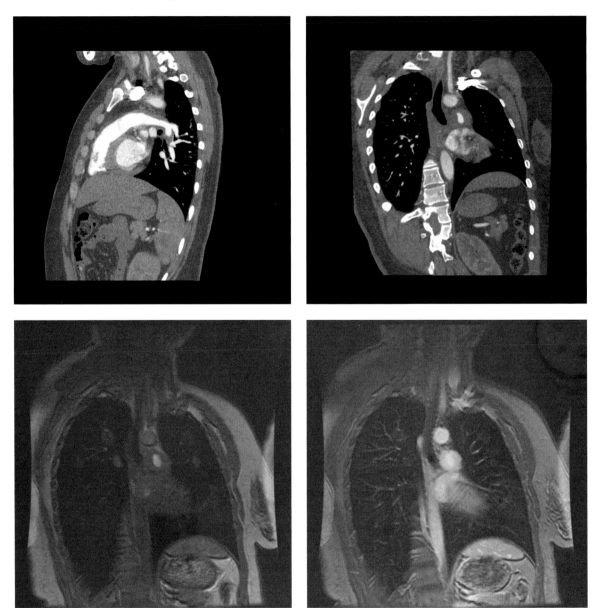

A. Polyarteritis nodosa
B. Kawasaki disease
C. Wegener granulomatosis
D. Giant cell arteritis

31 In adults with Marfan syndrome, what is the typical size of aorta that would meet surgical indication?

A. 4.0 cm
B. 5.0 cm
C. 6.0 cm
D. 7.0 cm

32 What is the next best step for this patient?

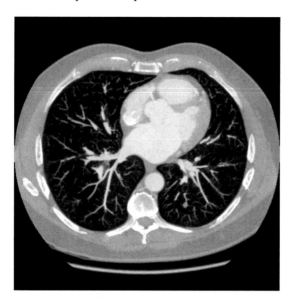

    A. Refer for embolization
    B. Refer for biopsy
    C. Close observation
    D. Look at thin axial images

33 Which of the following findings help identify the true lumen versus the false lumen on CTA?

    A. Larger luminal diameter
    B. Beak sign
    C. Lumen being wrapped by another lumen
    D. Inner wall calcification
    E. Cobweb sign

ANSWERS AND EXPLANATIONS

1 **Answer B.** There has been evolving use of thoracic endovascular aortic repair (TEVAR) in a number of aortic pathologies. Primary TEVAR indications include management of descending thoracic aortic aneurysms; penetrating atherosclerotic ulcer; type B aortic dissection; blunt trauma/thoracic aortic injury, and aortoesophageal and aortobronchial fistulas.

Thoracic aortic aneurysms exceeding 5.5 cm, symptomatic aneurysms, and aneurysms associated with a rapid growth rate of >1 cm per year are considered to be at increased risk for rupture and should be repaired. Penetrating atherosclerotic ulcers with depths >10 mm or diameters >20 mm are at a higher risk of progression and should be considered for repair. Open surgery for complicated acute type B dissection has been replaced by endovascular therapy in the current practice. Type B dissection is considered complicated when there is associated aneurysmal enlargement, rupture, or malperfusion.

In the setting of traumatic aortic transection, when the transection is contained and patients survive to treatment, endovascular repair has a significantly lower morbidity and mortality than open repair, even in the younger trauma patient population. Endovascular repair of infected fields are generally avoided. However, there is evolving experience that TEVAR may be useful as a temporizing measure in mycotic aneurysms and contaminated fields such as aortoesophageal fistula.

References: Manetta F, Newman J, Mattia A. Indications for thoracic endovascular aortic repair (TEVAR): a brief review. *Int J Angiol* 2018;27(4):177–184.

Nation DA, Wang GJ. TEVAR: endovascular repair of the thoracic aorta. *Semin Intervent Radiol* 2015;32(3):265–271.

Svensson LG, Kouchoukos NT, Miller DC, et al. Expert consensus document on the treatment of descending thoracic aortic disease using endovascular stent-grafts. *Ann Thorac Surg* 2008;85(1 Suppl):S1–S41.

2 **Answer A.** Usually, pulmonary artery dissection (PAD) is a complication of chronic pulmonary hypertension leading to a pulmonary artery (PA) aneurysm. PAD has also been associated with congenital heart defects leading to sustained high pulmonary artery flow and pulmonary hypertension. Dissection of the pulmonary artery, similar to aortic pathologies, occur as a result of formation of an intimal tear, which subsequently propagates along medial planes.

PAD occurs at the site of maximal dilatation of the pulmonary artery. The false lumen tends to rupture rather than propagate distally or develop a reentry site. Usually in younger patients, PAD is associated with congenital heart defects, whereas in older patients, it is associated with a variety of acquired diseases.

Rare causes include chronic inflammation of the pulmonary arteries, right heart endocarditis, amyloidosis, connective tissue disorders, trauma, and severe atherosclerosis.

References: Fernando DMG, Thilakarathne SMNK, Wickramasinghe CU. Pulmonary artery dissection-A review of 150 cases. *Heart Lung* 2019;48(5):428–435.

Perrotta S, Lentini S. Pulmonary artery dissection. *J Card Surg* 2015;30(5):442–427.

3 **Answer D.** Most common cause of aortic aneurysm is atherosclerosis and accounts for approximately 70% of cases. The other answer choices are all less common causes of ascending thoracic aortic aneurysm.

Reference: Agarwal PP, Chughtai A, Matzinger FR, et al. Multidetector CT of thoracic aortic aneurysms. *Radiographics* 2009;29(2):537–552. doi:10.1148/rg.292075080. Review.

4 **Answer C.** Hypertension is the most common risk factor for aortic dissection, occurring in a majority of patients with dissection. All of the other answer choices are less common risk factors for dissection.

Reference: McMahon MA, Squirrell CA. Multidetector CT of aortic dissection: a pictorial review. *Radiographics* 2010;30(2):445–460. doi:10.1148/rg.302095104. Review.

5 **Answer A.** The case illustrates a contrast entering the excluded lumen secondary to incomplete seal of the proximal endograft, characterized as a Type 1a endoleak. Despite recent advances in endovascular technology, endoleaks after endovascular repair of thoracic aortic aneurysms (TAA) remain one of the primary limitations of TAA repair.

- *Type I endoleaks* result from blood flow that originates from either proximal (type Ia) or distal (type Ib) endograft attachment sites.
- *Type II endoleaks* occur as a result of retrograde blood flow into the aneurysm sac from aortic branch vessels (most commonly intercostal and bronchial arteries and the left subclavian artery) as blood flows through branches from the nonstented segment of the aorta through the anastomotic connections and into vessels with a direct communication with the aneurysm sac. The most common branches involved in type II endoleaks are the intercostal and bronchial arteries and the left subclavian artery.
- *Type III endoleaks* occur when there is a structural defect within the endograft, such as fabric disruption or tear, or when disconnection occurs between two endografts in modular devices.
- *Type IV endoleaks* are caused by endograft porosity and are frequently identified at the time of graft implantation on the postimplantation.
- *Type V endoleaks* also called "endotension," refer to expansion of the aneurysm sac without the presence of an identifiable endoleak.

Management has generally consisted of aggressive endovascular repair of type I and III endoleaks and observation of type II endoleaks.

Reference: Ricotta JJ. Endoleak management and postoperative surveillance following endovascular repair of thoracic aortic aneurysms. *J Vasc Surg* 2010;52(4):91S–99S.

6 **Answer A.** Pulmonary arteriovenous malformations (AVMs) are the abnormal connections between a pulmonary artery and a pulmonary vein, which bypass the capillary bed and lead to right-to-left shunting of blood.

The etiology of pulmonary arteriovenous malformations (AVMs) can be congenital or acquired. Most patients with pulmonary AVMs have the autosomal dominant disease hereditary hemorrhagic telangiectasia (HHT) also known as Rendu-Osler-Weber disease.

Life-threatening complications of PAVM include stroke, transient ischemic attack, cerebral abscess, massive hemoptysis, and spontaneous hemothorax.

CT pulmonary angiography is considered the gold standard for diagnosis of PAVMs, and transcatheter embolization considered the gold standard for treatment.

References: Majumdar S, McWilliams JP. Approach to pulmonary arteriovenous malformations: a comprehensive update. *J Clin Med Res* 2020;9(6):1927.

Tellapuri S, Park HS, Kalva SP. Pulmonary arteriovenous malformations. *Int J Cardiovasc Imaging* 2019;35(8):1421–1428.

7 **Answer B.** Pulmonary artery sarcoma (PAS) a rare malignancy that can be misdiagnosed as pulmonary thromboembolism. PAS is commonly divided into mural and intimal sarcomas. The first is usually the typical leiomyosarcoma that develops along the medial smooth muscle of the large veins involving mainly the vena cava. The second affects the intimal layer of the large blood vessels along the pulmonary artery and the aorta. The distinction is difficult from imaging alone since grossly, both types of the tumor form a mass in the lumen and grow along the involved vessel. MR and PET may help differentiate PAS from regular thromboembolic disease with demonstration of gadolinium enhancement or FDG avidity.

Pulmonary arterial IMH is a rare event and an unusual complication of aortic dissection. Because ascending aorta and the pulmonary trunk have a common adventitia at the root of the great vessels, blood from ruptured IMH in ascending aorta can extend along the pulmonary artery and subsequently lead to luminal narrowing.

References: Assi T, Kattan J, Rassy E, et al. A comprehensive review on the diagnosis and management of intimal sarcoma of the pulmonary artery. *Crit Rev Oncol Hematol* 2020;147:102889.

Kang E-J, Lee K-N, Kim I, et al. Spontaneously developed pulmonary arterial intramural hematoma that mimicked thromboembolism. *Korean J Radiol* 2012;13(4):496–499.

8 **Answer D.** Annuloaortic ectasia is classically associated with Marfan syndrome. Other causes include Ehlers-Danlos syndrome, homocystinuria, and osteogenesis imperfecta. It can also be idiopathic without underlying genetic abnormality. Syphilitic aneurysm does not often involve the aortic root. Bicuspid aortopathy does not typically dilate the sinotubular junction. Takayasu arteritis tends to narrow the aorta.

Reference: Agarwal PP, Chughtai A, Matzinger FR, et al. Multidetector CT of thoracic aortic aneurysms. *Radiographics* 2009;29(2):537–552. doi:10.1148/rg.292075080. Review.

9a **Answer A.** The image demonstrates thickening of pulmonary valve leaflets and enlargement of the main pulmonary artery consistent with pulmonic stenosis. Aliasing within the pulmonary artery is also present on velocity-encoded images consistent with accelerated flow velocities that are beyond the selected Venc of the acquisition. The other pathologies would not apply.

The described murmur is classic for pulmonary stenosis. Aortic stenosis also presents with a similar sounding murmur and radiates to the region of the right clavicle and both carotids.

Reference: Porter RS, Kaplan JL, Lynn RB, et al. *The merck manual of diagnosis and therapy*, 20th ed. Whitehouse Station, NJ: Merck Sharp & Dohme Corp, 2018.

9b **Answer C.** Velocity aliasing artifact occurs when the chosen Venc of the acquisition is lower than the maximum velocities in the prescribed plane. In addition to misrepresenting the speed of flow, direction of flow is also erroneously mapped.

The peak gradient is estimated using the modified Bernoulli equation and as such, errors in peak velocity measurements will adversely be adversely affected. Diastolic flow volume is the total volume that occurs during the diastolic period of the cardiac cycle. Being much smaller in velocity, it will not be affected by aliasing artifact and sum measurement of this volume would not be affected. Aortic distensibility is calculated using minimum and maximum diameters of the aorta at the level of the sinotubular junction, in conjunction with maximal and minimal systolic and diastolic blood pressure (mm Hg). Aortic valve area is determined using planimetry of the valve opening and also would not be reliant on venc parameters.

References: Ibrahim E-SH, Johnson KR, Shaffer JM, et al. Comparison of different MRI techniques for measuring aortic compliance. *J Cardiovasc Magn Reson* 2010;12(1):P137.

Nayak KS, Nielsen J-F, Bernstein MA, et al. Cardiovascular magnetic resonance phase contrast imaging. *J Cardiovasc Magn Reson* 2015;17:71.

10 **Answer B.** Although the image demonstrates poor opacification of the pulmonary arteries, contrast is present in the SVC suggesting continued administration of contrast. In contrast, opacification on the systemic arterial system appears more uniform.

The phenomenon, transient interruption of contrast, occurs as unopacified blood entering the right heart from the IVC mixes with the administered intravenous contrast and results in dilution of overall contrast density. Deep inspiration which increases venous return is considered the most significant contributor to this artifact. Active coaching patients to minimize deep inspiration during the acquisition is recognized strategy to mitigate this phenomenon.

Increasing the contrast volume or injection rate does far less to remove the artifact and potentially compromising the study.

References: Renne J, von Falck C, Ringe KI, et al. CT angiography for pulmonary embolism detection: the effect of breathing on pulmonary artery enhancement using a 64-row detector system. *Acta Radiol* 2014;55(8):932–937.

Wittram C, Yoo AJ. Transient interruption of contrast on CT pulmonary angiography. *J Thorac Imaging* 2007;22(2):125–129.

11 **Answer B.** Dissection at the arch is considered a type B Stanford dissection. Type A involves the ascending aorta. Type B is any other type of dissection that does not involve the ascending aorta. There is no Stanford type C or D dissection.

Reference: McMahon MA, Squirrell CA. Multidetector CT of aortic dissection: a pictorial review. *Radiographics* 2010;30(2):445–460. doi:10.1148/rg.302095104. Review.

12 **Answer C.** A penetrating atherosclerotic ulcer (PAU) is among the spectrum of acute aortic syndromes. Pathologically it develops as a result of atherosclerotic change with ulceration of the vessel intima and slow progression to media layer. These typically result in intramural hematoma and can also lead to aortic dissection. Classically they appear as small contrast-filled outpouchings with jagged margins extending beyond the aortic wall contour, usually associated with severe atheromatous disease.

Most patients with PAU are at a higher risk from surgical intervention because of their advanced age and comorbidities. As such, patients can be managed conservatively with aggressive medical therapy and close observation, similar to a descending aortic dissection. For patients with continued pain or progression of disease, thoracic endovascular repair has been proved to yield excellent short-term and mid-term results in PAU of the descending aorta and has become the first line of management when intervention is indicated.

References: D'Annoville T, Ozdemir BA, Alric P, et al. Thoracic endovascular aortic repair for penetrating aortic ulcer: literature review. *Ann Thorac Surg* 2016;101(6):2272–2278.

Liu Y-H, Ke H-Y, Lin Y-C, et al. A penetrating atherosclerotic ulcer rupture in the ascending aorta with hemopericardium: a case report. *J Cardiothorac Surg* 2016;11(1):103.

13a **Answer B.** Coronal reformatted image shows annuloaortic ectasia (effacement of the sinotubular junction with dilated aortic root). Some have described this as a "pear-shaped/tulip bulb" appearance of the aorta. This constellation of anatomical changes is a classic morphologic appearance for Marfan syndrome. While atherosclerosis is the most common cause of aortic aneurysm, there does not appear to be atherosclerosis in this young patient. Bicuspid aortopathy can also cause aneurysm but does not typically give this classic appearance of annuloaortic ectasia. The appearance of aortic aneurysm caused by hypertension will also typically not involve annuloaortic ectasia.

References: Agarwal PP, Chughtai A, Matzinger FR, et al. Multidetector CT of thoracic aortic aneurysms. *Radiographics* 2009;29(2):537–552. doi:10.1148/rg.292075080. Review.

Ha HI, Seo JB, Lee SH, et al. Imaging of Marfan syndrome: multisystemic manifestations. *Radiographics* 2007;27(4):989–1004. Review.

13b **Answer D.** Although largely sporadic, mitral valve prolapse has also been associated with congenital connective tissue disorders, such as Marfan syndrome, and is considered the second most common cardiac abnormality in Marfan's. The other valvular abnormalities listed are not associated with Marfan syndrome.

References: Agarwal PP, Chughtai A, Matzinger FR, et al. Multidetector CT of thoracic aortic aneurysms. *Radiographics* 2009;29(2):537–552. doi:10.1148/rg.292075080. Review.

Ha HI, Seo JB, Lee SH, et al. Imaging of Marfan syndrome: multisystemic manifestations. *Radiographics* 2007;27(4):989–1004. Review.

14 **Answer D.** Classic ductus diverticulum features include smooth margins and gently sloping shoulders. It should form obtuse angles with the preserved aortic wall. There should not be an intimal flap; that would favor traumatic pseudoaneurysm. They can both be located at the aortic isthmus so that will not be a differentiating feature. Calcification can also occur in both chronic pseudoaneurysm and ductus diverticulum.

Reference: Steenburg SD, Ravenel JG, Ikonomidis JS, et al. Acute traumatic aortic injury: imaging evaluation and management. *Radiology* 2008;248(3):748–762. doi:10.1148/radiol.2483071416. Review.

15 **Answer D.** The rapid progression of the aneurysm is most consistent with mycotic aneurysm. Atherosclerosis would not be this rapid in course. Saccular type of aneurysm seen here is also more common in mycotic aneurysms. Takayasu arteritis typically causes narrowing but can also cause aneurysm; in this case, it could be in the differential but is considered a less likely cause. Posttraumatic aneurysm is also possible, but the rapid enlargement and irregular borders are more consistent with mycotic than posttraumatic aneurysm.

References: Agarwal PP, Chughtai A, Matzinger FR, et al. Multidetector CT of thoracic aortic aneurysms. *Radiographics* 2009;29(2):537–552. doi:10.1148/rg.292075080. Review.

Macedo TA, Stanson AW, Oderich GS, et al. Infected aortic aneurysms: imaging findings. *Radiology* 2004;231(1):250–257. Erratum in: Radiology 2006;238(3):1078.

16 **Answer B.** The noncontrast image confirms high density surrounding the ascending aorta, which makes this a type A dissection equivalent with intramural hematoma versus retrograde extension of the dissection down the ascending thoracic aorta. The best next step is immediate surgery.

References: Karmy-Jones R, Aldea G, Boyle EM Jr. The continuing evolution in the management of thoracic aortic dissection. *Chest* 2000;117(5):1221–1223.

Mészáros I, Mórocz J, Szlávi J, et al. Epidemiology and clinicopathology of aortic dissection. *Chest* 2000;117(5):1271–1278.

17 **Answer B.** This is a patient with Marfan syndrome who had a Bentall composite aortic root replacement that developed large coronary button aneurysms. Note the dissection in the descending thoracic aorta. Due to the underlying aortic wall abnormality in Marfan patients, the reimplanted contrary buttons can be prone to aneurysm formation. While Takayasu and prior syphilis infection can give rise to aneurysms, they are not associated with coronary button aneurysms.

References: Bruschi G, Cannata A, Botta L, et al. Giant true aneurysm of the right coronary artery button long after aortic root replacement. *Eur J Cardiothorac Surg* 2013;43(5):e139–e140. doi: 10.1093/ejcts/ezt057.

Prescott-Focht JA, Martinez-Jimenez S, Hurwitz LM, et al. Ascending thoracic aorta: postoperative imaging evaluation. *Radiographics* 2013;33(1):73–85. doi:10.1148/rg.331125090. Review.

18 **Answer A.** Reformatted images at the aortic root show type A dissection with the dissection flaps prolapsing into the aortic root during diastole causing aortic regurgitation.

Reference: McMahon MA, Squirrell CA. Multidetector CT of aortic dissection: a pictorial review. *Radiographics* 2010;30(2):445–460. doi:10.1148/rg.302095104. Review.

19a **Answer C.** An outpouching is seen in the descending thoracic aorta, which is consistent with a penetrating aortic ulcer (PAU). In a penetrating aortic ulcer, there is disruption of the inner layer (intima) by the penetrating ulcer with subsequent bleed in the medial layer. In this case, there is focal dilation of the aorta at the site of PAU. The adventitial/outer layer is intact or else there would be aortic rupture.

Reference: Castañer E, Andreu M, Gallardo X, et al. CT in nontraumatic acute thoracic aortic disease: typical and atypical features and complications. *Radiographics* 2003;23:S93–S110. Review.

19b **Answer A.** Penetrating aortic ulcers typically occur in the descending aorta and is considered a type B aortic dissection equivalent. The most appropriate treatment in an asymptomatic patient is medical therapy (control blood pressure). It is only in patients who have aortic rupture/hemodynamic instability that surgery is considered. Endovascular treatment can be performed particularly given the high risk of surgical repair. Indications for treatment include symptomatic patients or if there is rapid enlargement of the ulcerating aneurysm.

Reference: Castañer E, Andreu M, Gallardo X, et al. CT in nontraumatic acute thoracic aortic disease: typical and atypical features and complications. *Radiographics* 2003;23:S93–S110. Review.

20 **Answer C.** Axial image shows a luminal thrombus in the descending thoracic aorta. There is no current role for aggressive management such as surgical or endovascular thrombectomy. Instead, patients are managed medically with anticoagulation.

Reference: Ferrari E, Vidal R, Chevallier T, et al. Atherosclerosis of the thoracic aorta and aortic debris as a marker of poor prognosis: benefit of oral anticoagulants. *J Am Coll Cardiol* 1999;33(5):1317–1322.

21 **Answer A.** Right ventricle to left ventricle short-axis ratio is the best measurement to obtain for assessment of right heart strain and the severity of the pulmonary embolism. A ratio of >1 is indicative of RV strain, while >1.5 indicates a severe episode of PE. Interventricular septal wall thickness and right ventricular wall thickness have not been reported to correlate with acute pulmonary embolism outcomes.

Reference: Ghaye B, Ghuysen A, Bruyere PJ, et al. Can CT pulmonary angiography allow assessment of severity and prognosis in patients presenting with pulmonary embolism? What the radiologist needs to know. *Radiographics* 2006;26(1):23–39; discussion 39–40. Review.

22a **Answer C.** Frontal chest radiograph shows enlarged pulmonary artery contour along with increased flow suggesting of underlying left to right shunt. This is therefore most consistent with pulmonary hypertension with underlying atrial or ventricular septal defect.

Reference: Peña E, Dennie C, Veinot J, et al. Pulmonary hypertension: how the radiologist can help. *Radiographics* 2012;32(1):9–32. doi:10.1148/rg.321105232.

22b **Answer B.** Volume-rendered image shows markedly enlarged pulmonary artery compressing the origin/proximal left coronary artery. This can be treated with surgery or stenting, but given the high mortality of pulmonary hypertension patients for surgery, stenting is now an accepted treatment.

References: Caldera AE, Cruz-Gonzalez I, Bezerra HG, et al. Endovascular therapy for left main compression syndrome. Case report and literature review. *Chest* 2009;135(6):1648–1650. doi:10.1378/chest.08-2922. Review.

Peña E, Dennie C, Veinot J, et al. Pulmonary hypertension: how the radiologist can help. *Radiographics* 2012;32(1):9–32. doi:10.1148/rg.321105232.

23 **Answer C.** Simple malformations are ones that originate from 1 single segmental artery. Complex malformations are from multiple segmental feeding arteries. There is no intermediate malformation that has been described.

Reference: White RI Jr, Mitchell SE, Barth KH, et al. Angioarchitecture of pulmonary arteriovenous malformations: an important consideration before embolotherapy. *AJR Am J Roentgenol* 1983;140(4):681–686.

24 **Answer A.** Pulmonary AVMs are a type of right to left shunt between the unoxygenated blood from the pulmonary artery into the oxygenated blood of the pulmonary veins.

Reference: Martinez-Jimenez S, Heyneman LE, McAdams HP, et al. Nonsurgical extracardiac vascular shunts in the thorax: clinical and imaging characteristics. *Radiographics* 2010;30(5):e41. doi:10.1148/rg.e41.

25 **Answer A.** Greater than 50% of patients with pulmonary AVM have HHT, while 5% to 15% of HHT patients have pulmonary AVM.

Reference: Martinez-Jimenez S, Heyneman LE, McAdams HP, et al. Nonsurgical extracardiac vascular shunts in the thorax: clinical and imaging characteristics. *Radiographics* 2010;30(5):e41. doi:10.1148/rg.e41.

26 **Answer C.** The traditional cutoff for treatment of pulmonary AVMs is a 3-mm feeding vessel. However, it is now accepted that treatment of smaller than 3-mm feeding arteries should also be considered given that the smaller AVMs may still cause paradoxical embolization.

Reference: Trerotola SO, Pyeritz RE. PAVM embolization: an update. *AJR Am J Roentgenol* 2010;195(4):837–845. doi:10.2214/AJR.10.5230. Review.

27 **Answer B.** The most common variant of pulmonary venous anatomy is common left trunk.

Reference: Porres DV, Morenza OP, Pallisa E, et al. Learning from the pulmonary veins. *Radiographics* 2013;33(4):999–1022. doi:10.1148/rg.334125043. Review.

28 **Answer C.** Coronal reformat shows narrowing of the left superior pulmonary vein and abnormal left upper lobe airspace opacities. This is consistent with pulmonary vein stenosis post left atrial ablation with pulmonary venous infarct.

Reference: Porres DV, Morenza OP, Pallisa E, et al. Learning from the pulmonary veins. *Radiographics* 2013;33(4):999–1022. doi:10.1148/rg.334125043. Review.

29 **Answer B.** Axial and oblique sagittal views of the aorta show flaps at the arch. This is consistent with an elephant trunk type repair with the arch graft projecting into the aortic lumen in anticipation of future aortic procedure. This patient subsequently received a thoracic endograft connecting to the arch graft to exclude the arch aneurysm. While residual dissection flaps can be present, the appearance of the flaps in continuity with the ascending graft is diagnostic of a normal postoperative appearance of an elephant trunk procedure. This is not a limited intimal tear. There are no findings here to suggest graft infection.

Reference: Sundaram B, Quint LE, Patel HJ, et al. CT findings following thoracic aortic surgery. *Radiographics* 2007;27(6):1583–1594. Review.

30 Answer D. Oblique images show abnormal left pulmonary artery with wall thickening and enhancement. This is suggestive of vasculitis. Takayasu arteritis and giant cell arteritis are large vessel vasculitis that can involve the main pulmonary artery branches. Although the imaging features may be similar, clinical history may be helpful to differentiate. Takayasu arteritis typically occurs in younger patients (<40 years old), while giant cell arteritis typically occurs in patients >50 years of age.

Reference: Castañer E, Alguersuari A, Gallardo X, et al. When to suspect pulmonary vasculitis: radiologic and clinical clues. *Radiographics* 2010;30(1):33–53. doi:10.1148/rg.301095103.

31 Answer B. In adult patients with Marfan syndrome, prophylactic surgery is recommended when the diameter exceeds 5.0 cm. However, earlier surgery may be indicated if there is rapid rate of growth (>1 cm per year).

References: Agarwal PP, Chughtai A, Matzinger FR, et al. Multidetector CT of thoracic aortic aneurysms. *Radiographics* 2009;29(2):537–552. doi:10.1148/rg.292075080. Review.

Ha HI, Seo JB, Lee SH, et al. Imaging of Marfan syndrome: multisystemic manifestations. *Radiographics* 2007;27(4):989–1004. Review.

32 Answer D. MIP axial image shows a nodule with apparent vessel connection. This may be a small simple pulmonary AVM or an artifact due to MIP technique. For the diagnosis of pulmonary AVM, there must be visualization of both a feeding branch and also the draining vein. This one image is not diagnostic so the source images should be consulted to see if this is a nodule versus AVM. The thin axial images show this to be a nodule rather than an AVM.

Reference: Martinez-Jimenez S, Heyneman LE, McAdams HP, et al. Nonsurgical extracardiac vascular shunts in the thorax: clinical and imaging characteristics. *Radiographics* 2010;30(5):e41. doi:10.1148/rg.e41.

33 Answer C. The false lumen is often the larger diameter lumen and shows the beak sign. In cases where there is the appearance of the lumen being wrapped by another lumen, the true lumen is the one wrapped by the false lumen. Inner wall calcification is not helpful. However, in acute dissection, the outer wall calcification is indicative of the true lumen. This would not be as helpful in chronic dissection since the false lumen can calcify. Cobweb sign indicates false lumen; it is a specific sign but is not always seen.

Reference: LePage MA, Quint LE, Sonnad SS, et al. Aortic dissection: CT features that distinguish true lumen from false lumen. *AJR Am J Roentgenol* 2001;177(1):207–211.

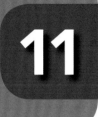

11 Devices and Postoperative Appearance

Jody Shen, MD • Joe Y. Hsu, MD • Amar B. Shah, MD, MPA •
Jean Jeudy, MD • Sachin Malik, MD

QUESTIONS

1a A 35-year-old male has a history of syncope. There is no family history of sudden death. The patient is scheduled for a cardiac MRI, and the technologist asks you to review a screening chest radiograph.

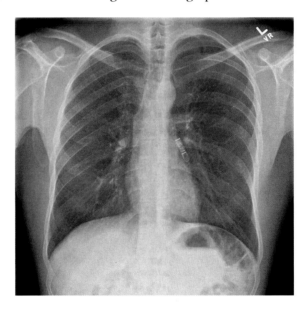

What is the finding on the radiograph?

A. Repeat CXR without device in patient's pocket.
B. Previous pacemaker with leads removed
C. Loop recorder
D. External ICD

1b After reviewing the previous screening chest radiograph, how would you proceed with the scheduled cardiac MRI?

A. The x-ray does not have any abnormalities to be concerned with.
B. Discuss the issue with the patient and proceed with the cardiac MRI.
C. Discuss the issue with the patient and postpone until you can discuss with the primary provider.
D. Discuss the issue with the patient and cancel the study because it is contra-indicated.

2a A chest radiograph was performed for a patient in the cardiac intensive care unit to check intra-aortic balloon pump (IABP) placement.

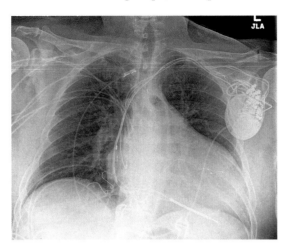

Which of the following are appropriate indications for IABP placement?

A. Aortic dissection
B. Acute tricuspid incompetence
C. Aortic insufficiency
D. Acute mitral incompetence

2b What is a potential complication related to the device positioning as shown?

A. Cerebrovascular accident
B. Acute tricuspid insufficiency
C. Pulmonary vein stenosis
D. Atrial septal perforation

3 A patient with ventricular assist device and worsening heart failure presents with the following CT

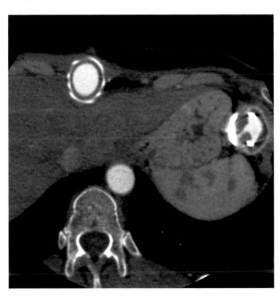

Which of the following is the best diagnosis?

A. LVAD infection
B. Cannula fracture
C. LVAD thrombosis
D. Myocardial infarction

4   A 74-year-old man with ischemic cardiomyopathy post left ventricular assist device placement presents with fever. Which component of the left ventricular assist device is most commonly associated with infection?

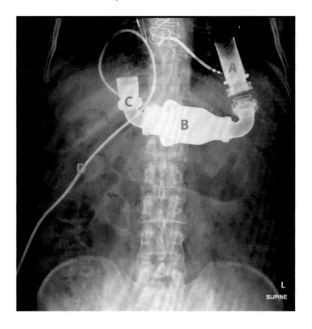

A. A
B. B
C. C
D. D

5   A 43-year-old male has a history of ventricular tachycardia and is status post ICD placement 4 months ago now complains of chest pain.

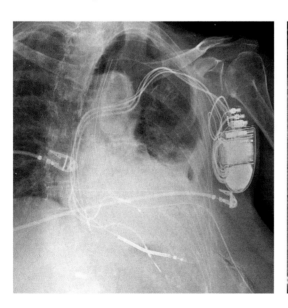
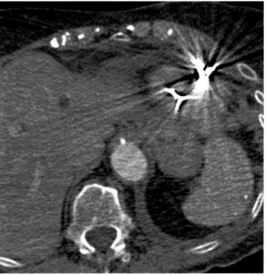

Which of the following is the most likely diagnosis?

A. Myocardial infarction
B. Lead perforation
C. Lead fracture
D. Pneumothorax

6a Which radiograph shows the appropriate positioning of an Impella Ventricular Support System?

A.

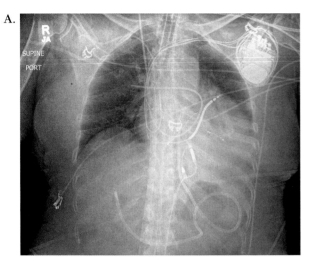

B.

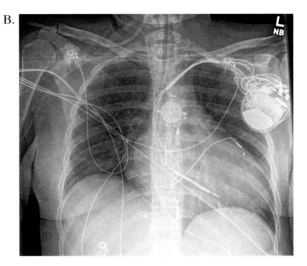

C.

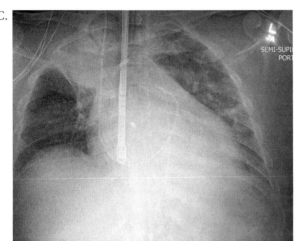

D.

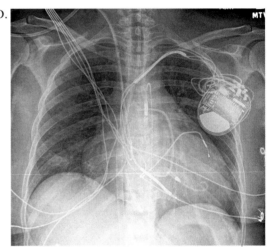

6b Which of the following is a potential complication of a malpositioned Impella device as shown?

A. Pulmonary embolism
B. Aortic wall injury
C. Acute tricuspid insufficiency
D. Pulmonary vein stenosis

7 After orthotopic heart transplantation where do the recipient's pulmonary veins most likely come from?

A. Donor
B. Recipient
C. Xenograft
D. Polytetrafluoroethylene (PTFE) graft

8   A 27-year-old female with a history of heart block presents for routine chest x-ray evaluation after implantable cardioverter–defibrillator (ICD) placement. Which letter best localizes the acute abnormality on the image shown?

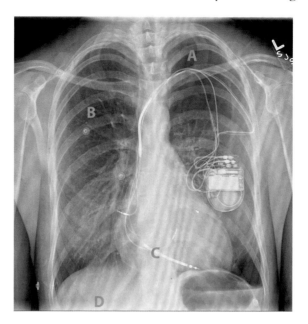

A. A
B. B
C. C
D. D

9   A 57-year-old man presents with shortness of breath. Which of the following best characterizes the device seen on the chest radiograph and CT?

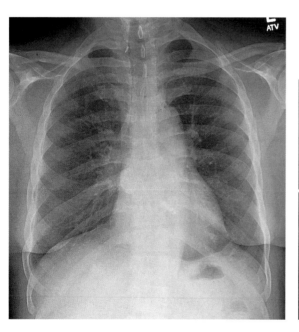
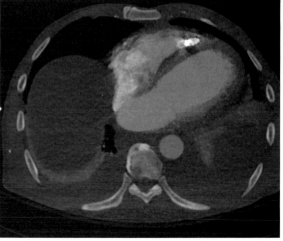

A. Pacemaker
B. Loop recorder
C. External cardiac defibrillator
D. Zio patch

10 A radiopaque device overlies the cardiac silhouette on a routine chest radiograph. Which of the following best describes the device?

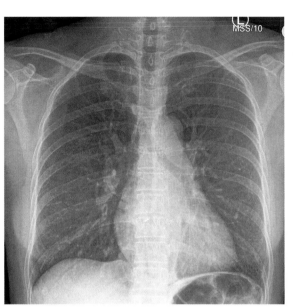
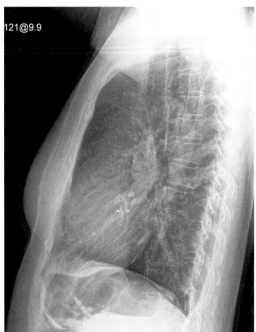

A. Atrial septal occluder device
B. Displaced prosthetic mitral valve
C. Atrial pacing device
D. Left atrial appendage closure device

11 Which of the following is an appropriate indication for the devices shown?

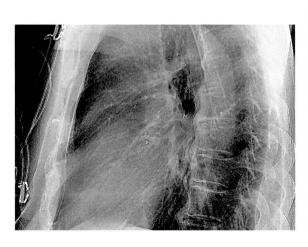
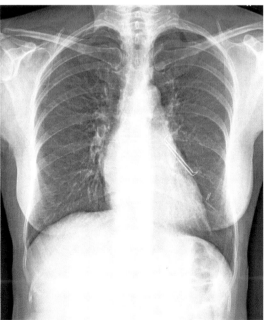

A. Pulmonary hypertension
B. Pulmonary edema
C. Pulmonary vein stenosis
D. Atrial fibrillation

12 A 46-year-old female underwent recent revision of her ICD for abnormal lead positioning and failure to capture. She presents for a chest radiograph 2 months after her revision for follow-up.

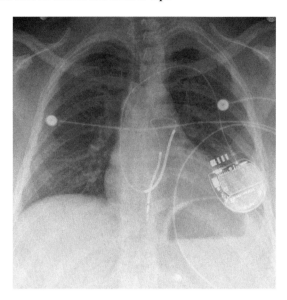

Which of the following best describes the diagnosis?

A. Persistent left superior vena cava
B. Twiddler syndrome
C. Atrial septal defect
D. Arterial placement

13 You are asked to read these postpacemaker chest radiographs. What is the best next step?

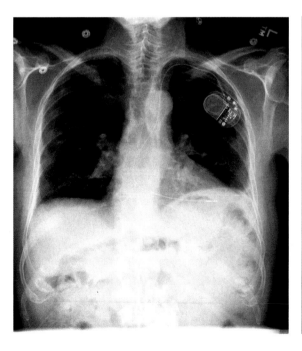
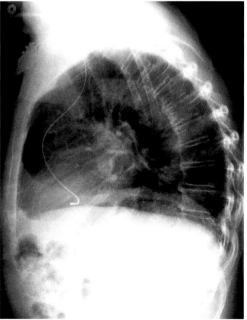

A. Do nothing; pacemaker is in a left-sided superior vena cava.
B. Recommend a CT of the chest.
C. Recommend a chest tube.
D. Recommend surgery.

14 A 60-year-old woman has a device (arrow) placed 12 days after aortic valve and root replacement. What is the indication for placement of this device?

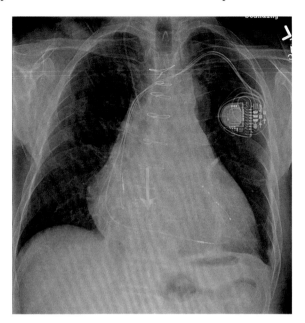

A. Severe pulmonary hypertension
B. Hypotension
C. Atrial fibrillation
D. Uncorrected bleeding diathesis

15 The below patient underwent surgery to repair a type A aortic dissection. The arrow indicates which of the following?

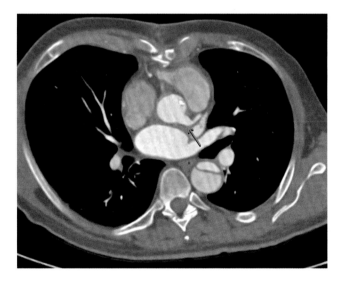

A. Aneurysm of the left main coronary artery
B. Dissection in the left main coronary artery
C. Thrombus in the left main coronary artery
D. Reimplanted left main coronary artery

16 A 57-year-old male underwent a composite aortic valve and root graft repair and coronary artery reimplantation for a type A dissection. Which of the following is seen on the axial and volume-rendered image from the postoperative CT angiogram shown below?

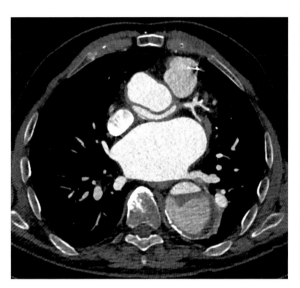
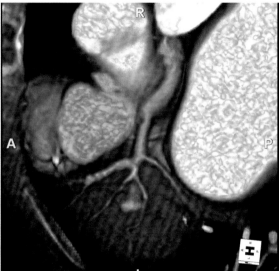

A. Ascending aortic aneurysm
B. Ascending aortic dissection
C. Ascending aortic thrombus
D. Reimplanted left coronary artery

17 The below images show which of the following?

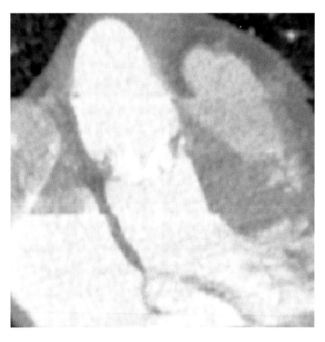
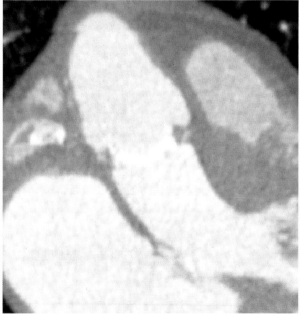

A. Aortic root dissection
B. Paravalvular leak
C. Postsurgical ventriculoseptal leaflet
D. Stuck leaflet

18 A 75-year-old woman with a history of bioprosthetic aortic valve replacement 4 years earlier for aortic stenosis presents with fevers and chills. Which of the following best describes the abnormality seen in the image below?

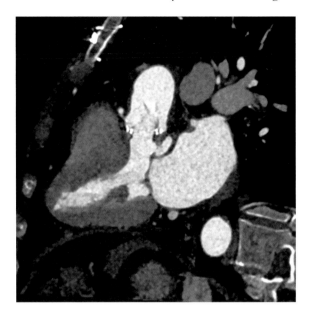

A. Pseudoaneurysm
B. Valve dehiscence
C. Paravalvular leak
D. Stuck leaflet

19 The below images show a patient who has had what type of treatment?

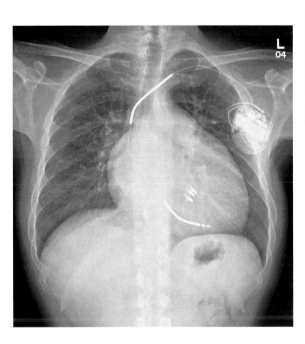 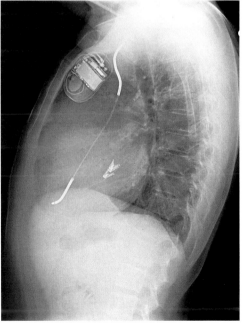

A. Mitral annuloplasty ring
B. Mitral clip
C. Mitral valve in valve replacement
D. Mitral valve replacement

20   Which of the following is the primary indication for use of the implanted device seen in the images below?

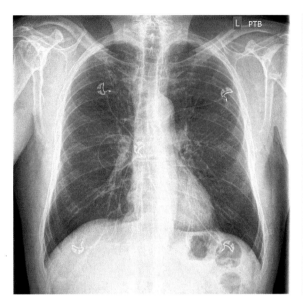 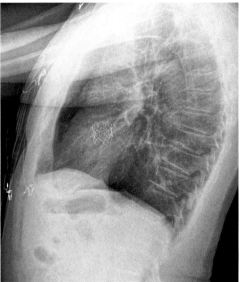

   A. Mitral stenosis
   B. Mitral regurgitation
   C. Aortic stenosis
   D. Aortic regurgitation

21   A 66-year-old male with a history of four-vessel coronary artery bypass grafting undergoes a coronary CT angiogram. What is a complication associated with the abnormality seen?

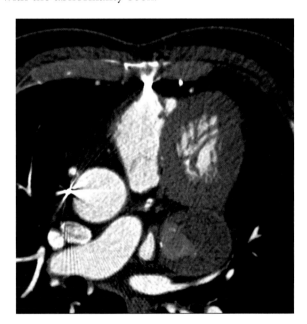

   A. Cerebrovascular accident
   B. Pulmonary embolism
   C. Atrial fibrillation
   D. Aortic dissection

22 A 62-year-old man with a history of coronary artery bypass graft surgery and severe mitral regurgitation undergoes a CT angiogram for preprocedural mitral valve repair evaluation.

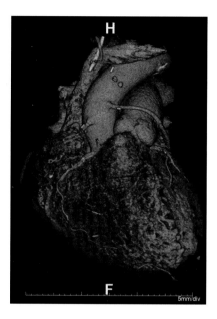

What is the abnormality shown?

A. Occluded left internal mammary artery graft
B. Occluded saphenous vein graft
C. Left internal mammary artery graft aneurysm
D. Saphenous vein graft aneurysm

23 A 72-year-old male with a history of endovascular stent graft repair of a thoracic aortic aneurysm presents for a follow-up CT examination. Volume-rendered images from 1 month and 6 months after the repair are shown below. Which of the following best describes the findings?

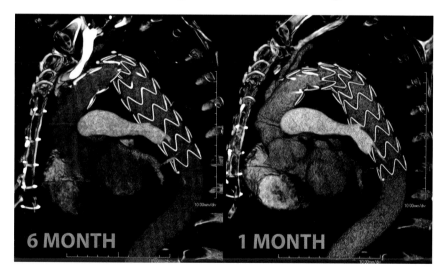

A. Expected appearance
B. Type III endoleak
C. Aortic perforation
D. Stent graft kinking

ANSWERS AND EXPLANATIONS

1a **Answer C.** The chest radiograph demonstrates an implantable loop recorder, which is typically contained in the anterior soft tissues of the chest.

Implantable loop recorders (ILRs) are useful in detecting undiagnosed recurrent arrhythmic episodes, particularly in unexplained syncope, with a significantly higher diagnostic rate than other conventional tests.

ILRs allow for prolonged monitoring without external electrodes (up to 3 years) and have the ability to autoactivate when an arrhythmia is present. Once an episode is recorded, the memory is archived by the patient or a relative by applying a nonmagnetic handheld activator. Given prolonged electrocardiographic monitoring, loop recorders can provide more accurate correlations between a patient's symptoms and documented abnormalities in heart rhythm.

Reference: Subbiah RN, Gula LJ, Klein GJ, et al. Ambulatory monitoring (Holter, event recorders, external, and implantable loop recorders and wireless technology). In: Gussak I, Antzelevitch C, Wilde AAM, et al. (eds.). *Electrical diseases of the heart*. London, UK: Springer, 2008:344–352.

1b **Answer B.** Studies investigating the effect of scanning implantable loop recorders (ILRs) in an MRI environment demonstrate no significant translational movement or dislodgement of ILRs in relation to exposure to long-bore and short-bore 1.5 T MRI systems. Thus, MRI scanning of ILR patients can be performed without harm to the patient or device. However, artifacts that could be mistaken for a tachyarrhythmia are seen frequently and should not be interpreted as pathology.

References: Shellock FG, Tkach JA, Ruggieri PM, et al. Cardiac pacemakers, ICDs, and loop recorder: evaluation of translational attraction using conventional ("long-bore") and "short-bore" 1.5 and 3.0 Tesla MRI systems: safety. *J Cardiovasc Magn Reson* 2003;5(2):387–397.

Wong JA, Yee R, Gula LJ, et al. Feasibility of magnetic resonance imaging in patients with an implantable loop recorder. *Pacing Clin Electrophysiol* 2008;31(3):333–337.

2a **Answer D.** Intra-aortic balloon pumps (IABP), initially introduced in the 1960s, remain the most widely used form of mechanical circulatory support for patients with critical cardiac disease. As the IABP balloon expands, the volume displacement of blood, which occurs both proximally and distally in the ascending and proximal descending aorta, is termed "counterpulsation." Effectively, balloon inflation in diastole and then rapid deflation in systole results in a decrease in systolic blood pressure and an increase in diastolic pressure. The result is afterload reduction in systole and augmentation of aortic root and coronary artery pressure in diastole, when coronary perfusion pressure is maximal.

The available clinical evidence supports intra-aortic balloon pump placement in cases of cardiogenic shock or refractory angina. Other indications such as mechanical complications of myocardial infarction (i.e., acute mitral regurgitation and ventricular septal defect), intractable arrhythmia, and refractory heart failure are less common but generally accepted indications for IABP support.

IABP placement is contraindicated in patients with aortic insufficiency because it worsens the magnitude of regurgitation. IABP insertion should not be attempted in case of suspected or known aortic dissection because inadvertent balloon placement in the false lumen may result in extension of the dissection or even aortic rupture. Similarly, aortic rupture can occur if IABP is inserted in patients with sizable abdominal aortic aneurysms. Patients with end-stage cardiac disease should not be considered for IABP unless as a bridge to ventricular assist device or cardiac transplantation.

References: Tsagalou EP, Drakos SG, Tsolakis E, et al. Intraaortic balloon pump in the management of acute heart failure syndromes. In: Mebazaa A, Gheorghiade M, Zannad FM (eds.). *Acute heart failure.* London, UK: Springer London, 2008:671–683.

White JM, Ruygrok PN. Intra-aortic balloon counterpulsation in contemporary practice—where are we? *Heart Lung Circulation* 2015;24(4):335–341.

2b **Answer A.** Chest radiograph shows the radiopaque tip of the IABP projecting over the aortic arch (arrow). This places the patient at risk for cerebral ischemia as it may obstruct the great vessels.

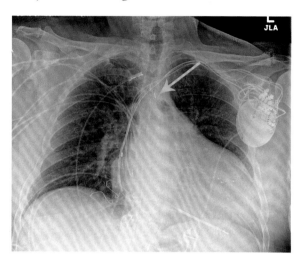

If the tip is too distally placed, then the IABP may not be effective enough in increasing coronary blood flow and may also obstruct the splanchnic vessels. Other IABP-associated complications include limb ischemia, aortic dissection, and infection.

IABP placement is important for successful diastolic augmentation of coronary perfusion. The IABP catheter is inserted percutaneously into the femoral artery through an introducer sheath with a modified Seldinger technique. Once vascular access is obtained, the balloon catheter is inserted and advanced, usually under fluoroscopic guidance, into the proximal descending thoracic aorta, with its radiopaque tip 2 to 3 cm distal to the origin of the left subclavian artery (at the level of the carina).

References: Godoy MC, Leitman BS, de Groot PM, et al. Chest radiography in the ICU: part 2, evaluation of cardiovascular lines and other devices. *AJR Am J Roentgenol* 2012;198(3): 572–581.

Krishna M, Zacharowski K. Principles of intra-aortic balloon pump counterpulsation. *Cont Educ Anaesth Crit Care Pain* 2009;9(1):24–28.

Mohamed I, Lau CT, Bolen MA, et al. Building a bridge to save a failing ventricle: radiologic evaluation of short- and long-term cardiac assist devices. *Radiographics* 2015;35(2):327–356.

White JM, Ruygrok PN. Intra-aortic balloon counterpulsation in contemporary practice—where are we? *Heart Lung Circulation* 2015;24(4):335–341.

3 **Answer C.** Axial image from a cardiac CT demonstrates the inflow (patient left) and outflow (patient right) cannulas of a ventricular assist device inferior to the base of the heart. Thrombus obstructs the inflow cannula.

The development of left ventricular assist devices (LVADs), first as a bridge to transplant and then as destination therapy, has significantly improved survival and quality of life of patients with end-stage heart failure.

LVAD thrombosis occurs in 2% to 13% of adult patients with a continuous-flow LVAD. This thrombus may form as an acute event or insidiously over a prolonged period of time. Thrombus in the left ventricle, inflow cannula, pump housing, outflow cannula, outflow graft, or aortic root may produce devastating events that include thromboembolic stroke, peripheral thromboembolism, LVAD malfunction with reduced systemic flows, LVAD failure with life-threatening hemodynamic impairment, cardiogenic shock, and death. For this reason, patients are placed on anticoagulation and antiplatelet therapy.

The definitive therapy for LVAD thrombosis is explantation of the device and cardiac transplantation. Unfortunately, the immediate availability of a compatible donor heart leaves this option as a last resort.

References: Bartoli CR, Ailawadi G, Kern JA. Diagnosis, nonsurgical management, and prevention of LVAD thrombosis: LVAD thrombosis. *J Cardiac Surg* 2014;29(1):83–94.

Lima B, Mack M, Gonzalez-Stawinski GV. Ventricular assist devices: the future is now. *Trends Cardiovasc Med* 2015;25(4):360–369.

4 **Answer D.** Frontal radiograph of the lower chest and upper abdomen obtained for LVAD line evaluation demonstrates the components of a HeartMate II, which is a continuous-flow LVAD for destination therapy. The percutaneous driveline (letter D) is most commonly associated with LVAD infection. This exits from the right upper quadrant of the abdomen and extends from the pump to an external controller and power source (not shown).

LVAD infections remain among the most frequently encountered adverse events and often lead to significant morbidity and mortality. LVAD-specific infections may be of the hardware itself or the body surfaces that contain them. This includes infections of the pump, cannula, anastomoses, pocket, and the percutaneous driveline or tunnel. LVAD driveline infections are the most common type of LVAD-associated infection and may reflect the presence of a deeper infection of the pocket space, pump, and/or cannula. The inflow conduit (letter A), pump (letter B), and outflow graft snap ring (letter C) are less commonly associated with infection.

LVAD-related infections include infective endocarditis, mediastinitis, and sternal wound infection. Evaluation with CT may reveal large vegetations and cannula insertion infections. CT may also play a role in characterizing sternal wound infections, particularly to define the extent of a deep-seated infection.

References: Mohamed I, Lau CT, Bolen MA, et al. Building a bridge to save a failing ventricle: radiologic evaluation of short- and long-term cardiac assist devices. *Radiographics* 2015;35(2):327–356.

Sigakis CJG, Mathai SK, Suby-Long TD, et al. Radiographic review of current therapeutic and monitoring devices in the chest. *Radiographics* 2018;38(4):1027–1045.

5 **Answer B.** Portable AP radiograph demonstrates multiple implanted cardiac leads with tips overlying the right ventricle. Further evaluation by CT shows that the tip has migrated beyond the myocardium and terminates outside the heart.

Cardiac perforation after pacemaker or implantable cardioverter–defibrillator (ICD) implantation is an infrequent complication, more frequently seen in the right ventricle but also in the right atrium. Cardiac perforations may present as acute (events occurring within 24 hours after implantation), subacute (occurring 5 days to 1 month after implantation), or delayed manifestations (occurring more than 1 month after implantation).

The most common symptom is pacing or sensing failure. If a lead perforates the myocardium, capture threshold will be increased, and sensing threshold will be reduced in general. In some asymptomatic patients with delayed perforation, pacemaker function and electro-physiologic parameters appear normal and thus cannot exclude cardiac perforation. Hemodynamic stability is mainly determined by the development of hemopericardium.

Sharp chest pain during the insertion, evidence of cardiac tamponade with breathlessness, raised jugular venous pressure, falling systemic blood pressure, and cyanosis, is suggestive of hemopericardium that requires emergency pericardiocentesis and possibly cardiac surgical repair. Echocardiography or computed tomography should confirm hemopericardium and may even show the electrode tip in the pericardial space. Signs and symptoms of pericarditis, including a pericardial friction rub, are also suggestive.

References: Oh S. Cardiac perforation associated with a pacemaker or ICD lead. In: Das MR (ed.). *Modern pacemakers—present and future*. InTech, 2011. Available from: http://www.intechopen.com/books/modern-pacemakers-present-and-future/cardiac-perforation-associatedwith-a-pacemaker-or-icd-lead

Ramsdale DR, Rao A. Complications of pacemaker implantation. In: *Cardiac pacing and device therapy*. London, UK: Springer London, 2012:249–282. Available from: https://doi.org/10.1007/978-1-4471-2939-4_12

6a **Answer D.** The Impella Ventricular Support System is a catheter-based blood pump that is placed retrograde across the aortic valve via femoral arterial access. The device rapidly draws blood from the left ventricle and returns blood into the ascending aorta. Ideally, the distal tip of the device should be positioned centrally over the left ventricle about 3 to 4 cm past the aortic valve. This is seen in Image D (arrow at the distal tip/inflow portion of the cannula).

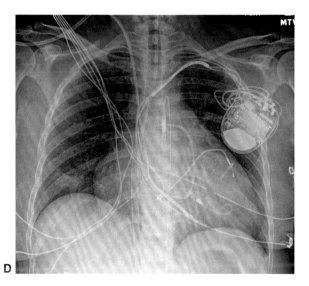

In Image A, the device is coiled in the upper abdominal aorta (arrow). In Image B, the device is malpositioned in the descending thoracic aorta (arrow). In Image C, the device tip/inflow portion of the cannula lies just past the aortic valve (arrow).

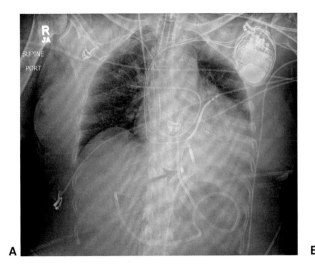

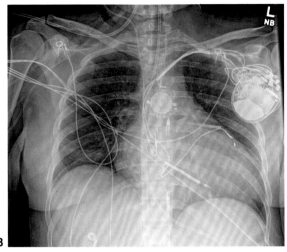

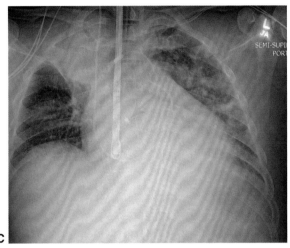

6b **Answer B.** Complications include aortic wall injury, diminished flow and damage to the aortic valve, arrhythmia, poor flow augmentation, ventricular perforation, thrombosis, device fracture, limb ischemia, and cerebrovascular accidents.

Reference: Mohamed I, Lau CT, Bolen MA, et al. Building a bridge to save a failing ventricle: radiologic evaluation of short- and long-term cardiac assist devices. *Radiographics* 2015;35(2):327–356.

Sigakis CJG, Mathai SK, Suby-Long TD, et al. Radiographic review of current therapeutic and monitoring devices in the chest. *Radiographics* 2018;38(4):1027–1045.

7 **Answer B.** The posterior aspect of the left atrium and pulmonary veins are from the native heart (recipient).

With the Lower and Shumway technique of orthotopic heart transplantation, the atrial anastomoses are typically created by connecting the posterior halves of the recipient's atria with the anterior parts of the donor's atria. The bicaval technique excises most of the recipient's atria and connects the donor heart to the recipient's superior and inferior vena caval cuffs, posterior wall of the left atrium, and pulmonary veins.

Reference: Bogot NR, Durst R, Shaham D, et al. Cardiac CT of the transplanted heart: Indications, technique, appearance, and complications. *Radiographics* 2007;27(5):1297–1309.

8 **Answer A.** The chest radiograph shows a left pneumothorax best localized by the letter A. Letters B, C, and D do not overlie any acute abnormalities.

Some of the immediate complications of cardiac conduction device placement include arrhythmia, pneumothorax, myocardial/venous perforation, valvular damage, and lead damage. An immediate postprocedural chest radiograph is obtained routinely to evaluate for pneumothorax or hemothorax, which can occur secondary to venous access.

Reference: Aguilera AL, Volokhina YV, Fisher KL. Radiography of cardiac conduction devices: a comprehensive review. *Radiographics* 2011;31(6):1669–1682.

9 **Answer A.** The chest radiograph and axial image from a thoracic CT angiogram demonstrate a leadless pacemaker in the right ventricular apex. Leadless pacemakers are affixed to the right ventricular apex by a transcatheter approach. The Nanostim and Micra systems are battery-shaped devices that overlie the right ventricle on a chest radiograph and should not be confused for a loop recorder, which is implanted subcutaneously.

Reference: Sigakis CJG, Mathai SK, Suby-Long TD, et al. Radiographic review of current therapeutic and monitoring devices in the chest. *Radiographics* 2018;38(4):1027–1045.

10 **Answer A.** Frontal and lateral chest radiographs demonstrate an atrial septal occluder device (arrows), which in this case was used to close a patent foramen ovale (PFO).

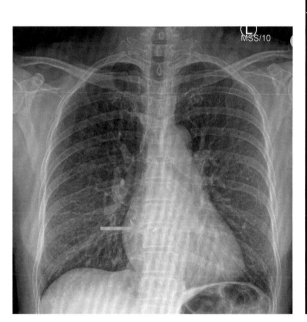 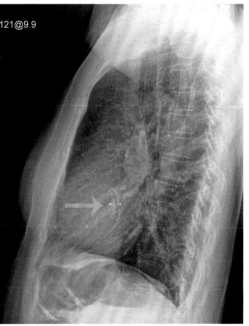

PFO is the most frequent congenital defect of the atrial septum found in approximately 20% to 30% of adults. The foramen ovale corresponds to an opening between the embryologic septum primum and septum secundum interatrial membranes. In some individuals, the septum primum and septum secundum fail to fuse. In combination with predisposing morphologic and hemodynamic conditions, this remnant interatrial communication promotes thromboembolic events, which have been linked to cryptogenic stroke, systemic hypoxemia, and migraine headaches. Transcatheter closure of a PFO has proven to be a very safe and effective technique with high success and low complication rates. Though infrequent, complications are serious and include cardiac perforation, air embolization, induced atrial fibrillation, nonspecific malaise attributed to nickel allergy, and access site problems.

A displaced prosthetic mitral valve would be rare and possibly seen in the setting of valve dehiscence related to endocarditis or penetrating trauma (likely deadly if the valve is displaced). Regardless, this device is not a prosthetic mitral valve. This is not an atrial pacing device (or cardiac lead). This device is not in the correct location to be in the left atrial appendage. The left atrial appendage can be closed surgically, endovascularly, or through a combined percutaneous pericardial and endovascular approach.

References: Franke J, Wunderlich N, Bertog SC, et al. Patent foramen ovale closure. In: Lanzer P (ed.). *Catheter-based cardiovascular interventions*. Berlin, Heidelberg: Springer, 2013:679–685.

Rohrhoff N, Vavalle JP, Halim S, et al. Current status of percutaneous PFO closure. *Curr Cardiol Rep* 2014;16(5):477.

11 Answer D. The zoomed in and edge-enhanced lateral chest radiograph demonstrates a Watchman device, which is a percutaneous left atrial appendage closure device. The frontal chest radiograph shows a surgical left atrial appendage ligation clip. These can be alternatives to anticoagulation in patients with atrial fibrillation.

Reference: Sigakis CJG, Mathai SK, Suby-Long TD, et al. Radiographic review of current therapeutic and monitoring devices in the chest. *Radiographics* 2018;38(4):1027–1045.

12 Answer B. The chest radiograph demonstrates coiling and migration of the ICD lead tips, consistent with Twiddler syndrome.

Twiddler syndrome is an uncommon complication of device implantation with a frequency of 0.07% to 7%. It occurs when the device rotates in the pocket and the leads coil around the generator. It is usually a painless phenomenon and may occur spontaneously or by willful manipulation by the patient.

Twiddler syndrome is more common in the elderly, presumably due to the laxity of their subcutaneous tissues. The disorder may induce lead dislodgment or lead fracture and cause life-threatening symptoms in case of pacemaker dependency. Lead displacement can also produce muscle stimulation or phrenic/brachial plexus stimulation.

Treatment consists of pocket revision, suturing the device to the pectoral muscle, or placing the generator in a subpectoral location. Sometimes, replacement of the leads or entire pacemaker system will be necessary.

References: Bhatia V, Kachru R, Parida AK, et al. Twiddler's syndrome. *Int J Cardiol* 2007;116(3):e82.

Ramsdale DR, Rao A. Complications of pacemaker implantation. In: *Cardiac pacing and device therapy*. London, UK: Springer London, 2012:249–282.

13 Answer B. Single-lead pacemaker has an abnormal course. It appears to course directly down the aortic arch and the ascending aorta. Of all the choices offered, a CT of the chest is most helpful to further define the course. CT later shows the pacemaker coursing through the left subclavian artery and through the aortic root to end up in the LV apex. A left-sided SVC would be more posterior in course as it goes through the coronary sinus. There is no pneumothorax to warrant a chest tube. Definitive diagnosis of lead malposition should be done before recommending surgery.

References: Bauersfeld UK, Thakur RK, Ghani M, et al. Malposition of transvenous pacing lead in the left ventricle: radiographic findings. *AJR Am J Roentgenol* 1994;162(2):290–292.

Mazzetti H, Dussaut A, Tentori C, et al. Transarterial permanent pacing of the left ventricle. *Pacing Clin Electrophysiol* 1990;13(5):588–592.

14 Answer B. The arrow on the chest radiograph identifies a percutaneous pigtail pericardial drain, which was placed in this case due to cardiac tamponade. Hypotension is a common presenting symptom of tamponade.

According to the 2015 European Society of Cardiology Guidelines for the diagnosis and management of pericardial diseases, pericardial drainage is indicated for cardiac tamponade, symptomatic moderate-to-large pericardial effusions refractory to medical therapy, and suspected bacterial or neoplastic etiology. Severe pulmonary hypertension and uncorrected bleeding diathesis are relative contraindications to catheter pericardiocentesis. Atrial fibrillation is not an indication for placement of a pericardial drain.

Pericardiocentesis is performed through a subxiphoid approach under fluoroscopic or echocardiographic guidance with hemodynamic and ECG monitoring. The most common complications are arrhythmias, coronary artery or cardiac chamber puncture, hemothorax, pneumothorax, pneumopericardium, and hepatic injury. A surgical approach is preferred when the pericardial fluid is loculated, <10 mm thick, or located in a lateral or posterior position.

Reference: Adler Y, Charron P, Imazio M, et al. 2015 ESC Guidelines for the diagnosis and management of pericardial diseases: the task force for the diagnosis and management of pericardial diseases for the European Society of Cardiology (ESC) Endorsed by: the European Association for Cardio-Thoracic Surgery (EACTS). *Eur Heart J* 2015;35(42):2921–2964.

15 Answer D. The image shows a dissection in the descending thoracic aorta. The left main coronary artery has been reimplanted. The implanted coronary artery has a bulbous origin secondary to a coronary button procedure. In the button procedure, a segment of the native aorta is used to attach the aortic graft in the root, creating a slightly enlarged origin.

Reference: Platis IE, Kopf GS, Dwar MS, et al. Composite graft with coronary button reimplantation: procedure of choice for aortic root replacement. *Int J Angiol* 1998;7(1):41–45.

16 Answer D. The axial image from the postoperative CT angiogram demonstrates a retroaortic conduit (arrows). The conduit connects to the left main coronary artery. In the images shown, the connection is only fully visualized on the volume-rendered image (arrows).

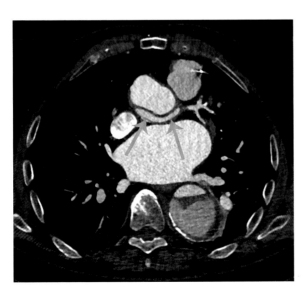
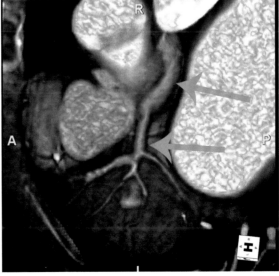

This is the normal postsurgical appearance of a composite aortic valve and root graft repair using the hemi-Cabrol technique. Severe proximal coronary artery disease, postoperative changes (in the setting of a redo procedure), and grossly displaced coronary ostia present a challenge for coronary artery button formation. In some cases, it may not be possible to fully mobilize the coronary ostia for direct reimplantation without tension. The Cabrol mustache graft and the Kay-Zubiate end-to-end saphenous vein graft extension are surgical techniques that address this problem. In the Cabrol procedure, the coronary ostia are anastomosed to a prosthetic conduit with an end-to-end anastomosis. The retroaortic conduit is then connected to the ascending aortic graft with a side-to-side anastomosis. The imaging appearance of the retroaortic conduit could easily be mistaken for a dissection flap.

References: Chiu P, Miller DC. Evolution of surgical therapy for Stanford acute type A aortic dissection. *Ann Cardiothorac Surg* 2016;5(4):275–295.

Hanneman K, Chan FP, Mitchell RS, et al. Pre- and postoperative imaging of the aortic root. *Radiographics* 2016;36(1):19–37.

17 **Answer D.** The image shows a patient who has undergone aortic valve repair with a St. Jude type valve. The valve leaflets are closed during ventricular diastole; however, only one of the leaflets opens during systole, while the other is stuck/frozen. The leaflet may be frozen secondary to tissue material at the valve attachment.

Reference: Chen JJ, Mannin MA, Frazier AA, et al. CT angiography of the cardiac valves: normal, diseased, and postoperative appearances. *Radiographics* 2009;29(5):1393–1412.

18 **Answer A.** Three-chamber view from a CT angiogram demonstrates a subvalvular left ventricular outflow tract pseudoaneurysm extending toward the left atrium. Given the history of fevers and chills, this is most likely related to infective endocarditis.

Prosthetic heart valve endocarditis complications include paravalvular abscess, pseudoaneurysm, dehiscence, and extension to adjacent structures. Dehiscence is defined as separation of the prosthetic heart valve from the annulus due to suture breakdown. A paravalvular leak is characterized by an abnormal channel between the prosthesis and the valve annulus due to an inadequate seal. Limited mobility or immobility of a prosthetic heart valve leaflet would be seen in the setting of a stuck leaflet. This is not shown here.

Reference: Raijiah P, Moore A, Saboo S, et al. Multimodality imaging of complications of cardiac valve surgeries. *Radiographics* 2019;39(4):932–956.

19 **Answer B.** Frontal and lateral chest radiographs demonstrate three mitral clips. Note that the patient also has a single chamber ICD. Mitral clips are used to percutaneously repair mitral regurgitation. Patients who have severe mitral regurgitation due to degenerative mitral valve disease may be candidates for the procedure. The clip is placed via a percutaneous approach and creates a functionally bicuspid mitral valve with two openings, allowing for blood to transit through the mitral valve.

Reference: Yuksel UC, Kapadia SR, Tuzcu EM. Percutaneous mitral repair: patient selection, results, and future directions. *Curr Cardiol Rep* 2011;13(2):100–106. doi: 10.1007/211886-010-0158-x.

20 **Answer C.** Frontal and lateral views of the chest show a valved stent in the aortic position consistent with a transcatheter aortic valve replacement (TAVR). The FDA-approved indication for use is to repair aortic stenosis.

Aortic stenosis is an obstruction of the left ventricular outflow tract at or near the level of the valve with a stenotic jet velocity of more than 4 m/s, a mean gradient of over 40 to 50 mm Hg, and a valve area of <1.0 cm². A TAVR is deployed via a minimally invasive approach—usually endovascular (transfemoral or transaxillary), transaortic, or transapical.

Mitral stenosis and regurgitation are incorrect because the device shown is a valve in the aortic position. A TAVR device can be used off-label for repair of aortic regurgitation, but this was not the original FDA-approved indication for use.

Reference: Salgado RA, Leipsic JA, Shivalkar B, et al. Preprocedural CT evaluation of transcatheter aortic valve replacement: what the radiologist needs to know. *Radiographics* 2014;34(6):1491–1514.

21 **Answer A.** Axial image from a coronary CT angiogram shows a large, partially thrombosed saphenous vein graft aneurysm in the left atrioventricular groove (arrow). Cerebrovascular accident is a known complication related to thromboembolism.

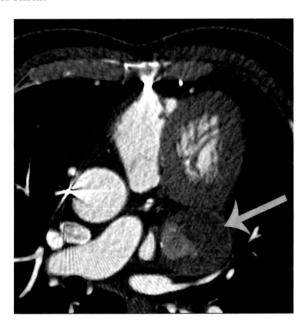

Bypass graft aneurysm is a late complication of coronary artery bypass graft surgery. They typically occur in the body of the graft more than 5 years after the initial bypass. The mechanism is thought to be related to accelerated atherosclerosis. Surgical correction is generally indicated for aneurysms exceeding 2 cm.

In contrast, graft pseudoaneurysms occur earlier (usually within 6 months after surgery) and arise at proximal or distal anastomotic sites.

Complications of graft aneurysms include thrombosis, thromboembolism, fistulization to a cardiac chamber, aneurysm rupture, and myocardial infarction.

Reference: Frazier AA, Qureshi F, Read KM, et al. Coronary artery bypass grafts: assessment with multidetector CT in the early and late postoperative settings. *Radiographics* 2005;25(4):881–896.

22 **Answer B.** Volume-rendered image demonstrates an occluded saphenous vein graft (SVG) to the right coronary artery (arrow). Note that a patent SVG-LCX graft is also seen (arrowhead).

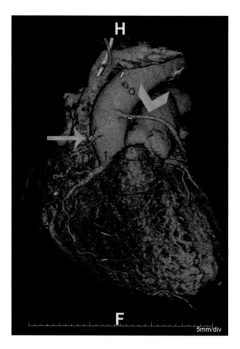

Saphenous vein conduits are harvested from the legs and grafted from the ascending aorta to the distal coronary artery past the obstructive coronary lesion. Chest pain is common after CABG surgery and can be due to many different causes, including recurrent angina secondary to graft occlusion. Early graft occlusion occurs primarily due to vascular damage during surgical retrieval and attachment, whereas late occlusion results from vessel wall changes ("arterialization") in response to systemic blood pressure.

Internal mammary artery (IMA) grafts have higher long-term patency rates than SVGs. Late IMA graft failure typically occurs from progressive atherosclerotic disease of the native vessel distal to the anastomosis.

Reference: Frazier AA, Qureshi F, Read KM, et al. Coronary artery bypass grafts: assessment with multidetector CT in the early and late postoperative settings. *Radiographics* 2005;25(4):881–896.

23 **Answer D.** Serial volume-rendered images of the thoracic aorta show progressive kinking of the endograft across an angulated segment in the proximal descending aorta.

Potential complications of endovascular stent grafts include endoleaks, stent migration, pseudoaneurysm formation, dissection, aortic perforation, kinking, thrombosis, and coverage of branch vessels. Variation in tortuosity and angulation of the aortic arch may be an anatomic feature that increases the risk of endoleak and graft migration.

References: Bean MJ, Johnson PT, Roseborough GS, et al. Thoracic aortic stent-grafts: utility of multidetector CT for pre- and post-procedure evaluation. *Radiographics* 2008;28(7):1835–1851.

Saremi F, Hassani C, Lin LM, et al. Image predictors of treatment outcome after thoracic aortic dissection repair. *Radiographics* 2018;38(7):1949–1972.

INDEX

A

Acute myocardial infarction, 65, 77
  with cardiogenic shock, 67, 78
  and delayed enhancement associated with
    wall motion abnormalities, 38, 50
  indication, 69, 79
AE. *See* Annuloaortic ectasia (AE)
Amplatzer septal occluder
  complication, 193, 212
  rims requirement, 212
Amyloidosis, 89, 96, 99, 106–107, 114
Anatomic structure
  anterolateral papillary muscle, 26, 34
  left atrial appendage, 18, 30
  membranous septum, 23, 33
  middle cardiac vein, 23, 32
  obtuse marginal, 24, 33
  right atrial appendage, 21, 32
Aneurysm, 61, 73–74
Angiosarcoma, cardiac, 119, 128, 138–139,
  142
Annuloaortic ectasia (AE), 103, 154, 166,
  222, 236
Anterior wall, delayed enhancement
  sequence, 62, 74–75
Anterolateral papillary muscle, anatomic
  structure, 26, 34
Aortic dissection, 220, 235, 243, 254–255
Aortic insufficiency, 41, 44, 52, 55, 201, 216
Aortic nipple, 31
Aortic regurgitation, 145, 156, 227, 239
  phase-contrast sequence, 150, 162
Aortic root, 19, 30
Aortic stenosis, 252, 262
Aortic ulceration, 224, 237
Aortic valve, 16, 28
  trileaflet, 18, 29
Aortic wall, 227, 239
Arch abnormality, 231, 240–241
Arrhythmias, 204, 217
Arrhythmogenic right ventricular dysplasia
  (ARVD), 82, 98
Arteriovenous malformation, 230, 240
Artifact, incorrect encoding velocity range,
  41, 52
ARVD. *See* Arrhythmogenic right
  ventricular dysplasia (ARVD)
ASD. *See* Atrial septal defects (ASD)
Atherosclerosis, 64, 75, 220, 234
Atherosclerotic plaque, 60, 73
Atrial fibrillation, 44, 54, 247, 260
Atrial septal defects (ASD), 192, 212
  complications, 212
  secundum, 212–213, 217
  sinus venosus, 193, 212–213

surgical treatment, 193, 212–213
  types of, 194, 213
Atrial septal occluder device, 247, 259–260
Atrioventricular valves, 152, 165

B

Balanced steady-state free precession
    sequence
  cardiac function, 5, 12
  cardiac MRI, 7, 13
  longitudinal magnetization and
    transverse magnetization, 7, 13
Basal septal hypertrophy (BSH), 103
BAV. *See* Bicuspid aortic valve (BAV)
Beck triad, cardiac tamponade complexes,
  183
Beta-blockers, 3, 10
Bicuspid aortic valve (BAV), 149, 153, 160,
    165
  associated with aortic coarctation, 150,
    161
  "fish-mouth" appearance, 161, 165
  incidence, 167
  prevalence, 165
  Sievers classification system, 161
Body mass index (BMI), 7, 14, 60, 73
Bolus geometry, 6, 12
Brachiocephalic vein, 19, 30
Breast cancer, cardiac MRI role in, 136
Bright blood imaging, 157

C

Calcium score, 60, 73
Carcinoid heart disease, 153, 165–166
Cardiac amyloidosis
  cardiac MR imaging, 89, 106–107
  classification, 106
  diagnosis of, 106
  difficulty nulling the myocardium in, 91,
    109
  feature of, 106–107
  99m-Technetium pyrophosphate SPECT
    imaging, 91, 109
  types, 109
Cardiac arrhythmia, 44, 54
Cardiac CTA (CCTA)
  abnormal nuclear medicine stress test,
    42, 53
  body mass index (BMI), 7, 14
  cardiac cycle, 7, 14
  flow-limiting stenosis, 43, 53
  intravenous beta blockers, 41, 52–53
  metoprolol, 39, 51
  obstructed pulmonary vein, 45, 55
  open mitral valve, 37, 49

reduced radiation dose, 37, 49
  reducing kVp, 38, 50
  sublingual nitroglycerin (SL-NTG), 43,
    54, 57, 71
Cardiac cycle
  cardiac CTA, 7, 14
  definition, 46
  phase of, 37, 49
  temporal windows within, 48
Cardiac magnetic resonance imaging
    (CMRI), 104
  adenosine stress perfusion, 67, 70, 78,
    80–81
  anatomical planes, 26, 34
  angular phase shift, 39, 51
  aortic insufficiency, 41, 44, 52, 55
  aortic stenosis, 149, 160
  aortic stenosis evaluation, 36, 47
  balanced steady-state free precession
    sequence, 5, 7, 12–13
  Bernoulli equation, 36–37, 47, 49
  cardiac amyloidosis, 89, 106–107
  cardiac pacemaker device for, 6, 12
  for cardiac thrombus assessment,
    116, 136
  cardiovascular shunts assessment, 37, 49
  cavity size, 44, 55
  decreased atrial contractility, 35, 46
  diastolic dysfunction, 44, 55
  diastolic function evaluation, 35, 46
  difficulty nulling the myocardium in,
    91, 109
  dilated cardiomyopathy evaluation,
    44, 55
  E/A wave, 35, 46
  ECG editing, 36, 48
  ECV with underlying myocardial fibrosis,
    36, 47–48
  ejection fraction, 38, 44, 50, 54
  hypertrophic cardiomyopathy, 84,
    100–101
  incomplete blood suppression, 2, 9–10
  intensive athlete's heart condition, 36, 47
  left ventricular (LV) mass, 37, 48–49
  magnitude image and phase velocity
    map, 41, 52
  morphologic changes in heart, 45, 56
  MR conditional device, 6, 12
  myocardial mass, 44, 55
  myocardial nulling, 5, 11–12
  myocardial viability on, 70, 80
  phase-contrast, 39, 51
  pressure gradient, 40, 51
  pseudomass in right atrium, 135, 144
  Qp/Qs, 42, 53

Cardiac magnetic resonance imaging
   (CMRI) (*Continued*)
   role in breast carcinoma, 136
   single radiofrequency inversion pulses,
      8, 14
   spatial resolution, 7, 14
   superior–inferior frequency encoding
      direction, 5, 12
   velocity, 37, 49
   ventricular filling, 35, 46
   ventricular interdependence, 93, 111
   zone, 7, 13
Cardiac masses
   anticoagulation, 120, 139
   atrial wall mass, 125, 141
   breast cancer, cardiac MRI role in,
      116, 136
   cardiac angiosarcoma, 119, 128, 138–139,
      142
   cardiac fibroma, 119, 127, 138, 141, 143
   cardiac lipomas, 116, 137
   central line placement, 132, 143
   chemical fat suppression, 126, 141
   chest pain
      catheter angiography, 122, 140
      right heart border, 123, 140
   constrictive pericarditis (CP), 118, 138
   contrast-enhanced CTA, 134, 143
   echinococcus infection, 133, 143
   fossa ovalis, sparing of, 125, 141
   hepatic PEComa with metastases,
      116, 136
   interatrial septum, 128, 142
   between left and right coronary cusps,
      130, 142
   left atrial appendage, 121, 139
      thrombus, 121, 139–140
   left atrium
      osteosarcoma, 117, 137
      surgical treatment for, 129, 142
   left ventricle abnormality, 126, 141
   left ventricular cavity, 120, 139
   lipomatous hypertrophy (LH), 116, 137
   lymphoma, 132, 143
   metastasis, 122, 140
   pericardium, 120, 139
   PET imaging studies, 116, 137
   primary cardiac lymphoma, 116, 136
   primary pericardial mesothelioma (PPM),
      118, 138
   pseudomass in right atrium, 135, 144
   renal angiomyolipomas, 117, 131, 138,
      142
   rhabdomyoma, 126, 141
   right atrial mass, 124, 140
   right coronary artery, 134, 144
   right pericardial cyst, 123, 140
   short tau inversion recovery (STIR),
      126, 141
   thrombus, 120, 139
      delayed enhancement sequences for,
         116, 136
      diagnosis of, 130, 142
      left ventricular, 139
      lobulated, 117, 137
   transient ischemic attack, 131, 142

   transvenous, 116, 136
Cardiac MRI (CMRI). *See* Cardiac magnetic
      resonance imaging (CMRI)
Cardiac pacemaker device, 6, 12
Cardiac rhabdomyomas, 117, 138
Cardiac valve
   brachiocephalic vein, 19, 30
   mitral valve, 16, 27
   pulmonic, 16, 28
   thebesian, 16, 28
Cardiomyopathy
   amyloidosis, 89, 91, 96, 106–107, 109,
      114
   arrhythmogenic right ventricular
      dysplasia (ARVD), 82, 98
   cardiac sarcoidosis
      clinical and histologic diagnosis of,
         96, 114
      decrease glucose uptake by normal
         myocardium, 96, 114
      FDG-PET uptake for, 96, 113
   hemochromatosis, 86, 103
   hypertrophic cardiomyopathy (HCM)
      (*see* Hypertrophic cardiomyopathy
      (HCM))
   ICD, 87, 104
   interstitial fibrosis, for increased ECV,
      95, 113
   intramyocardial fat, 92, 110
   iron overload, 94, 112
   left ventricular noncompaction (VNC),
      84, 101
   Loeffler endocarditis, 87, 104–105
   myocardial–pericardial adhesions,
      94, 111
   myocarditis, 85, 90, 101–102, 107–108
   myotonic dystrophy, 93, 110
   nonischemic dilated cardiomyopathy,
      88, 106
   palpitations and dizziness, 82, 98
   peripartum/postpartum cardiomyopathy
      (PPCM), 94, 113
   and peripheral eosinophilia, 87,
      104–105
   pulmonary hypertension, 83, 98–99
   restrictive, 88, 105
      vs. constrictive pericarditis, 94, 112
   right ventricular dyskinesia, 82, 98
   RV wall, 97, 115
   severe aortic stenosis, 86, 103
   stress-induced cardiomyopathy, 85, 102
   T2* relaxation by cardiac MR sequence,
      94, 112
   turbulent flow, 89, 107
   ventricular compliance and diastolic
      volume, 94, 112
   ventricular interdependence, 92–93,
      110–111
   ventricular noncompaction (*see*
      Ventricular noncompaction (VNC))
Cardiotoxicity, 136
CCTA. *See* Cardiac CTA (CCTA)
CHD. *See* Congenital heart disease (CHD)
Circumflex coronary artery, 42, 53
Cobweb sign, 233, 241
Codominant anatomy, 15, 27

Computed tomography (CT). *See also*
      Cardiac CTA (CCTA)
   curved multiplanar reformation, 4, 11
   FDG-PET, for cardiac sarcoidosis, 96,
      113–114
   filtered-back projection (FBP), 1, 9
Computed tomography angiography (CTA)
   cardiac (*see* Cardiac CTA (CCTA))
   coronary (*see* Coronary CTA)
   true lumen *vs.* false lumen, 233, 241
Congenital heart disease (CHD)
   abnormal vertical linear opacity, 194, 213
   anomalous pulmonary venous return,
      194–195, 213
   aortic insufficiency, 201, 216
   arrhythmias, 204, 217
   associated with left VNC, 109
   atrial fibrillation, surgical repair for, 197,
      214
   atrial septal defects (ASD) (*see* Atrial
      septal defects (ASD))
   atrial switch procedure, 209
   bronchial anatomy to pulmonary artery,
      191, 212
   chest CTA imaging, 194, 213
   commissures, 202, 217
   complication of, 193, 212
   congenital aortic arch malformations,
      190, 210
   conotruncal anomalies, 190, 210
   coronary sinus, 202, 216–217
   dextrocardia, situs inversus, 191, 211
   double aortic arch with dominant right
      arch, 205, 218
   D-TGA, 188, 209
   Ebstein's anomaly, 209
   erosion of device, 193, 212
   hypoplastic left heart syndrome, 189, 209
   Kawasaki disease, 207, 218
   lack of adequate rims, 192, 212
   left to right shunt, 195, 213
   levotransposition of the great arteries
      (L-TGA), 199, 215
   main pulmonary trunk, shortness of
      breath, 197, 215
   membranous ventricular septal defect
      with Eisenmenger syndrome, 196,
      214
   membranous *vs.* muscular ventricular
      septal defects (VSD), 194, 213
   moderator band characteristics, 16, 28
   multiple aortopulmonary collateral
      arteries (MAPCAs), 206, 218
   Mustard/Senning procedure, 200, 216
   Norwood procedure, surgical palliation
      stage, 189, 209
   parachute mitral valve, 195, 214
   patent ductus arteriosus, 190, 211
   polysplenia, 198, 215
   primum atrial septal defect, 203, 217
   pulmonary atresia with ventricular septal
      defect (PA-VSD), 206, 218
   pulmonary regurgitation, 211
   pulmonary vein, 197, 214
   retroaortic left circumflex artery, 199,
      216

right ventricular dysfunction, 204, 217
right ventricular outflow tract, rupture of, 208, 219
Ross procedure, 195, 214
sail-like anterior leaflet, 203, 217
Shone complex/syndrome, 195, 214
shunt, 198, 215
    left to right, 195, 201, 213, 216
sinus venosus atrial septal defect (ASD), 193, 212–213
stress test, 205, 217–218
supravalvular aortic stenosis, 191, 211
tetralogy of Fallot, 209
transposition of great arteries (TGA), 188, 209
tricuspid atresia, 189, 210
tricuspid valve, 201, 216
tricuspid valvular abnormality, 203, 217
truncus arteriosus, 201, 216
unroofed coronary sinus, 193–194, 213
Constrictive pericarditis (CP)
    characteristics, 112
    clinical presentation, 118, 138
    constellation of findings, 105, 108
    physiologic and morphologic changes, 170, 182
    vs. restrictive cardiomyopathy, 112, 173, 184
    setting of, 186
    ventricular interdependence with, 110–111
Contrast bolus
    geometry, 6, 12
    transient interruption of, 6, 13
Contrast flow rate, 4, 11
Coronary arteries, 20, 31, 42–43, 53
    aneurysms, 64, 76
    atherosclerotic plaque, 60, 73
    bypass grafts, 66, 78
    left circumflex, 25, 33–34
    left main artery, 68, 79
    obtuse marginal, 24, 33
    prognosis, 68, 79
    RAO caudal position, 25, 33–34
    right, 20, 24, 30–31, 33, 43, 53
Coronary Artery Disease—Reporting and Data System (CAD-RADS), 59, 72
    scores, 66, 77
Coronary artery dominance, codominant anatomy, 15, 27
Coronary CTA
    atypical chest pain, 67, 79
    with CT-derived fractional flow reserve (FFR$_{CT}$) analysis, 62, 75
    indication for, 61, 74
    pitch, reduced radiation dose, 8, 14
    retrospective ECG-gated image, 36, 48
Coronary sinus, 16, 28
Coronary venogram, 42, 53
Crista terminalis, 17, 29
Curved multiplanar reformation, 4, 11

D
Dark blood imaging, 157
Dark rim artifact, 80–81
Devices and postoperative appearance

aortic dissection, 243, 254–255
aortic stenosis, 252, 262
atrial fibrillation, 247, 260
atrial septal occluder, 247, 259–260
cardiac conduction device placement complications, 259
cardiac MRI, 242, 254
cerebrovascular accident, 252, 263
endovascular stent grafts repair, 253, 264
hypotension, 249, 261
Impella Ventricular Support System
    aortic wall injury, 245, 258
    radiographs, 245, 257
implantable cardioverter–defibrillators (ICDs), 244, 246, 256–257, 259
intra-aortic balloon pumps (IABP), 243, 254–255
    cerebrovascular accident, 243, 255
lead perforation, 244, 256–257
leadless pacemaker, 246, 259
left atrium and pulmonary veins from recipient, 245, 258
left pneumothorax, 246, 259
left ventricular assist devices (LVADs)
    infection, 244, 256
    thrombosis, 243, 255–256
loop recorder, 242, 254
mitral clip, 251, 262
occluded saphenous vein graft, 253, 264
orthotopic heart transplantation, 245, 258
postpacemaker chest radiographs, 248, 260
pseudoaneurysm, 251, 262
reimplanted left main coronary artery, 249, 261
    axial and volume-rendered image, 250, 261–262
stent graft kinking, 253, 264
stuck leaflet, 250, 262
Twiddler syndrome, 248, 260
volume-rendered image studies, 253, 264
Watchman device, 260
Diastolic dysfunction, left ventricular filling rate, 44, 55
Dilated cardiomyopathy (DCM), 55
Dose length product (DLP), 1, 9
Double-inversion recovery sequence, 1–2, 9–10
Dressler syndrome, 74
Dual antiplatelet therapy, 65, 76

E
Effective dose, 3, 10
Ehlers-Danlos syndrome, 222, 236
Eisenmenger syndrome, 165, 196, 214
Endomyocardial fibrosis, 99, 105, 110
End-ventricular systole, 40, 51
Eosinophil-mediated myocarditis, 104
Epicardial fat necrosis, acute chest pain, 176, 186

F
False lumen, 233, 241
FDG-PET CT, for cardiac sarcoidosis, 96, 113–114

Filtered-back projection (FBP), 1, 9
    reconstruction algorithm/kernel, 1, 9
Flail leaflet, 160
Fontan procedure, reconstructive open heart procedure, 210
Fontan-associated liver disease (FALD), 210
Four-chamber plane, 21, 31
Four-dimensional flow MRI
    aortic regurgitation, 145, 156
    principles and applications, 145–146, 156–157
    pulmonic regurgitation, 146, 157

G
Gadolinium
    intravascular injection—extracellular space, 6, 13
    paramagnetic properties, 7, 13
Giant cell arteritis, 232, 241
Graft patency rates, 59, 73

H
HCM. *See* Hypertrophic cardiomyopathy (HCM)
Heart rate, 51–53
    decreased, 35, 46
    elevated, 39, 51
Hemi-Fontan operation, reconstructive open heart procedure, 209–210
Hemochromatosis, 86, 103
Hemopericardium, 174, 184
Hereditary hemorrhagic telangiectasia (HHT), 230, 240
Heyde syndrome, 166
Hibernating myocardium, 70, 80
Hyparterial, pulmonary artery to trachea, 16, 27
Hypertension, 220, 235
Hypertensive cardiomyopathy, 99
Hypertrophic cardiomyopathy (HCM), 99, 105, 108
    cardiac MRI, 84, 90, 100–101, 107
    characteristics, 83, 99–100
    late gadolinium enhancement (LGE) in, 104
    vs. physiologic cardiac hypertrophy, 47
    prevalence, 104
    related-sudden death, 104
    septal variant, 95, 113
Hypertrophic obstructive cardiomyopathy (HOCM), 39, 50
Hypoplastic left heart syndrome (HLHS), 189, 209
Hypotension, 3, 11, 249, 261

I
IABP. *See* Intra-aortic balloon pumps (IABP)
ICDs. *See* Implantable cardioverter–defibrillators (ICDs)
Idiopathic dilated cardiomyopathy, 103
Image acquisition time, 7, 14
Impella Ventricular Support System
    aortic wall injury, 245, 258
    radiographs, 245, 257

Implantable cardioverter–defibrillators (ICDs), 244, 246, 256–257, 259
Implantable loop recorders (ILR), 242, 254
Infective endocarditis, 151, 162–163
Inflammatory cardiomyopathy, 108
In-stent restonsis, 65, 76
Interatrial septum, 22, 32
Internal mammary artery (IMA) grafts, 264
Interventricular septum, 33
Intra-aortic balloon pumps (IABP), 243, 254–255
   cerebrovascular accident, 243, 255
Inversion time, 64, 76
Iodine flux, 4, 11
Iron overload cardiomyopathy (IOC), 103
Ischemic cardiomyopathy, 105, 110
Ischemic heart disease
   acute myocardial infarction, 69, 79–80
   adenosine stress perfusion MRI, 67, 78
   anteroseptal myocardial segment, 69, 80
   atherosclerosis, 64, 75–76
   body mass index (BMI), 60, 73
   bypass grafting, 66, 78
   CAD-RADS 5 score, 66, 77
   CAD-RADS 4A lesion, 59, 72
   chest pain, noncardiac causes of, 63, 75
   dual antiplatelet therapy, 65, 76
   ECG tracing, 68, 79
   ER with chest pain, 63, 75
   FFR_{CT} values, 62, 75
   hibernating myocardium, 70, 80
   inversion time for imaging, 64, 76
   LAD territory, 69, 80
   left internal mammary artery origin, 66, 78
   microvascular obstruction, 69, 80
   myocardial infarction, 61, 65, 73, 76
   occluded RCA stent, 64, 76
   patent LAD stent, 64, 76
   percutaneous coronary intervention (PCI), 67, 78
   right coronary artery (RCA), 65, 77
     coronary angiographic images, 58, 71
     inferior wall, significant restriction of blood flow, 57, 71
     severe stenosis, 57, 71
     territory, five myocardial segments of, 58, 71–72
   sildenafil, 57, 71
   stable anginal symptoms, with ECG stress test, 61, 74
   three-vessel ischemia, 70, 80–81
   ventricular aneurysms, 61, 73–74
   vulnerability modifier, 59, 72
   wavefront phenomenon, 77
Isovolumetric contraction, ventricles, 38, 50

K
Kawasaki disease, 207, 218
Kussmaul sign, cardiac tamponade complexes, 183

L
Late gadolinium enhancement imaging, 157
Left anterior descending artery, 22, 32
Left atrial appendage, 18, 30

Left circumflex, 15, 27
   RAO caudal position, 25, 33–34
Left superior vena cava (SVC), 20, 31
Left ventricular assist devices (LVADs)
   infection, 244, 256
   thrombosis, 243, 255–256
Left ventricular end-diastolic pressure (LVEDP)., 35, 46
Left ventricular outflow tract, 39, 50
Left ventricular systolic ejection fraction, 38, 50
Levotransposition of the great arteries (L-TGA), 199, 215
Ligament of Marshall, 25, 33
Lipomatous hypertrophy (LH), 116, 137
Lipomatous hypertrophy of the interatrial septum (LHIAS), 141
Loeffler endocarditis, 87, 104–105
Loeys-Dietz syndrome (LDS), 154, 166
Longitudinal magnetization (LM), 7, 13
Lower and Shumway technique, 258
Lung adenocarcinoma, 177, 186

M
Marfan syndrome, 154, 165–166, 222, 224, 226, 232, 236–238, 241
Membranous septum, anatomic structure, 23, 33
Metoprolol, 39, 51
Microvascular obstruction (MVO), 62, 69, 74–75, 79–80
Middle cardiac vein, anatomic structure, 23, 32
Mitral annular calcifications, 152, 164
Mitral valve, 16, 28
Mitral valve prolapse (MVP), 148, 160, 162, 224, 238
   definition, 148, 160
   Marfan syndrome, 154, 165
   myxomatous degeneration in, 158, 160
Mitral valves, 16, 27
Multiple aortopulmonary collateral arteries (MAPCAs), 206, 218
Mustard/Senning procedure, 200, 216
MVO. See Microvascular obstruction (MVO)
MVP. See Mitral valve prolapse (MVP)
Mycotic aneurysm, 225, 238
Myocardial infarction, 61, 65, 73, 76–77, 108
   wall motion abnormalities, 38, 50
Myocardial mass, 44, 55
Myocardial nulling, 5, 11–12, 64, 76
Myocarditis, 80, 85, 90, 99, 101–102, 107–108
Myotonic dystrophy, 93, 110

N
Nephrogenic systemic fibrosis (NSF), 3, 11
Noncompaction cardiomyopathy, 103
Nonischemic dilated cardiomyopathy, 88, 99, 106
Norwood procedure, reconstructive open heart procedure, 189, 209

O
Obtuse marginal, anatomic structure, 24, 33
Occluded saphenous vein graft, 253, 264

Oreo cookie sign, 187
Orthotopic heart transplantation, 245, 258

P
Papillary fibroelastoma, 150, 161, 163
Papillary muscle infarction, 65, 76
Parachute mitral valve, 195, 214
Paravalvular pseudoaneurysm, 151, 163
Patent ductus arteriosus (PDA), 190, 211
Patent foramen ovale (PFO), 259–260
PAVMs. See Pulmonary arteriovenous malformations (PAVMs)
Penetrating atherosclerotic ulcer (PAU), 237, 239
Percutaneous coronary intervention (PCI), 67, 78
Pericardial disease
   calcific pericarditis, 170, 181
   calcifications, 169, 181
   cardiac MRI
     fat fluid interface, chemical shift artifact, 168, 181
     pericardial effusion, 168, 181
   cardiac tamponade, physiologic findings of, 173, 183
   congenital absence of pericardium, 177, 186
   constrictive pericarditis, 173, 184
   CT vs. MRI, 175, 185
   decreased right ventricular volume, 170, 182
   EKG changes, 173, 184
   epicardial and pericardial fat, separation of, 170, 182
   epicardial fat, 180, 187
     deposition, cardiovascular disease, 175, 185
     necrosis, 176, 186
   fluid in pericardial recess, 177, 186
   hemopericardium, 174, 184
   increased ventricular interdependence, causes of, 178, 186
   lymphangitic extension, 174, 184
   malignant cytology, 175, 185
   malignant pericardial effusion, 171, 182
   metastatic disease, 175, 185
   pericardectomy, 172, 182
   pericardial fluid volume, 175, 185
   pericardial lipoma, 169, 181
   pericardial thickness, 176, 185
   pericardial window, 173, 184
   physiologic and morphologic changes, 170, 182
   pneumopericardium, 173, 178, 183, 186
   positive pressure ventilation, 178, 186
   restrictive cardiomyopathy, 173, 184
   right cardiophrenic angle, mass, 171, 182
   septations, pericardial cyst, 176, 186
   superior aortic pericardial recess, 179, 187
   with thickened pericardium and late gadolinium enhancement, 172, 183
   ventricular interdependence, 172, 179, 183, 186
Pericardial effusion, 168, 181
Pericardial lymphangioma, 169, 181

Pericardiocentesis, 261
Peri-infarct ischemia, 80–81
Peripartum/postpartum cardiomyopathy (PPCM), 94, 113
PET imaging
    cardiac amyloidosis, 109
    cardiac masses, 116, 137
    lipomatous hypertrophy of the interatrial septum (LHIAS), 141
Phase-contrast images
    bipolar gradients, 2, 10–11
    three-dimensional, 146, 156
    velocity and flow, measure and quantify, 157
    velocity-encoding gradient, 3, 11
Pitch, definition of, 8, 14
Pneumopericardium, 173, 183
Polysplenia, 198, 215
Posteromedial papillary muscle, 20, 31, 34
Premature ventricular complexes (PVCs), 97, 115
Primary cardiac lymphoma, 116, 136
Primary pericardial mesothelioma (PPM), 118, 138
Primum atrial septal defect, 203, 217
Pseudoaneurysm, 251, 262
Pulmonary arteriovenous malformations (PAVMs), 221, 235
    complications, 235
    CT pulmonary angiography, 235
    etiology, 235
    and hereditary hemorrhagic telangiectasia, 230, 240
    shunt type, 230, 240
    traditional cutoff for treatment of, 230, 240
Pulmonary artery (PA) aneurysm, 146, 157, 234
Pulmonary artery dissection (PAD), 220, 234
Pulmonary artery sarcoma (PAS), 222, 236
Pulmonary atresia with ventricular septal defect (PA-VSD), 206, 218
Pulmonary valve stenosis, 146, 157–158
Pulmonary vein, 17, 29, 197, 214
Pulmonary venous anatomy, 230, 240
Pulmonary venous wedge pressure, 45, 56
Pulmonic regurgitation, 146, 157
Pulmonic stenosis, 222, 236
Pulmonic valve, 16, 28
Pulsus paradoxus, cardiac tamponade complexes, 183

R

RCA. *See* Right coronary artery (RCA)
Reduce radiation dose, cardiac CTA (CCTA), 37, 49
Renal angiomyolipomas, 117, 138
Rendu-Osler-Weber disease, 235
Restrictive cardiomyopathy, 88, 105
Retroaortic left circumflex artery, 199, 216
Rheumatic heart disease (RHD), 148, 159, 165–166
    associated with aortic stenosis, 147, 158
    characteristics, 158

mitral valve stenosis, causes of, 146, 148, 158–159
Rheumatic mitral valve disease, 151, 162
Right atrial appendage, 21, 32
Right atrium, 17, 29
Right coronary artery (RCA)
    angiographic images, 24, 33
    ischemic heart disease, 65, 77
        coronary angiographic images, 58, 71
        inferior wall, significant restriction of blood flow, 57, 71
        severe stenosis, 57, 71
        territory, five myocardial segments of, 58, 71–72
    noncalcified plaque, 43, 53
    posteromedial papillary muscle, 20, 31
    sinoatrial nodal artery from, 20, 30
Right inferior pulmonary vein, 17, 29
Right superior pulmonary vein (RSPV), 197, 214
Right ventricular outflow tract aneurysm, 109
Ross procedure, 195, 214

S

Saphenous vein grafts (SVG), 78
    vs. left internal mammary artery grafts, 59, 73
Sarcoidosis, 80, 99
Scimitar sign, 213
Scimitar syndrome, 213–214
Septal bounce sign, 110–111
Severe aortic stenosis, 86, 103
Shone complex/syndrome, 195, 214
Shone syndrome, 166
Short tau inversion recovery (STIR), 126, 141
Sildenafil, 57, 71
Sinoatrial nodal artery, 20, 30
Sinoatrial node, 44, 54
Sinus of Valsalva (SOV) aneurysm, 208, 219
Sinus venosus atrial septal defect, 193, 212–213
Skin thickening of extremities, nephrogenic systemic fibrosis (NSF), 3, 11
SL-NTG. *See* Sublingual nitroglycerin (SL-NTG)
Spatial modulation of magnetization (SPAMM) tagging, 94, 111
Specific absorption rate (SAR), 6, 13
Spongiform cardiomyopathy. *See* Ventricular noncompaction (VNC)
Spotty calcifications, 72
Stanford classification
    type A, 237
    type B, 223, 237
Stress test, 205, 217–218
Subaortic stenosis (SAS), 167
Sublingual nitroglycerin (SL-NTG), 43, 54, 57, 71
Supravalvular aortic stenosis (SVAS), 167

T

Takayasu arteritis, 232, 241
Takotsubo cardiomyopathy (TTC), 102
TAVI. *See* Transcatheter aortic valve implantation (TAVI)

TAVR. *See* Transcatheter aortic valve replacement (TAVR)
Territories, 42–43, 53
Tetralogy of Fallot (TOF), 146, 157–158, 191, 211
TEVAR. *See* Thoracic endovascular aortic repair (TEVAR)
Thebesian valve, 16, 28
Thoracic aorta and great vessels
    annuloaortic ectasia, 222, 236
    aortic dissection, 220, 235
    aortic regurgitation, 227, 239
    aortic ulceration, 224, 237
    aortic wall, 227, 239
    arch abnormality, 231, 240–241
    arteriovenous malformation, 230, 240
    ascending aorta, noncontrast image, 226, 238
    asymptomatic patient, medical therapy for, 228, 239
    atherosclerosis, 220, 234
    axial images, 233, 241
    complex malformation, 230, 240
    Ehlers-Danlos syndrome, 222, 236
    false lumen, 233, 241
    giant cell arteritis, 232, 241
    hereditary hemorrhagic telangiectasia (HHT), 230, 240
    hypertension, 220, 235
    intimal flap, 225, 238
    lumen being wrapped by another lumen, 233, 241
    luminal thrombus, 228, 239
    Marfan syndrome, 222, 224, 226, 232, 236–238, 241
    mitral valve prolapse, 224, 238
    mycotic aneurysm, 225, 238
    peak gradient, 223, 236
    pulmonary artery dissection, 220, 234
    pulmonary artery sarcoma, 222, 236
    pulmonary AVMs (*see* Pulmonary arteriovenous malformations (PAVMs))
    pulmonary embolism, 228, 239
    pulmonary hypertension, due to left to right shunting, 229, 239
    pulmonary vein stenosis, 231, 240
    pulmonary venous anatomy, 230, 240
    pulmonic stenosis, 222, 236
    small breath hold without deep inspiration, 223, 237
    Stanford classification
        type A, 237
        type B, 223, 237
    stent, 229, 240
    Takayasu arteritis, 232, 241
    thoracic endovascular aortic repair, 220, 234
    traumatic pseudoaneurysm *vs.* ductus diverticulum, 225, 238
    true lumen, 233, 241
    type 1a endoleak, 221, 235
Thoracic aortic aneurysms (TAA), 235
Thoracic endovascular aortic repair (TEVAR), 220, 234

Three-dimensional phase-contrast image, 145, 156
TM. *See* Transverse magnetization (TM)
Transcatheter aortic valve implantation (TAVI), 152, 163
Transcatheter aortic valve replacement (TAVR), 262–263
Transesophageal echocardiogram (TEE), 139–140
Transient interruption, of contrast bolus, 6, 13
Transverse magnetization (TM), 7, 13
Tricuspid aortic valve, 40, 51
Tricuspid atresia, 189, 210
Tricuspid regurgitation, 147, 159
Tricuspid valve, 16, 28
   and mitral valves, 16, 27
Tricuspid valvular abnormality, 203, 217
Trileaflet aortic valve, 18, 29
True lumen, 233, 241
Twiddler syndrome, 248, 260
Two-dimensional phase contrast through plane, 145, 156

U
Uhl anomaly, 103
Unroofed coronary sinus, 193, 213
   left-sided SVC, 194, 213

V
Valvular disease
   annular dilation, 147, 158
   annuloaortic ectasia, 154, 166
      aortic peak velocity, 154, 167
      aortic regurgitation, 145, 150, 156, 162
      aortic stenosis, 149, 160
      atrioventricular valves, 152, 165
      bicuspid aortic valve, 149, 153, 160, 165
         associated with aortic coarctation, 150, 161
         "fish-mouth" appearance, 161, 165
         incidence, 167
         prevalence, 165
         Sievers classification system, 161
      carcinoid heart disease, 153, 165
      congenital stenosis, 146, 158
      four-dimensional flow MRI, 145, 156
      infarcted papillary muscle with rupture, 145, 156–157
      infective endocarditis, 151, 162–163
         pseudoaneurysm in, 151, 163
      Loeys-Dietz syndrome (LDS), 154, 166
      mitral annular calcifications with caseous necrosis, 152, 164
      mitral stenosis, 148, 159
      mitral valve prolapse (MVP), 148, 154, 160, 165
      papillary fibroelastoma, 150, 161, 163
      pulmonary artery aneurysm, 146, 157
      pulmonary valve stenosis, 146, 157–158
      pulmonic regurgitation, 146, 157
      rheumatic disease, aortic stenosis, 147, 158
      rheumatic heart disease, 146, 148, 158–159
      rheumatic mitral valve disease, 151, 162
      subvalvular aortic stenosis, 155, 167
      transcatheter aortic valve implantation (TAVI), 152, 163
      transcatheter pulmonary valve replacement, 152, 164
      tricuspid regurgitation, 147, 159
Vascular territory, 42, 53
Velocity-encoding gradient (VENC), 3, 11
Ventricles, isovolumetric contraction, 38, 50
Ventricular aneurysms, 61, 73–74
Ventricular diastole, end-diastolic volume, 40, 52
Ventricular interdependence, 92–93, 110–111
Ventricular noncompaction (VNC), 84, 101
   cardiac MR, 91, 108
   cardiac transplantation, 101
   characteristics, 91, 101, 108
   complication, 91, 108–109
   computed tomography imaging, 108
   diagnostic studies, 101
   morbidity and mortality, 101
Ventricular preload, 39
Ventricular pseudoaneurysms, 74
Ventricular septal defects (VSD), 194, 213
Verapamil, 3, 10
VNC. *See* Ventricular noncompaction (VNC)

W
Wall motion abnormalities, 38, 50
Williams syndrome, 166–167

CCS0921